PSYCHOLOGY OF THE FUTURE

SUNY series in Transpersonal and Humanistic Psychology

Richard D. Mann, editor

PSYCHOLOGY OF THE FUTURE

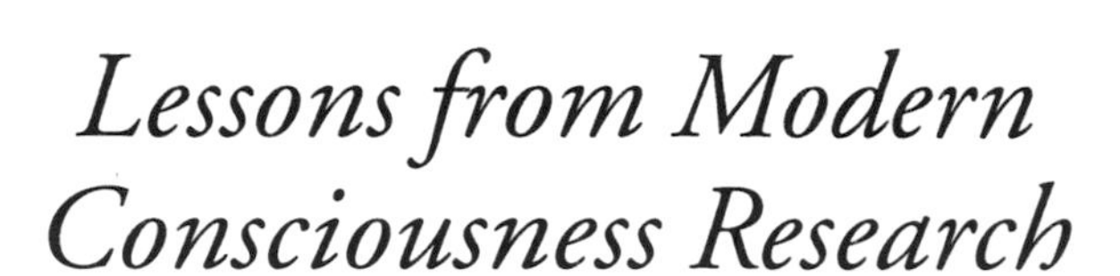

Lessons from Modern Consciousness Research

STANISLAV GROF

STATE UNIVERSITY OF NEW YORK PRESS

Published by
State University of New York Press, Albany

Printed in the United States of America

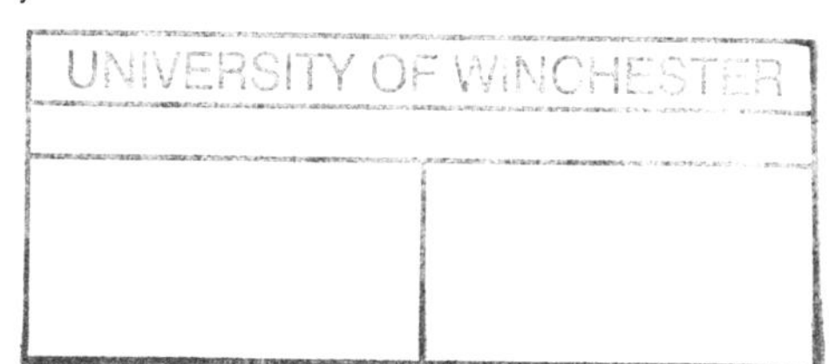

For information, address State University of New York Press,
194 Washington Avenue, Suite 305, Albany, NY 12210-2384

Production by Marilyn P. Semerad
Marketing by Fran Keneston

Library of Congress Cataloging-in-Publication Data

Grof, Stanislav, 1931–

Psychology of the future : lessons from modern consciousness research / Stanislav Grof.

p. cm. — (SUNY series in transpersonal and humanistic psychology)

Includes bibliographical references and index.

ISBN 0-7914-4621-2 (alk. paper) — ISBN 0-7914-4622-0 (pbk. : alk. paper)

1. Altered states of consciousness. 2. Consciousness. 3. Spirituality. 4. Psychology—Philosophy. 5. Psychiatry—Philosophy. 6. Transpersonal psychology. I. Title. II. Series.

BF1045.A48 G76 2000

154.4—dc21 00-025255

10 9 8 7 6 5 4 3 2 1

To Christina

with much love and deep appreciation
for your contributions to the ideas
expressed in this book

CONTENTS

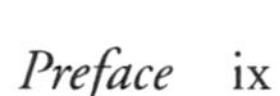

PREFACE

More than forty years ago, a powerful experience lasting only several hours of clock-time profoundly changed my personal and professional life. As a young psychiatric resident, only a few months after my graduation from medical school, I volunteered for an experiment with LSD, a substance with remarkable psychoactive properties that had been discovered by the Swiss chemist Albert Hofmann in the Sandoz pharmaceutical laboratories in Basel.

This session, particularly its culmination period during which I had an overwhelming and indescribable experience of cosmic consciousness, awakened in me an intense lifelong interest in nonordinary states of consciousness. Since that time, most of my clinical and research activities have consisted of systematic exploration of the therapeutic, transformative, and evolutionary potential of these states. The four decades that I have dedicated to consciousness research have been for me an extraordinary adventure of discovery and self-discovery.

I spent approximately half of this time conducting therapy with psychedelic substances, first in Czechoslovakia in the Psychiatric Research Institute in Prague and then in the United States, at the Maryland Psychiatric Research Center in Baltimore, where I participated in the last surviving American psychedelic research program. Since 1975, I have worked with holotropic breathwork, a powerful method of therapy and self-exploration that I have developed jointly with my wife Christina. Over the years, I have also supported many people undergoing psychospiritual crises, or "spiritual emergencies" as Christina and I call them.

The common denominator of these three situations is that they involve nonordinary states of consciousness or, more specifically, an important subcategory of them that I call holotropic. In psychedelic therapy, these states are induced by administration of mind-altering substances, such as LSD, psilocybin, mescaline, ibogain, and tryptamine or amphetamine derivatives. In holotropic breathwork, consciousness is changed by a combination of faster breathing, evocative music, and energy-releasing bodywork. In spiritual emergencies, holotropic states occur spontaneously, in the middle of everyday life, and their cause is usually unknown.

In addition, I have been more peripherally involved in many disciplines that are, more or less directly, related to nonordinary states of consciousness. I have participated in sacred ceremonies of native cultures in different parts of the world, had contact with North American, Mexican, and South American shamans, and exchanged information with many anthropologists. I have also had extensive contact with representatives of various spiritual disciplines, including Vipassana, Zen, and Vajrayana Buddhism, Siddha Yoga, Tantra, and the Christian Benedictine order.

Another area that has received much of my attention has been thanatology, the young discipline studying near-death experiences and the psychological and spiritual aspects of death and dying. I participated in the late 1960s and early 1970s in a large research project studying the effects of psychedelic therapy in individuals dying of cancer. I should also add that I have had the privilege of personal acquaintance and experience with some of the great psychics and parapsychologists of our era, pioneers of laboratory consciousness research, and therapists who developed and practiced powerful forms of experiential therapy that induce nonordinary states of consciousness.

My initial encounter with nonordinary states was very difficult and intellectually, as well as emotionally, challenging. In the early years of my laboratory and clinical research with psychedelics, I was daily bombarded with experiences and observations, for which my medical and psychiatric training had not prepared me. As a matter of fact, I was experiencing and seeing things which, in the context of the scientific worldview I was brought up with, were considered impossible and were not supposed to happen. And yet, those obviously impossible things were happening all the time.

After I had overcome my initial conceptual shock and doubts about my own sanity, I began to realize that the problem might not be in my capacity to observe, or in my critical judgment, but in the limitations of current psychological and psychiatric theory and of the monistic materialistic paradigm of Western science. Naturally, it was not easy for me to come to this realization, since I had to struggle with the awe and respect a medical student or a beginning psychiatrist feels toward the academic establishment, scientific authorities, and impressive credentials and titles.

Over the years, my initial suspicion about the inadequacy of academic theories concerning consciousness and the human psyche has gradually turned into certainty, nourished and reinforced by thousands of clinical observations, as well as personal experiences. At this point, I have no doubts that the data from the research of nonordinary states of consciousness represent a critical conceptual challenge for the scientific paradigm that currently dominates psychology, psychiatry, psychotherapy, and many other disciplines.

This book is an attempt to point out in a systematic and comprehensive way the areas that require a radical revision and to suggest the direction and nature of the necessary changes. The conceptual challenges presented by consciousness research are very fundamental and cannot be resolved by a minor conceptual patchwork or a few ad hoc hypotheses. In my opinion, the nature and scope of the conceptual crisis facing psychology and psychiatry is comparable to the situation introduced at the beginning of the twentieth century into physics by the results of the Michelson-Morley experiment.

The opening chapter of the book offers a general discussion of nonordinary states of consciousness, the role they have played in the ritual, spiritual, and cultural life of humanity, and of the challenges they present for the monistic materialistic worldview of Western science. This chapter closes with an outline of the areas in which major conceptual changes are necessary and briefly sketches the nature of the suggested alternatives. These are then explored at some length and depth in the following sections of the book.

The next chapter focuses on the first of these areas—the nature and origin of consciousness and the dimensions of the human psyche. The observations from consciousness research dispel the current myth of materialistic science that consciousness is an epiphenomenon of matter, a product of neurophysiological processes in the brain. They show that consciousness is a primary attribute of existence and that it is capable of many activities that the brain could not possibly perform. According to the new findings, human consciousness is a part of and participates in a larger universal field of cosmic consciousness that permeates all of existence.

Traditional academic psychiatry and psychology also use a model of the psyche that is limited to biology, postnatal biography, and to the

Freudian individual unconscious. To account for all the phenomena occurring in holotropic states, our understanding of the dimensions of the human psyche would have to be drastically extended. The new cartography of the psyche outlined in the book includes two additional domains: *perinatal* (related to the trauma of birth) and *transpersonal* (comprising ancestral, racial, collective, and phylogenetic memories, karmic experiences, and archetypal dynamics).

As the book continues, this expanded understanding of the psyche is applied to various emotional and psychosomatic disorders that do not have an organic basis ("psychogenic psychopathology"). To explain these conditions, traditional psychiatry uses a model that is limited to postnatal biographical traumas in infancy, childhood, and later life. The new understanding suggests that the roots of such disorders reach much deeper and include significant contributions from the perinatal level and from the transpersonal domains of the psyche.

One of the most important consequences of this new understanding of the dimensions of the human psyche is the realization that many states that modern psychiatry considers pathological and treats with suppressive medication are actually "spiritual emergencies," psychospiritual crises that have a healing and transformative potential. A special chapter is dedicated to the discussion of the nature of these conditions, situations that trigger them, their forms of manifestation, and new therapeutic strategies.

The following chapter then explores the practical implications of the new observations concerning the human psyche. It discusses the principles of psychotherapy using holotropic states and the healing mechanisms that become available when the process of experiential self-exploration reaches the perinatal and transpersonal levels. A special section of this chapter discusses the theory and practice of holotropic breathwork and shows how the new principles manifest and are utilized in this form of experiential therapy.

The observations from holotropic states seriously undermine the fundamental cornerstone of materialistic thinking, the belief in the primacy of matter and in the absence of the spiritual dimension in the fabric of existence. They bring direct experiential and empirical evidence that spirituality is a critical and legitimate attribute of the human psyche and of the universal scheme of things. This important topic is given special attention in the book. It is argued that, properly understood, spirituality and science are not and cannot be in conflict, but represent two complementary approaches to existence.

A special chapter in the book is dedicated to psychological, philosophical, and spiritual aspects of death and dying. It explores such problems as the significance of death for psychology, near-death experiences, the possibility of survival of consciousness after death, karma and reincarnation, the ancient books of the dead, and preparation and experiential training for death. The observations on which this chapter is based are drawn, among others, from an extensive study of psychedelic therapy with terminal cancer patients that is described and discussed in this chapter in some detail.

The most far-reaching metaphysical insights from the research of holotropic states are summarized in the chapter on the "cosmic game." They concern such issues as the nature of reality, the cosmic creative principle and our relationship to it, the dynamics of creation, the taboo against knowing our true identity, and the problem of good and evil. It is fascinating that the answers to these fundamental questions of human existence, which spontaneously emerge in holotropic states, are surprisingly similar not only to those found in the literature on "perennial philosophy," as described by Aldous Huxley, but also to revolutionary findings of new paradigm science.

The closing chapter of the book focuses on the implications of the new findings for the understanding of the current global crisis and of the ways in which consciousness research and transpersonal psychology can contribute to its alleviation. It explores the psychospiritual roots of malignant aggression and insatiable greed, two forces that have dominated human history and that, because of rapid technological progress, have become a serious threat to survival of life on our planet. The work with holotropic states of consciousness provides not only a new understanding of these dangerous elements in the human psyche, but also effective ways of confronting and transforming them.

Forty years of intensive and systematic research of holotropic states have led me to the conclusion that radical inner transformation of humanity and rise to a higher level of consciousness might be our only real hope for the future. I would like to believe that those who are about to embark on the inner journey, or are traveling it already, will find this book and the information presented in it to be useful companions in this challenging adventure.

I feel deeply indebted and very grateful to Jane Bunker, acquisitions editor for State University of New York Press, without whom this book would not have been written. It was she who suggested that my readers might appreciate a work that would cover in one volume the most important insights that had emerged from my research of nonordinary states of consciousness. Following her guidance, I have written this book in such a way that it provides comprehensive information about all the major areas that I have explored in my research.

Those readers who will become interested in some particular subject discussed in one of the chapters can use this general overview as an introduction to my other books, which offer a more in-depth discussion of various specific topics. The following is a list of references to my writings or their parts that can be used as sources of additional information about the themes explored in the individual chapters.

Chapter 1. More detailed information about the heuristic and therapeutic potential of psychedelics can be found in my book *LSD Psychotherapy,* a comprehensive manual specifically dedicated to this topic, and in the appendix to *The Adventure of Self-Discovery,* focusing on the ritual and therapeutic use of psychedelic substances. The role of nonordinary states of consciousness in shamanism, rites of passage, the ancient mysteries of death and rebirth, and the great spiritual traditions is discussed in *The Stormy Search for the Self,* co-authored by my wife Christina.

Chapter 2. The new cartography of the human psyche is explored in detail particularly in *Realms of the Human Unconscious* and *The Adventure of Self-Discovery.* These books describe the dynamics of COEX systems, the perinatal matrices, and various forms of transpersonal experiences with many illustrative examples. *The Holotropic Mind,* co-authored by Hal Zina Bennett, is a very elementary introduction to the expanded map of the psyche, written for newcomers to the transpersonal field.

Chapter 3. The implications of my research for the diagnosis and treatment of emotional and psychosomatic disorders and for psychiatry and psychology in general are explored in *Beyond the Brain.* This book also contains a discussion of various revolutionary developments in modern science with which these new findings are compatible. Although accessible to interested lay persons, this book is primarily addressed to professional audiences.

Chapter 4. Those who are specifically interested in the concept of spiritual emergency and in the implications of consciousness research for the understanding and therapy of psychoses will find more information in two books that I have co-authored with my wife Christina, *The Stormy Search for the Self* and *Spiritual Emergency.* The first one is our own detailed and comprehensive discussion of alternative approaches to psychoses, the second is a compendium of articles by various other authors addressing this subject.

Chapter 5. The therapeutic potential of nonordinary states is the subject of many of my books. Of special interest might be the second half of *The Adventure of Self-Discovery* that describes the practice of holotropic breathwork and the therapeutic mechanisms operating in nonordinary states of consciousness. Relevant are also the passages in *Beyond the Brain* that discuss the pros and cons of various schools of psychotherapy and compare the uncovering and covering methods of therapy. *LSD Psychotherapy* is a manual discussing specifically the use of psychedelics in psychotherapy and *The Stormy Search for the Self* explores alternative therapeutic strategies in psychotic states.

Chapter 6. The relationship between spirituality and religion is discussed most comprehensively in *The Cosmic Game.* Information relevant to this subject can also be found in *The Stormy Search for the Self.*

Chapter 7. The psychological philosophical, and spiritual aspects of death and dying are discussed in *The Human Encounter with Death,* coauthored by Joan Halifax, describing a research project of psychedelic therapy with over two hundred cancer patients that we conducted at the Maryland Psychiatric Research Center in Baltimore. I have also written two richly illustrated quality paperbacks, exploring the cultural ramifications of this work—*Books of the Dead* and *Beyond Death,* the latter coauthored by my wife Christina.

Chapter 8. The philosophical, metaphysical, and spiritual aspects of my research are the subject of a separate volume, *The Cosmic Game.* This book explores the understanding of human nature and the nature of reality based on experiences and insights in holotropic states of consciousness. It points out the surprising similarity of this vision with Aldous Huxley's "perennial philosophy," as well as the revolutionary advances in modern science known as the new or emerging paradigm.

Chapter 9. Additional information on broader global implications of the work with holotropic states can be found in the epilogue to *Beyond the Brain* and in *The Cosmic Game.* I have also edited the book *Human Survival and Consciousness Evolution,* a compendium of articles by various prominent authors on this important subject.

All the above books that I have referred to also have extensive bibliographies that will direct interested readers to literature on related subjects written by other authors.

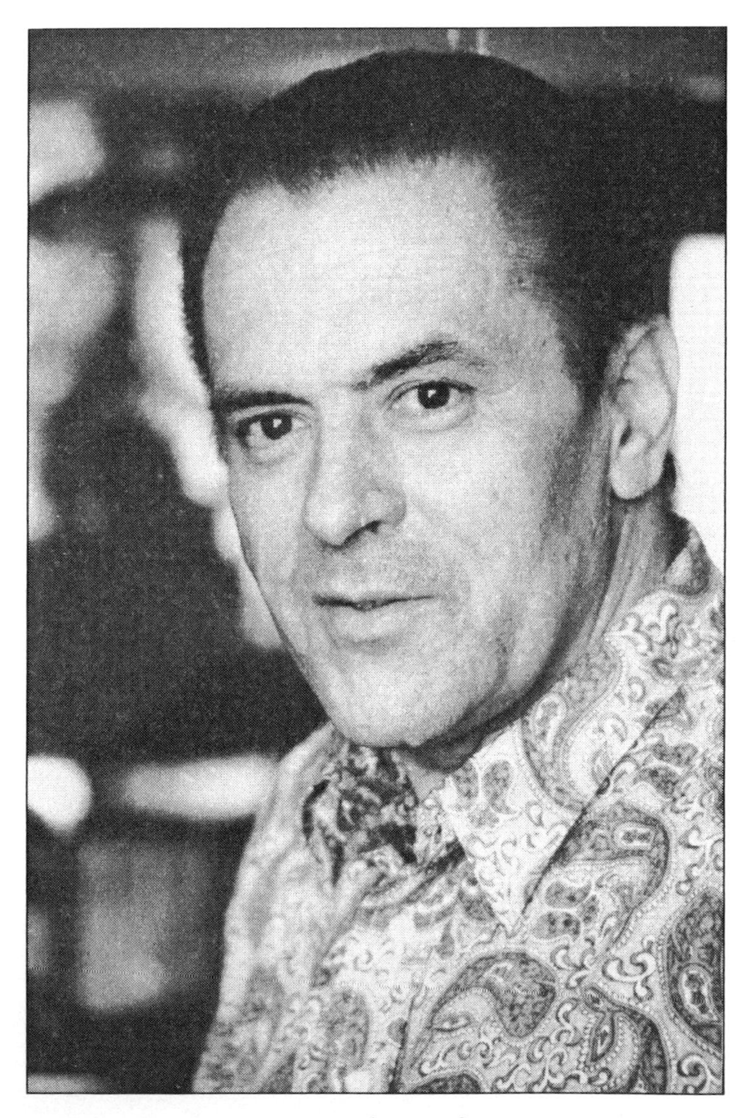

Stanislav Grof

CHAPTER ONE

Healing and Heuristic Potential of Nonordinary States of Consciousness

This book summarizes my experiences and observations from more than forty years of research of nonordinary states of consciousness. My primary interest is to focus on the heuristic aspects of these states; that is, on what they can contribute to our understanding of the nature of consciousness and of the human psyche. Since my original training was as clinical psychiatrist, I will also pay special attention to the healing, transformative, and evolutionary potential of these experiences. For this purpose, the term *nonordinary states of consciousness* is too broad and general. It includes a wide range of conditions that are of little or no interest from a heuristic or therapeutic perspective.

Consciousness can be profoundly changed by a variety of pathological processes—by cerebral traumas, by intoxications with poisonous chemicals, by infections, or by degenerative and circulatory processes in the brain. Such conditions can certainly result in profound mental changes that would relegate them to the category of "nonordinary states of consciousness." However, such impairments cause "trivial deliria" or "organic psychoses," states that are very important clinically, but are not relevant for our discussion. People suffering from such states are typically disoriented; they do not know who and where they are and what date it is. In addition, their intellectual functions are significantly impaired and they typically have subsequent amnesia for their experiences.

In this book, I will focus on a large and important subgroup of nonordinary states of consciousness which significantly differ from the rest and represent an invaluable source of new information about the human psyche in health and disease. They also have a remarkable therapeutic and transformative potential. Over the years, daily clinical observations convinced me about the extraordinary nature of these experiences and about the far-reaching implications they have for the theory and practice of psychiatry. I found it difficult to believe that contemporary psychiatry does not recognize their specific features and does not have a special name for them.

Because I feel strongly that they deserve to be distinguished from the rest and placed into a special category, I have coined for them the name *holotropic* (Grof 1992). This composite word literally means "oriented toward wholeness" or "moving in the direction of wholeness" (from the Greek *holos* = whole and *trepein* = moving toward or in the direction of something). The full meaning of this term and the justification for its use will become clear later in this book. It suggests that in our everyday state of consciousness we identify with only a small fraction of who we really are. In holotropic states, we can transcend the narrow boundaries of the body ego and reclaim our full identity.

Holotropic States of Consciousness

In holotropic states, consciousness is changed qualitatively in a very profound and fundamental way, but it is not grossly impaired like in the organically caused conditions. We typically remain fully oriented in terms of space and time and do not completely lose touch with everyday reality. At the same time, our field of consciousness is invaded by contents from other dimensions of existence in a way that can be very intense and even overwhelming. We thus experience simultaneously two very different realities, "have each foot in a different world."

Holotropic states are characterized by dramatic perceptual changes in all sensory areas. When we close our eyes, our visual field can be flooded with images drawn from our personal history and from the individual and collective unconscious. We can have visions and experiences portraying various aspects of the animal and botanical kingdoms, nature in general, or of the cosmos. Our experiences can take us into the realm of archetypal beings and mythological regions. When we open the eyes, our perception of the environment can be illusively transformed by vivid projections of this unconscious material. This can be accompanied by a wide range of experiences engaging other senses—various sounds, physical sensations, smells, and tastes.

The emotions associated with holotropic states cover a very broad spectrum that typically extends far beyond the limits of our everyday experience, both in their nature and intensity. They range from feelings of ecstatic rapture, heavenly bliss, and "peace that passeth all understanding" to episodes of abysmal terror, murderous anger, utter despair, consuming guilt, and other forms of unimaginable emotional suffering. Extreme forms of these emotional states match the descriptions of the paradisean or celestial realms and of hells described in the scriptures of the great religions of the world.

A particularly interesting aspect of holotropic states is their effect on thought processes. The intellect is not impaired, but functions in a way that is significantly different from its everyday mode of operation. While we might not be able to rely on our judgment in ordinary practical matters, we can be literally flooded with remarkable valid information on a variety of subjects. We can reach profound psychological insights concerning our personal history, unconscious dynamics, emotional difficulties, and interpersonal problems. We can also experience extraordinary revelations concerning various aspects of nature and of the cosmos that by a wide margin transcend our educational and intellectual background. However, by far the most interesting insights that become available in holotropic states revolve around philosophical, metaphysical, and spiritual issues.

We can experience sequences of psychological death and rebirth and a broad spectrum of transpersonal phenomena, such as feelings of oneness with other people, nature, the universe, and God. We might uncover what seem to be memories from other incarnations, encounter powerful archetypal figures, communicate with discarnate beings, and visit numerous mythological landscapes. Holotropic experiences of this kind are the main source of cosmologies, mythologies, philosophies, and religious systems describing the spiritual nature of the cosmos and of existence. They are the key for understanding the ritual and spiritual life of humanity from shamanism and sacred ceremonies of aboriginal tribes to the great religions of the world.

Holotropic States of Consciousness and Human History

When we examine the role that holotropic states of consciousness have played in human history, the most surprising discovery is a striking difference between the attitude toward these states characterizing the Western industrial society and those of all the ancient and pre-industrial cultures. In sharp contrast with modern humanity, all the indigenous cultures held holotropic states in great esteem and spent much time and effort developing safe and effective ways of inducing them. They used them as a principal vehicle in their ritual and spiritual life and for several other important purposes.

In the context of sacred ceremonies, nonordinary states mediated for the natives direct experiential contact with the archetypal dimensions of reality—deities, mythological realms, and numinous forces of nature. Another area where these states played a crucial role was diagnosing and healing of various disorders. Although aboriginal cultures often possessed impressive knowledge of naturalistic remedies, they put primary emphasis on metaphysical healing. This typically involved induction of holotropic states of consciousness—for the client, for the healer, or both of them at the same time. In many instances, a large group or even an entire tribe entered a healing trance together, as it is, for example, until this day among the !Kung Bushmen in the African Kalahari Desert.

Holotropic states have also been used to cultivate intuition and extrasensory perception (ESP) for a variety of practical purposes, such as finding lost persons and objects, obtaining information about people in remote locations, and for following the movement of the game. In addition, they served as a source of artistic inspiration, providing ideas for rituals, paintings, sculptures, and songs. The impact that the experiences encountered in these states had on the cultural life of pre-industrial societies and the spiritual history of humanity has been enormous.

The importance of holotropic states for ancient and aboriginal cultures is reflected in the amount of time and energy dedicated to the development of "technologies of the sacred," various mind-altering procedures capable of inducing holotropic states for ritual and spiritual purposes. These methods combine in various ways drumming and other forms of percussion, music, chanting, rhythmic dancing, changes of breathing, and cultivation of special forms of awareness. Extended social and sensory isolation, such as a stay in a cave, desert, arctic ice, or in high mountains, also play an important role as means of inducing holotropic states. Extreme physiological interventions used for this purpose include fasting, sleep deprivation, dehydration, and even massive bloodletting, use of powerful laxatives and purgatives, and infliction of severe pain.

A particularly effective technology for inducing holotropic states has been ritual use of psychedelic plants and substances. The legendary divine

TABLE 1.1 **Ancient and Aboriginal Techniques for Inducing Holotropic States**

Work with breath, direct or indirect (pranayama, yogic bastrika, Buddhist "fire breath," Sufi breathing, Balinese ketjak, Inuit Eskimo throat music, etc.)

Sound technologies (drumming, rattling, use of sticks, bells, and gongs, music, chanting, mantras, didjeridoo, bull-roarer)

Dancing and other forms of movement (whirling of the dervishes, lama dances, Kalahari Bushmen trance dance, hatha yoga, tai chi, chigong, etc.)

Social isolation and sensory deprivation (stay in the desert, in caves, on mountain tops, in the snow fields, vision quest, etc.)

Sensory overload (a combination of acoustic, visual, and proprioceptive stimuli during aboriginal rituals, extreme pain, etc.)

Physiological means (fasting, sleep deprivation, purgatives, laxatives, blood letting [Mayas], painful physical procedures (Lakota Sioux sun dance, subincision, filing of teeth)

Meditation, prayer, and other spiritual practices (various yogas, Tantra, Soto and Rinzai Zen practice, Tibetan Dzogchen, Christian hesychasm (Jesus prayer), the exercises of Ignatius of Loyola, etc.)

Psychedelic animal and plant materials (hashish, peyote, teonanacatl, ololiuqui, ayahuasca, eboga, Hawaian woodrose, Syrian rue, secretion from the skin of the toad Bufo alvarius, Pacific fish Kyphosus fuscus, etc.)

---

potion referred to as *haoma* in the ancient Persian Zend Avesta and as *soma* in India was used by the Indoiranian tribes several millenia ago and was probably the most important source of the Vedic religion and philosophy. Preparations from different varieties of hemp have been smoked and ingested under various names (*hashish, charas, bhang, ganja, kif, marijuana*) in the Oriental countries, in Africa, and in the Caribbean area for recreation, pleasure, and during religious ceremonies. They have represented an important sacrament for such diverse groups as the Brahmans, certain Sufi orders, ancient Skythians, and the Jamaican Rastafarians.

Ceremonial use of various psychedelic materials also has a long history in Central America. Highly effective mind-altering plants were well known in several Pre-Hispanic Indian cultures—among the Aztecs, Mayans, and Toltecs. Most famous of these are the Mexican cactus *peyote* (Lophophora williamsii), the sacred mushroom *teonanacatl* (Psilocybe mexicana), and *ololiuqui,* seeds of different varieties of the morning glory plant (Ipomoea violacea and Turbina corymbosa). These materials have been used as sacraments until this day by the Huichol, Mazatec, Chichimeca, Cora, and other Mexican Indian tribes, as well as the Native American Church.

The famous South American yajé or ayahuasca is a decoction from a jungle liana (Banisteriopsis caapi) combined with other plant additives.

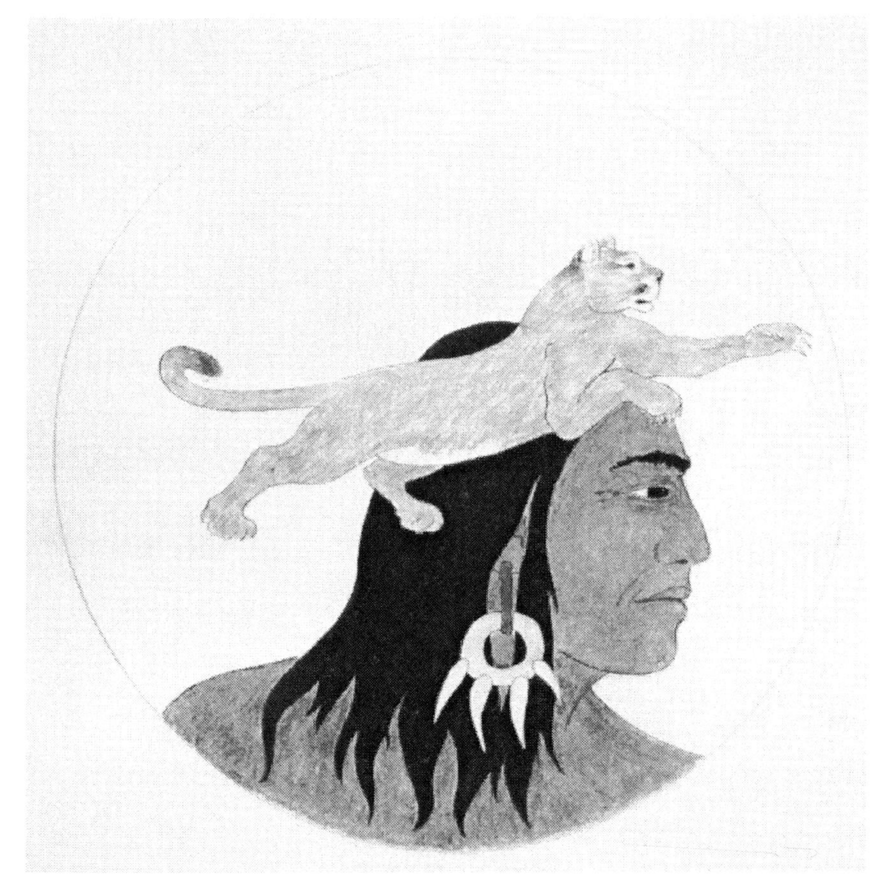

Painting from a holotropic breathwork session reflecting the experience of the shaman's transformation into a mountain lion (Tai Ingrid Hazard).

The Amazonian area and the Caribbean islands are also known for a variety of psychedelic snuffs. Aboriginal tribes in Africa ingest and inhale preparations from the bark of the eboga shrub (Tabernanthe iboga). They use them in small quantities as stimulants and in larger dosages in initiation rituals for men and women. The psychedelic compounds of animal origin include the secretions of the skin of certain toads (Bufo alvarius) and the meat of the Pacific fish Kyphosus fuscus. The above list represents only a small fraction of psychedelic materials that have been used over many centuries in ritual and spiritual life of various countries of the world.

The practice of inducing holotropic states can be traced back to the dawn of human history. It is the most important characteristic feature of *shamanism,* the oldest spiritual system and healing art of humanity. The career of many shamans begins with a spontaneous psychospiritual crisis ("shamanic illness"). It is a powerful visionary state during which the future shaman experiences a journey into the underworld, the realm of the dead, where he or she is attacked by evil spirits, subjected to various ordeals, killed, and dismembered. This is followed by an experience of rebirth and ascent into the celestial realms.

Shamanism is connected with holotropic states in yet another way. Accomplished and experienced shamans are able to enter into a trance state at will and in a controlled way. They use it for dignosing diseases,

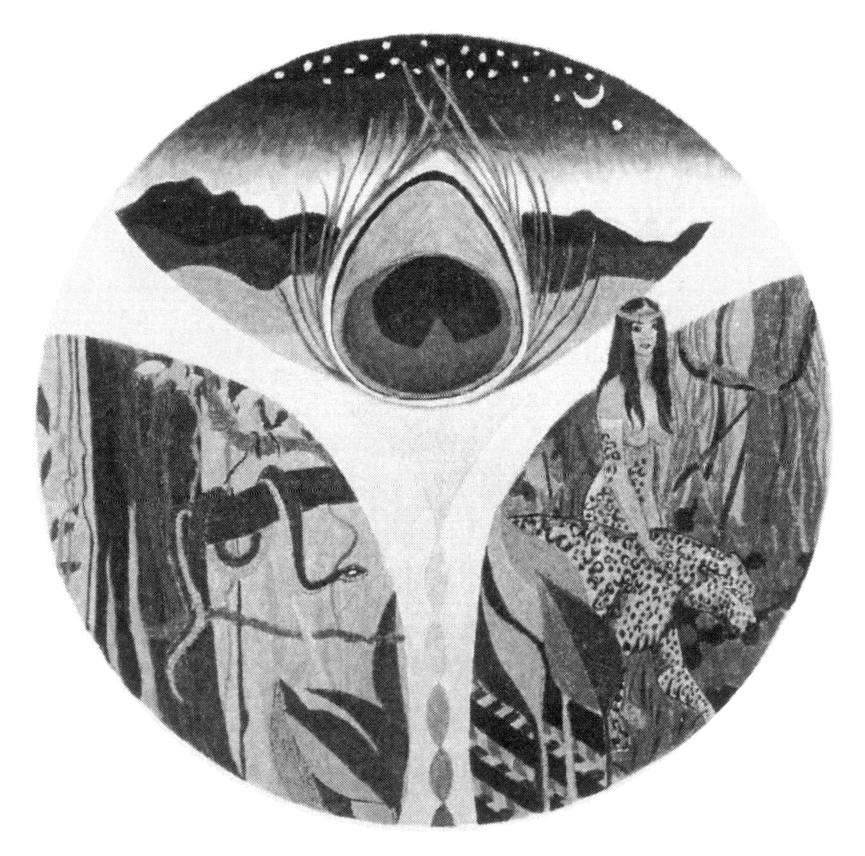

Painting from a holotropic breathwork session in which the artists identified with an adolescent girl from a South American tribe participating in a puberty rite. An important part of the ritual was experiential identification with a jaguar (Kathleen Silver).

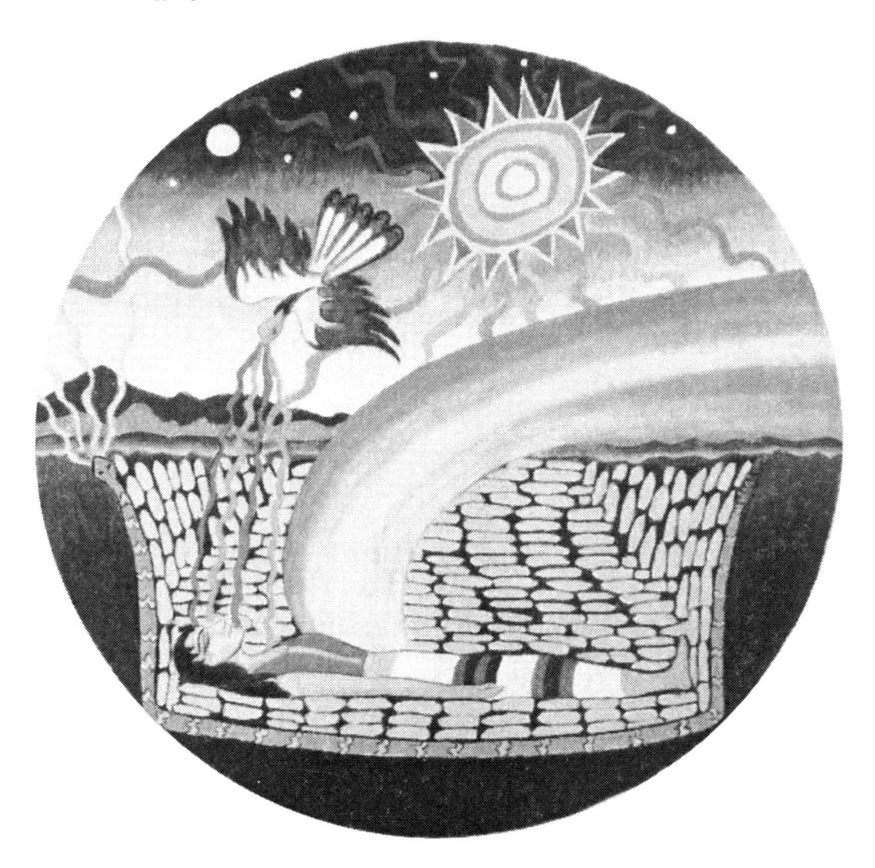

Painting from a holotropic breathwork session representing identification with a virgin from the Yucatan part of Mexico used as sacrificial victim in a ritual celebrating the Corn Goddess. A period of suffocation, panic, and sexual arousal was followed by a beautiful rainbow bringing light and peace (Kathleen Silver).

healing, extrasensory perception, exploration of alternate dimensions of reality, and other purposes. They also often induce holotropic states in other members of their tribes and play the role of "psychopomps"—provide the necessary support and guidance for those traversing the complex territories of the Beyond.

Shamanism is extremely ancient, probably at least thirty to forty thousand years old; its roots can be traced far back into the Paleolithic era. The walls of the famous caves in Southern France and northern Spain, such as Lascaux, Font de Gaume, Les Trois Frères, Altamira, and others, are decorated with beautiful images of animals. Most of them represent species that actually roamed the Stone Age landscape—bisons, wild horses, stags, ibexes, mammoths, wolves, rhinos, and reindeers. However, others like the "Wizard Beast" in Lascaux are mythical creatures that clearly have magical and ritual significance. And in several of these caves are paintings and carvings of strange figures combining human and animal features, who undoubtedly represent ancient shamans.

The best known of these images is the "Sorcerer of Les Trois Frères," a mysterious composite figure combining various male symbols. He has the antlers of a stag, eyes of an owl, tail of a wild horse or wolf, human beard, and paws of a lion. Another famous carving of a shaman in the same cave complex is the "Beast Master," presiding over the Happy Hunting Grounds teeming with beautiful animals. Also well known is the hunting scene on the wall in Lascaux. It shows a wounded bison and a lying figure of a shaman with an erect penis. The grotto known as La Gabillou harbors a carving of a shamanic figure in dynamic movement whom the archeologists call "The Dancer."

On the clay floor of one of these caves, Tuc d'Audoubert, the discoverers found footprints in circular arrangement around two clay bison effigies suggesting that its inhabitants conducted dances, similar to those that are still being performed by many aboriginal cultures for the induction of trance states. The origins of shamanism can be traced back to a yet older Neanderthal cult of the cave bear as exemplified by the animal shrines from the interglacial period found in the grottoes in Switzerland and southern Germany.

Shamanism is not only ancient, it is also universal; it can be found in North and South America, in Europe, Africa, Asia, Australia, Micronesia, and Polynesia. The fact that so many different cultures throughout human history have found shamanic techniques useful and relevant suggests that the holotropic states engage what the anthropologists call the "primal mind," a basic and primordial aspect of the human psyche that transcends race, sex, culture, and historical time. In cultures that have escaped the disruptive influence of the Western industrial civilization, shamanic techniques and procedures have survived to this day.

Another example of culturally sanctioned psychospiritual transformation involving holotropic states are ritual events that the anthropologists call *rites of passage*. This term was coined by the Dutch anthropologist Arnold van Gennep, the author of the first scientific treatise on the subject (van Gennep 1960). Ceremonies of this kind existed in all known native cultures and are still being performed in many pre-industrial societies. Their main purpose is to redefine, transform, and consecrate individuals, groups, and even entire cultures.

Rites of passage are conducted at times of critical change in the life of an individual or a culture. Their timing frequently coincides with major physiological and social transitions, such as childbirth, circumcision, puberty, marriage, menopause, and dying. Similar rituals are also associated with initiation into warrior status, acceptance into secret societies, calendrical festivals of renewal, healing ceremonies, and geographical moves of human groups.

Rites of passage involve powerful mind-altering procedures that induce psychologically disorganizing experiences resulting in a higher level of integration. This episode of psychospiritual death and rebirth is then interpreted as dying to the old role and being born into the new one. For example, in the puberty rites the initiates enter the procedure as boys or girls and emerge as adults with all the rights and duties that come with this status. In all these situations, the individual or social group leaves behind one mode of being and moves into totally new life circumstances.

The person who returns from the initiation is not the same as the one who entered the initiation process. Having undergone a deep psychospiritual transformation, he or she has a personal connection with the numinous dimensions of existence, as well as a new and much expanded worldview, a better self-image, and a different system of values. All this is the result of a deliberately induced crisis that reaches the very core of the initiate's being and is at times terrifying, chaotic, and disorganizing. The rites of passage thus provide another example of a situation in which a period of temporary disintegration and turmoil leads to greater sanity and well-being.

The two examples of "positive disintegration" I have discussed so far—the shamanic crisis and the experience of the rite of passage—have many features in common, but they also differ in some important ways. The shamanic crisis invades the psyche of the future shaman unexpectedly and without warning; it is spontaneous and autonomous in nature. In comparison, the rites of passage are a product of the culture and follow a predictable time schedule. The experiences of the initiates are the result of specific "technologies of the sacred," developed and perfected by previous generations.

In cultures that venerate shamans and also conduct rites of passage, the shamanic crisis is considered to be a form of initiation that is much superior to the rite of passage. It is seen as intervention of higher power and thus indication of divine choice and special calling. From another perspective, rites of passage represent a further step in cultural appreciation of the positive value of holotropic states. Shamanic cultures accept and hold in high esteem holotropic states that occur spontaneously during initiatory crises and the healing trance experienced or induced by recognized shamans. Rites of passage introduce holotropic states into the culture on a large scale, institutionalize them, and make them an integral part of ritual and spiritual life.

Holotropic states of consciousness also played a critical role in the *mysteries of death and rebirth,* sacred and secret procedures that were widespread in the ancient world. These mysteries were based on mythological stories about deities symbolizing death and transfiguration. In ancient Sumer it was Inanna and Tammuz, in Egypt Isis and Osiris, and in Greece the deities Attis, Adonis, Dionysus, and Persephone. Their Mesoamerican counterparts were the Aztec Quetzalcoatl, or the Plumed Serpent, and the Mayan Hero Twins known from the Popol Vuh. These mysteries were particularly popular in the Mediterranean area and in the Middle East, as exemplified by the Sumerian and Egyptian temple initiations, the Mithraic mysteries, or the Greek Korybantic rites, Bacchanalia, and the mysteries of Eleusis.

An impressive testimony for the power and impact of the experiences involved is the fact that the mysteries conducted in the Eleusinian sanctuary near Athens took place regularly and without interruption every five years for a period of almost two thousand years. Even then they did not simply cease to attract the attention of the antique world. The ceremonial activities in Eleusis were brutally interrupted when the Christian Emperor Theodosius interdicted participation in the mysteries and all other pagan cults. Shortly afterward, in 395 A.D., the invading Goths destroyed the sanctuary.

In the telestrion, the giant initiation hall in Eleusis, over three thousand neophytes at a time experienced powerful experiences of psychospiritual transformation. The cultural importance of these mysteries for the ancient world and their as yet unacknowledged role in the history of European civilization becomes evident when we realize that among their initiates were many famous and illustrious figures of antiquity. The list of neophytes included the philosophers Plato, Aristotle, and Epictetus, the military leader Alkibiades, the playwrights Euripides and Sophocles, and the poet Pindaros. Another famous initiate, Marcus Aurelius, was fascinated by the eschatological hopes offered by these rites. Roman statesman and philosopher Marcus Tullius Cicero took part in these mysteries and wrote an exalted report about their effects and their impact on the antique civilization (Cicero 1977).

Another example of the great respect and influence the ancient mystery religions had in the antique world is Mithraism. It began to spread throughout the Roman Empire in the first century A.D., reached its peak in the third century, and succumbed to Christianity at the end of the fourth century. At the cult's height, the underground Mithraic sanctuaries (*mithraea*), could be found from the shores of the Black Sea to the mountains of Scotland and to the border of the Sahara Desert. The Mithraic mysteries represented the sister religion of Christianity and its most important competitor (Ulansey 1989).

The specifics of the mind-altering procedures involved in these secret rites have remained for the most part unknown, although it is likely that the sacred potion *kykeon* that played a critical role in the Eleusinian mysteries was a concoction containing alkaloids of ergot similar to LSD. It is also highly probable that psychedelic materials were involved in the bacchanalia and other types of rites. Ancient Greeks did not know distillation of alcohol and yet, according to the reports, the wines used in Dionysian rituals had to be diluted three to twenty times and a mere three cups brought some initiates "to the brink of insanity" (Wasson, Hofmann, and Ruck 1978).

In addition to the above ancient and aboriginal technologies of the sacred, many great religions developed *sophisticated psychospiritual procedures* specifically designed to induce holotropic experiences. Here belong, for example, different techniques of yoga, meditations used in Vipassana, Zen, and Tibetan Buddhism, as well as spiritual exercises of the Taoist tradition and complex Tantric rituals. We could also add various elaborate approaches used by the Sufis, the mystics of Islam. They regularly used in their sacred ceremonies, or *zikers,* intense breathing, devotional chants, and trance-inducing whirling dance.

From the Judeo-Christian tradition, we can mention here the breathing exercises of the Essenes and their baptism involving half-drowning, the Christian Jesus prayer (hesychasm), the exercises of Ignatius of Loyola, and various Cabalistic and Hassidic procedures. Approaches designed to induce or facilitate direct spiritual experiences are characteristic for the mystical branches of the great religions and for their monastic orders.

Holotropic States in the History of Psychiatry

The unambiguous acceptance of holotropic states in the preindustrial era stands in sharp contrast with the complex and confusing attitude toward these states in the industrial civilization. Holotropic states played a crucial role in the early history of depth psychology and psychotherapy. In psychiatric handbooks, the roots of depth psychology are usually traced back to hypnotic sessions with hysterical patients conducted by Jean Martin Charcot at the Salpetrière in Paris and to the research in hypnosis carried out by Hippolyte Bernheim and Ambroise Liébault at Nancy. Sigmund Freud visited both places during his study journey to France and learned the technique of inducing hypnosis. He used it in his initial explorations to access his patients' unconscious. Later, he radically changed his strategy and replaced this approach with the method of free associations.

In addition, Freud's early ideas were inspired by his work with a patient whom he treated jointly with his friend Joseph Breuer. This young woman, whom Freud called in his writings Miss Anna O., suffered from severe hysterical symptoms. During their therapeutic sessions, she experienced spontaneous holotropic states of consciousness in which she regressed to childhood and relived various traumatic memories underlying her neurotic disorder. She found these experiences very helpful and referred to them as "chimney sweeping." In *Studies in Hysteria,* the two therapists recommended hypnotic regression and belated emotional abreaction of traumas as the treatment for psychoneuroses (Freud and Breuer 1936).

In his later work, Freud moved from direct emotional experience in a holotropic state to free association in the ordinary state of consciousness. He also shifted emphasis from conscious reliving and emotional abreaction of unconscious material to analysis of transference and from actual trauma to Oedipal fantasies. In retrospect, these seem to have been unfortunate developments that sent Western psychotherapy in the wrong direction for the next fifty years (Ross 1989). While verbal therapy can be very useful in providing interpersonal learning and rectifying skewed interaction and communication in human relationships (e.g., couple and family therapy), it is ineffective in dealing with emotional and bioenergetic blockages and macrotraumas that underlie many emotional and psychosomatic disorders.

As a result of this development, psychotherapy in the first half of the twentieth century was practically synonymous with talking—face-to-face interviews, free associations on the couch, and the behaviorist deconditioning. At the same time holotropic states, initially seen as an effective therapeutic tool, became associated with pathology rather than healing.

This situation started to change in the 1950s with the advent of psychedelic therapy and radical innovations in psychology. A group of American psychologists headed by Abraham Maslow, who were dissatisfied with behaviorism and Freudian psychoanalysis, launched a new revolutionary movement, *humanistic psychology*. Within a very short time, this movement became very popular and provided the context for a broad spectrum of therapies based on entirely new principles.

While traditional psychotherapies used primarily verbal means and intellectual analysis, these new, so-called experiential, therapies emphasized direct experience and expression of emotions. Many of them also included various forms of bodywork as integral parts of the therapeutic process. Probably the most famous representative of these new approaches is Fritz Perls's Gestalt therapy (Perls 1976). In spite of their emphasis on emotional experience, most of these therapies still rely to a great degree on verbal communication and require that the client stay in the ordinary state of consciousness.

The most radical innovations in the therapeutic field have been approaches so powerful that they profoundly change the state of consciousness of the clients, such as psychedelic therapy, various neo-Reichian approaches, primal therapy, rebirthing, and a few others. My wife Christina and I have developed holotropic breathwork, a method that can facilitate profound holotropic states by very simple means—a combination of conscious breathing, evocative music, and focused bodywork (Grof 1988). We will explore the theory and practice of this powerful form of self-exploration and psychotherapy later in this book.

Modern psychopharmacological research enriched the armamentarium of methods for inducing holotropic states of consciousness by adding *psychedelic substances in pure chemical form,* either isolated from plants or synthetized in the laboratory. Here belong the tetrahydrocannabinols (THC), active principles from hashish and marijuana, mescaline from peyote, psilocybine and psilocine from the Mexican magic mushrooms, and various tryptamine derivatives from the psychedelic snuffs used in the Caribbean area and in South America. LSD, or diethylamid of lysergic acid, is a semisynthetic substance; lysergic acid is a natural product of ergot and its diethylamid group is added in the laboratory. The most famous synthetic psychedelics are the amphetamine derivatives MDA, MDMA (Adam or Ecstasy), STP, and 2-CB.

There also exist very effective laboratory techniques for altering consciousness. One of these is *sensory isolation,* which involves significant reduction of meaningful sensory stimuli (Lilly 1977). In its extreme form the individual is deprived of sensory input by submersion in a dark and soundproof tank filled with water of body temperature. Another well-known laboratory method of changing consciousness is *biofeedback,* where the individual is guided by electronic feedback signals into holotropic states of consciousness characterized by preponderance of certain specific frequencies of brainwaves (Green and Green 1978). We could also mention here the techniques of *sleep and dream deprivation* and *lucid dreaming* (LaBerge 1985).

It is important to emphasize that episodes of holotropic states of varying duration can also occur spontaneously, without any specific identifiable cause, and often against the will of the people involved. Since modern psychiatry does not differentiate between mystical or spiritual states and mental diseases, people experiencing these states are often labeled psychotic, hospitalized, and receive routine suppressive psychopharmacological treatment. My wife Christina and I refer to these states as *psychospiritual crises* or *spiritual emergencies.* We believe that properly supported and treated, they can result in emotional and psychosomatic healing, positive personality transformation, and consciousness evolution (Grof and Grof 1989, 1990). I will return to this important topic in a later chapter.

Although I have been deeply interested in all the categories of holotropic states mentioned above, I have done most of my work in the area of psychedelic therapy, holotropic breathwork, and spiritual emergency. This book is based predominantly on my observations from these three areas in which I have most personal experience. However, the general conclusions I will be drawing from my research apply to all the situations involving holotropic states.

Western Psychiatry:
Misconceptions and Urgent Need for Revision

The advent of psychedelic therapy and powerful experiential techniques reintroduced holotropic states into the therapeutic armamentarium of modern psychiatry. However, since the very beginning, the mainstream academic community has shown a strong resistance against these approaches and has not accepted them either as treatment modalities or as a source of critical conceptual challenges.

All the evidence published in numerous professional journals and books was not enough to challenge the deeply ingrained attitude toward holotropic states established in the first half of the twentieth century. The problems resulting from unsupervised self-experimentation of the young generation in the 1960s and the misconceptions spread by sensation-hunting journalists further complicated the picture and prevented a realistic evaluation of the potential of psychedelics, as well as the risks associated with their use.

In spite of the overwhelming evidence to the contrary, mainstream psychiatrists continue to view all holotropic states of consciousness as pathological, disregard the information generated in researching them, and do not distinguish between mystical states and psychosis. They also continue using various pharmacological means to suppress indiscriminately all spontaneously occurring nonordinary states of consciousness. It is remarkable to what extent mainstream science has ignored, distorted, and misinterpreted all the evidence concerning holotropic states, whether their source has been historical study, comparative religion, anthropology, or various areas of modern consciousness research, such as parapsychology, psychedelic therapy, experiential psychotherapies, hypnosis, thanatology, or work with laboratory mind-altering techniques.

The rigidity with which mainstream scientists have dealt with the information amassed by all these disciplines is something that one would expect from religious fundamentalists. It is very surprising when such attitude occurs in the world of science, since it is contrary to the very spirit of scientific inquiry. More than four decades that I have spent in consciousness research have convinced me that serious examination of the data from the study of holotropic states would have far-reaching consequences not only for the theory and practice of psychiatry, but for the Western scientific worldview. The only way modern science can preserve its monistic materialistic philosophy is by systematically excluding and censoring all the data concerning holotropic states.

As we have seen, utilization of the healing potential of holotropic states is the most recent development in Western psychotherapy, if we do not take into consideration the brief period at the turn of the century that we discussed earlier. Paradoxically, in a larger historical context, it is also the oldest form of healing, one that can be traced back to the dawn of humanity. The therapies using holotropic states thus represent a rediscovery and modern reinterpretation of the elements and principles that have been documented by anthropologists studying ancient and aboriginal forms of spiritual healing, particularly various shamanic procedures.

Implications of Modern Consciousness Research for Psychiatry

As I mentioned earlier, Western psychiatry and psychology do not see holotropic states (with the exception of dreams that are not recurrent or frightening) as having therapeutic and heuristic potential, but basically as pathological phenomena. Michael Harner, an anthropologist of good academic standing, who also underwent a shamanic initiation during his field work in the Amazonian jungle and practices shamanism, suggests that Western psychiatry is seriously biased in at least two significant ways. It is *ethnocentric,* which means that it considers its own view of the human psyche and of reality to be the only correct one and superior to all others. It is also *cognicentric* (a more accurate word might be *pragmacentric*), meaning that it takes into consideration only experiences and observations in the ordinary state of consciousness (Harner 1980).

Psychiatry's disinterest in holotropic states and disregard for them has resulted in a culturally insensitive approach and a tendency to pathologize all activities that cannot be understood in the narrow context of the monistic materialistic paradigm. This includes the ritual and spiritual life of ancient and preindustrial cultures and the entire spiritual history of humanity. At the same time, this attitude also obfuscated the critical conceptual challenge that the study of holotropic states brings for the theory and practice of psychiatry.

If we study systematically the experiences and observations associated with holotropic states, this leads inevitably to a radical revision of our basic ideas about consciousness and about the human psyche and to an entirely new approach to psychiatry, psychology, and psychotherapy. The changes we would have to make in our thinking fall into several large categories.

The Nature of the Human Psyche and the Dimensions of Consciousness

Traditional academic psychiatry and psychology use a model that is limited to biology, postnatal biography, and the Freudian individual unconscious. To account for all the phenomena occurring in holotropic states, we must drastically revise our understanding of the dimensions of the human psyche. Besides *the postnatal biographical level,* the new expanded cartography includes two additional domains: *perinatal* (related to the trauma of birth) and *transpersonal* (comprising ancestral, racial, collective, and phylogenetic memories, karmic experiences, and archetypal dynamics).

The Nature and Architecture of Emotional and Psychosomatic Disorders
To explain various disorders that do not have an organic basis ("psychogenic psychopathology"), traditional psychiatry uses a model that is limited to postnatal biographical traumas in infancy, childhood, and later life. The new understanding suggests that the roots of such disorders reach much deeper to include significant contributions from the perinatal level (trauma of birth) and from the transpersonal domains (as specified above).

Effective Therapeutic Mechanisms
Traditional psychotherapy knows only therapeutic mechanisms operating on the level of the biographical material, such as remembering of forgotten events, lifting of repression, reconstruction of the past from dreams or neurotic symptoms, reliving of traumatic memories, and analysis of transference. Holotropic research reveals many other important mechanisms of healing and personality transformation that become available when our consciousness reaches the perinatal and transpersonal levels.

Strategy of Psychotherapy and Self-Exploration
The goal in traditional psychotherapies is to reach an intellectual understanding as to how the psyche functions, why symptoms develop, and what they mean. This understanding then becomes the basis for developing a technique that therapists can use to treat their patients. A serious problem with this strategy is the striking lack of agreement among psychologists and psychiatrists concerning the most fundamental theoretical issues and the resulting astonishing number of competing schools of psychotherapy. The work with holotropic states shows us a surprising radical alternative—mobilization of deep inner intelligence of the clients that guides the process of healing and transformation.

The Role of Spirituality in Human Life
Western materialistic science has no place for any form of spirituality and, in fact, considers it incompatible with the scientific worldview. Modern consciousness research shows that spirituality is a natural and legitimate

dimension of the human psyche and of the universal scheme of things. However, in this context, it is important to emphasize that this statement applies to genuine spirituality and not to ideologies of organized religions.

The Nature of Reality: Psyche, Cosmos, and Consciousness

The necessary revisions discussed up to this point were related to the theory and practice of psychiatry, psychology, and psychotherapy. However, the work with holotropic states brings challenges of a much more fundamental nature. Many of the experiences and observations that occur during this work are so extraordinary that they cannot be understood in the context of the monistic materialistic approach to reality. Their conceptual impact is so far-reaching that it undermines the most basic metaphysical assumptions of Western science, particularly those regarding the nature of consciousness and its relationship to matter.

CHAPTER TWO

Cartography of the Human Psyche: Biographical, Perinatal, and Transpersonal Domains

The experiences in holotropic states of consciousness and the observations related to them cannot be explained in terms of the conceptual framework of academic psychiatry, that is limited to postnatal biography and to the Freudian individual unconscious. To account for the phenomenology of these states and for the events associated with them, we need a model with an incomparably larger and more encompassing image of the human psyche and a radically different understanding of consciousness. In the early years of my psychedelic research, I sketched a vastly expanded cartography of the psyche that seems to meet this challenge.

As mentioned earlier, this map contains, in addition to the usual *biographical level,* two transbiographical realms: *the perinatal domain,* related to the trauma of biological birth; and *the transpersonal domain,* which accounts for such phenomena as experiential identification with other people, animals, plants, and other aspects of nature. The latter realm is also the source of ancestral, racial, phylogenetic, and karmic memories, as well as visions of archetypal beings and mythological regions. The extreme experiences in this category are identification with the Universal Mind and with the Supracosmic and Metacosmic Void. Perinatal and transpersonal phenomena have been described throughout the ages in the religious, mystical, and occult literature of various countries of the world.

Postnatal Biography and the Individual Unconscious

The biographical domain of the psyche consists of our memories from infancy, childhood, and later life. This part of the psyche does not require much discussion, since it is well known from traditional psychiatry, psychology, and psychotherapy. As a matter of fact, the image of the psyche used in academic circles is limited exclusively to this domain and to the individual unconscious. And the unconscious, as described by Sigmund Freud, is closely related to this realm, since it consists mostly of postnatal biographical material that has been forgotten or actively repressed. But the description of the biographical level of the psyche in the new cartography is not identical with the traditional one. The work with holotropic states has revealed certain aspects of the dynamics of the biographical realm that remained hidden to researchers using verbal psychotherapy.

First, in holotropic states, unlike in verbal therapy, one does not just remember emotionally significant events or reconstruct them indirectly from dreams, slips of tongue, or from transference distortions. One experiences the original emotions, physical sensations, and even sensory perceptions in full age regression. That means that during the reliving of an important trauma from infancy or childhood, one actually has the body image, the naïve perception of the world, sensations, and the emotions corresponding to the age he or she was at that time. The authenticity of this regression is evident from the fact that the wrinkles in the face of these people temporarily disappear, giving them an infantile expression, and their postures, gestures, and behavior become childlike.

The second difference between the work on the biographical material in holotropic states, as compared with verbal psychotherapies, is that, besides confronting the usual psychotraumas known from handbooks of psychology, we often have to relive and integrate traumas that were primarily of a physical nature. Many people undergoing psychedelic or holotropic therapy have relived experiences of near drowning, operations, accidents, and children's diseases. Of particular importance seem to be insults that were associated with suffocation, such as diphtheria, whooping cough, strangling, or aspiration of a foreign object.

This material emerges quite spontaneously and without any programming. As it surfaces, we realize that these physical traumas had a strong psychotraumatic impact on us and that they played a significant role in the psychogenesis of our emotional and psychosomatic problems. A history of physical traumas can regularly be found in clients suffering from asthma, migraine headaches, psychosomatic pains, phobias, sadomasochistic tendencies, or depression and suicidal tendencies. Reliving of traumatic memories of this kind and their integration can have very far-reaching therapeutic consequences. This fact contrasts sharply with the position of academic psychiatry and psychology that do not recognize psychotraumatic impact of physical traumas.

Another new insight concerning the biographical/recollective level of the psyche that emerged from my research was the discovery that emotionally relevant memories are not stored in the unconscious as a mosaic of isolated imprints, but in the form of complex dynamic constellations. I have coined for these memory aggregates the name *COEX systems,* which is short for "systems of condensed experience." This concept is of such theoretical and practical importance that it deserves special discussion.

Systems of Condensed Experience (COEX Systems)

A COEX system consists of emotionally charged memories from different periods of our life that resemble each other in the quality of emotion or physical sensation that they share. Each COEX has a basic theme that permeates all its layers and represents their common denominator. The individual layers then contain variations on this basic theme that occurred at different periods of the person's life. The unconscious of a particular individual can contain several COEX constellations. Their number and the nature of the central themes varies considerably from one person to another.

The layers of a particular system can, for example, contain all the major memories of humiliating, degrading, and shaming experiences that have damaged our self-esteem. In another COEX system, the common denominator can be anxiety experienced in various shocking and terrifying situations or claustrophobic and suffocating feelings evoked by oppressive and confining circumstances. Rejection and emotional deprivation damaging the ability to trust men, women, or people in general, is another common motif. Situations that have generated profound feelings of guilt and a sense of failure, events that have resulted in a conviction that sex is dangerous or disgusting, and encounters with indiscriminate aggression and violence can be added to the above list as characteristic examples. Particularly important are COEX systems that contain memories of encounters with situations endangering life, health, and integrity of the body.

The above discussion could easily leave the impression that COEX systems always contain painful and traumatic memories. However, it is the intensity of the experience and its emotional relevance that determines whether a memory will be included into a COEX, not its unpleasant nature. In addition to negative constellations there are also those that comprise memories of very pleasant or even ecstatic moments and situations.

The concept of COEX dynamics emerged from psychotherapy with clients suffering from serious forms of psychopathology, where the work on traumatic aspects of life plays a very important role. This accounts for the fact that constellations involving painful experiences received relatively much more attention. The spectrum of negative COEX systems is also considerably richer and more variegated than that of the positive ones. It seems that the misery in our life can have many different forms, while happiness depends on the fulfillment of a few basic conditions. However, a general discussion requires emphasizing that the COEX dynamics is not limited to constellations of traumatic memories.

In the early stages of my psychedelic research, when I first discovered the existence of COEX systems, I described them as principles governing the dynamics of the biographical level of the unconscious. At that time, my understanding of psychology was based on a narrow biographical model of the psyche inherited from teachers, particularly my Freudian analyst. In addition, in the initial psychedelic sessions of a therapeutic series, particularly when lower dosages were used, the biographical material often dominated the picture. As my experience with holotropic states became richer and more extensive, it became clear that the roots of the COEX systems reach much deeper.

In my present understanding, each of the COEX constellations seems to be superimposed over and anchored in a particular aspect of the trauma of birth. The experience of biological birth is so complex and rich in emotions and physical sensations that it contains in a prototypical form the elementary themes of most conceivable COEX systems. However, a typical COEX system reaches even further and its deepest roots consist of various forms of transpersonal phenomena, such as past-life experiences, Jungian archetypes, conscious identification with various animals, and others.

I now see the COEX systems as general organizing principles of the human psyche. The concept of COEX systems resembles to some extent C. G. Jung's ideas about "psychological complexes" (Jung 1960b) and Hanskarl Leuner's notion of "transphenomenal dynamic systems" (*tdysts*) (Leuner 1962), but it has many features that differentiates it from both of them. The COEX systems play an important role in our psychological life. They can influence the way we perceive ourselves, other people, and the world and how we feel and act. They are the dynamic forces behind our emotional and psychosomatic symptoms, difficulties in relationships with other people, and irrational behaviors.

There exists a dynamic interplay between the COEX systems and the external world. Various events in our life can specifically activate corresponding COEX systems and, conversely, active COEX systems can make us perceive and behave in such a way that we recreate their core themes in our present life. This mechanism can be observed very clearly in experiential work. In holotropic states, the content of the experience, the perception of the environment, and the behavior of the client are determined in general terms by the COEX system that dominates the session and more specifically by the layer of this system that is momentarily emerging into consciousness.

All the characteristics of COEX systems can best be demonstrated by a practical example. I have chosen for this purpose Peter, a thirty-seven-year-old tutor who had been intermittently hospitalized and treated in our department in Prague without success prior to his psychedelic therapy.

> At the time we began with the experiential sessions, Peter could hardly function in his everyday life. He was almost constantly obsessed with the idea of finding a man with certain physical characteristics and preferably clad in black. He wanted to befriend this man and tell him about his urgent desire to be locked in a dark cellar and exposed to various diabolic physical and mental tortures. Unable to concentrate on anything else, he wandered aimlessly through the city, visiting public parks, lavatories, bars, and railroad stations searching for the "right man."
>
> He succeeded on several occasions to persuade or bribe various men who met his criteria to promise or do what he asked for. Having a special gift for finding persons with sadistic traits, he was twice almost killed, several times seriously hurt, and once robbed of all his money. On those occasions, where he was able to experience what he craved for, he was extremely frightened and actually strongly disliked the tortures. In addition to this main problem, Peter suffered from suicidal depressions, impotence, and infrequent epileptiform seizures.
>
> Reconstructing his history, I found out that his major problems started at the time of his involuntary employment in Germany during World War II. The Nazis used people brought to Germany from occupied territories for work in places threatened by air-raids, such as foundries and ammunition factories. They referred to this form of slave labor as *Totaleinsetzung*. At

that time, two SS officers repeatedly forced him at gun point to engage in their homosexual practices. When the war was over, Peter realized that these experiences created in him strong preference for homosexual intercourse experienced in the passive role. This gradually changed into fetishism for black male clothes and finally into the complex obsessive-compulsive masochistic behavior described above.

Fifteen consecutive psychedelic sessions revealed a very interesting and important COEX system underlying his problems. In its most superficial layers were Peter's more recent traumatic experiences with his sadistic partners. On several occasions, the accomplices whom he recruited actually bound him with ropes, locked him into a cellar without food and water, and tortured him by flagellation and strangulation according to his wish. One of these men hit him on his head, bound him with a string, and left him lying in a forest after stealing his money.

Peter's most dramatic adventure involved a man who claimed he had in his cabin in the woods just the kind of cellar Peter wanted and promised to take him there. When they were traveling by train to this man's weekend house, Peter was struck by a strange-looking bulky backpack of his companion. When the latter left the compartment and went to the bathroom, Peter stepped up on the seat and checked the suspect baggage. He discovered a complete set of murder weapons, including a gun, a large butcher knife, a freshly sharpened hatchet, and a surgical saw used for amputations. Panic-stricken, he jumped out of the moving train and suffered serious injuries. Elements of the above episodes formed the superficial layers of Peter's most important COEX system.

A deeper layer of the same system contained Peter's memories from the Third Reich. In the sessions where this part of the COEX constellation manifested, he relived in detail his experiences with the homosexual SS officers with all the complicated feelings involved. In addition, he relived several other traumatic memories from World War II and dealt with the entire oppressive atmosphere of this period. He had visions of pompous Nazi military parades and rallies, banners with swastikas, ominous giant eagle emblems, scenes from concentration camps, and many others.

Then came layers related to Peter's childhood, particularly those involving punishment by his parents. His alcoholic father was often violent when he was drunk and used to beat him in a sadistic way with a large leather strap. His mother's favorite method of punishing him was to lock him into a dark cellar without food for long periods of time. Peter recalled that throughout his childhood she always wore black dresses; he did not remember her ever wearing anything else. At this point, he realized that one of the roots of his obsession seemed to be craving for suffering that would combine elements of punishment inflicted on him by his parents.

However, that was not the whole story. As we continued with the sessions, the process deepened and Peter confronted the trauma of his birth with all its biological brutality. This situation had all the elements that he expected from the sadistic treatment he was so desperately trying to receive: dark enclosed space, confinement and restriction of the body movements, and exposure to extreme physical and emotional tortures. Reliving of the trauma of birth finally resolved his difficult symptoms to such an extent that he could again function in life.

In a holotropic state, when a COEX system is emerging into consciousness, it assumes a governing function and determines the nature and content of the experience. Our perceptions of ourselves and of the human and physical environment are distorted and illusively transformed in correspondence with the basic motif of the emerging COEX constellation and with the specific features of its individual layers. This mechanism can be illustrated by describing the dynamics of Peter's holotropic process.

When Peter was working through the most superficial layers of the described COEX system, he saw me transformed into his past sadistic partners or into figures symbolizing aggression, such as a butcher, murderer, medieval executioner, Inquisitor, or cowboy with a lasso. He perceived my fountain pen as an Oriental dagger and expected to be attacked with it. When he saw on the table a knife with a staghorn handle used for opening envelopes, he immediately saw me changing into a violent-looking forester. On several occasions he asked to be tortured and wanted to suffer "for the doctor" by withholding urination. During this period, the treatment room and the view from the window were illusively transformed into various settings where Peter's adventures with his sadistic partners took place.

When the older layer from World War II was in the focus of his experience, Peter saw me transformed into Hitler and other Nazi leaders, a concentration-camp commander, SS member, and Gestapo officer. Instead of ordinary noises outside the treatment room, he heard ominous sounds of parading soldiers' boots, music of the fascist parades by the Brandenburg Gate, and the national anthems of Nazi Germany. The treatment room was successively transformed into a room in the Reichstag with eagle emblems and swastikas, a barrack in a concentration camp, a jail with heavy bars in the window, and even a death row.

When the core experiences from childhood were emerging in these sessions, Peter perceived me as punishing parental figures. At this time, he tended to display toward me various anachronistic behavior patterns characteristic of his relationship with his father and mother. The treatment room was changing into various parts of his home setting in childhood, particularly into the dark cellar in which he was repeatedly locked up by his mother.

The mechanism described above has its dynamic counterpart, the tendency of external stimuli to activate corresponding COEX systems of persons in holotropic states and to facilitate emergence of the content of these systems into consciousness. This happens in those instances where specific external influences, such as elements of the physical setting, interpersonal environment, or therapeutic situation, bear a resemblance to the original traumatic scenes or contain identical components. This seems to be the clue for understanding the extraordinary significance of set and setting for the holotropic experience. The activation of a COEX system by specific external stimuli accidentally introduced into the therapeutic situation can be illustrated by a sequence from one of Peter's LSD sessions.

> One of the important core experiences that Peter uncovered in his LSD therapy was a memory of being locked by his mother into a dark cellar and denied food while the other members of the family were eating. The reliving of this memory was triggered quite unexpectedly by the angry barking of a dog that ran by the open window of the treatment room. The analysis of this event showed an interesting relationship between the external stimulus and the activated memory. Peter recalled that the cellar his mother used for punishment had a small window overlooking the neighbor's courtyard. The neighbor's German shepherd, chained to his doghouse, used to bark almost incessantly on the occasions when Peter was confined in the cellar.

In holotropic states, people often manifest seemingly inappropriate and highly exaggerated reactions to various environmental stimuli. Such overreacting is specific and selective and can be usually understood in terms of the dynamics of the governing COEX systems. Thus, patients are particularly sensitive to what they consider uninterested, cold, and "professional" treatment when they are under the influence of memory constellations that involve emotional deprivation, rejection, or neglect by their parents or other relevant figures in their childhood.

When working through the problems of rivalry with their siblings, patients attempt to monopolize the therapist and want to be the only or at least the favorite patient. They find it difficult to accept that the therapist has other patients, and can be extremely irritated by any sign of interest paid to somebody else. Patients, who on other occasions do not mind or even wish to be left alone during a session, cannot bear the therapist to leave the room for any reason when they are connecting with memories related to abandonment and childhood loneliness. These are just a few examples of situations in which oversensitivity to external circumstances reflect an underlying COEX systems.

The "Inner Radar" Operating in Holotropic States

Before we continue our discussion of the new extended cartography of the human psyche, it seems appropriate to mention a very important and extraordinary aspect of holotropic states that has played an important role in charting the experiential territories of the psyche. The same feature of holotropic states has also proved to be of invaluable help for the process of psychotherapy. Holotropic states tend to engage something like an "inner radar," that automatically brings into consciousnes the contents from the unconscious that have the strongest emotional charge, are most psychodynamically relevant at the time, and most readily available for conscious processing.

This represents a great advantage in comparison with verbal psychotherapy, where the client brings a rich array of information of various kinds and the therapist has to decide what is important, what is irrelevant, where the client is blocking, and so on. There exists a large number of schools of psychotherapy and they differ greatly in their opinions about the basic mechanisms of the human psyche, the causes and meaning of symptoms, and the nature of effective therapeutic mechanisms. Since there is no general agreement about these fundamental theoretical issues, many interpretations made during verbal psychotherapy are arbitrary and questionable. They will always reflect the personal bias of the therapist, as well as the specific views of his or her school.

Holotropic states save the therapist such problematic decision making and eliminate much of the subjectivity and professional idiosyncrasy of the verbal approaches. Once the client enters a holotropic state, the material for processing is chosen quite automatically. As long as the client keeps the experience internalized, the best we can do as therapists is to accept and support what is happening, whether or not it is consonant with our theoretical concepts and expectations.

It was this "inner radar" function of holotropic states that made it obvious that the memories of physical traumas carry a strong emotional and physical charge and play an important role in the genesis of emotional and psychosomatic disorders. This automatic selection of emotionally relevant material also spontaneously led the process to the perinatal and transpersonal levels of the psyche, transbiographical domains not recognized and acknowledged by academic psychiatry and psychology.

The Perinatal Level of the Unconscious

When our process of deep experiential self-exploration moves beyond the level of memories from childhood and infancy and reaches back to birth, we start encountering emotions and physical sensations of extreme intensity, often surpassing anything we previously considered humanly possible. At this point, the experiences become a strange mixture of the themes of birth and death. They involve a sense of a severe, life-threatening confinement and a desperate and determined struggle to free ourselves and survive.

Because of the close connection between this domain of the unconscious and biological birth, I have chosen for it the name *perinatal.* It is a Greek-Latin composite word where the prefix *peri-* means "near" or "around" and the root *natalis* signifies "pertaining to childbirth." This word is commonly used in medicine to describe various biological processes occurring shortly before, during, and immediately after birth. The obstetricians talk, for example, about perinatal hemorrhage, infection, or brain damage. However, since traditional medicine denies that the child can consciously experience birth and claims that this event is not recorded in memory, one never hears about perinatal experiences. The use of the term *perinatal* in connection with consciousness reflects my own findings and is entirely new (Grof 1975).

The strong representation of birth and death in our unconscious psyche and the close association between them might surprise mainstream psychologists and psychiatrists, since it challenges their deeply ingrained beliefs. According to the traditional medical view, only a birth so difficult that it causes irreversible damage to the brain cells can have psychopathological consequences, and even then mostly of a neurological nature, such as mental retardation or hyperactivity. Academic psychiatry generally denies the possibility that biological birth, whether or not it damages the brain cells, also has a strong psychotraumatic impact on the child. The cerebral cortex of the newborn is not fully myelinized; its neurons are not completely covered by protective sheaths of a fatty substance called *myelin.*

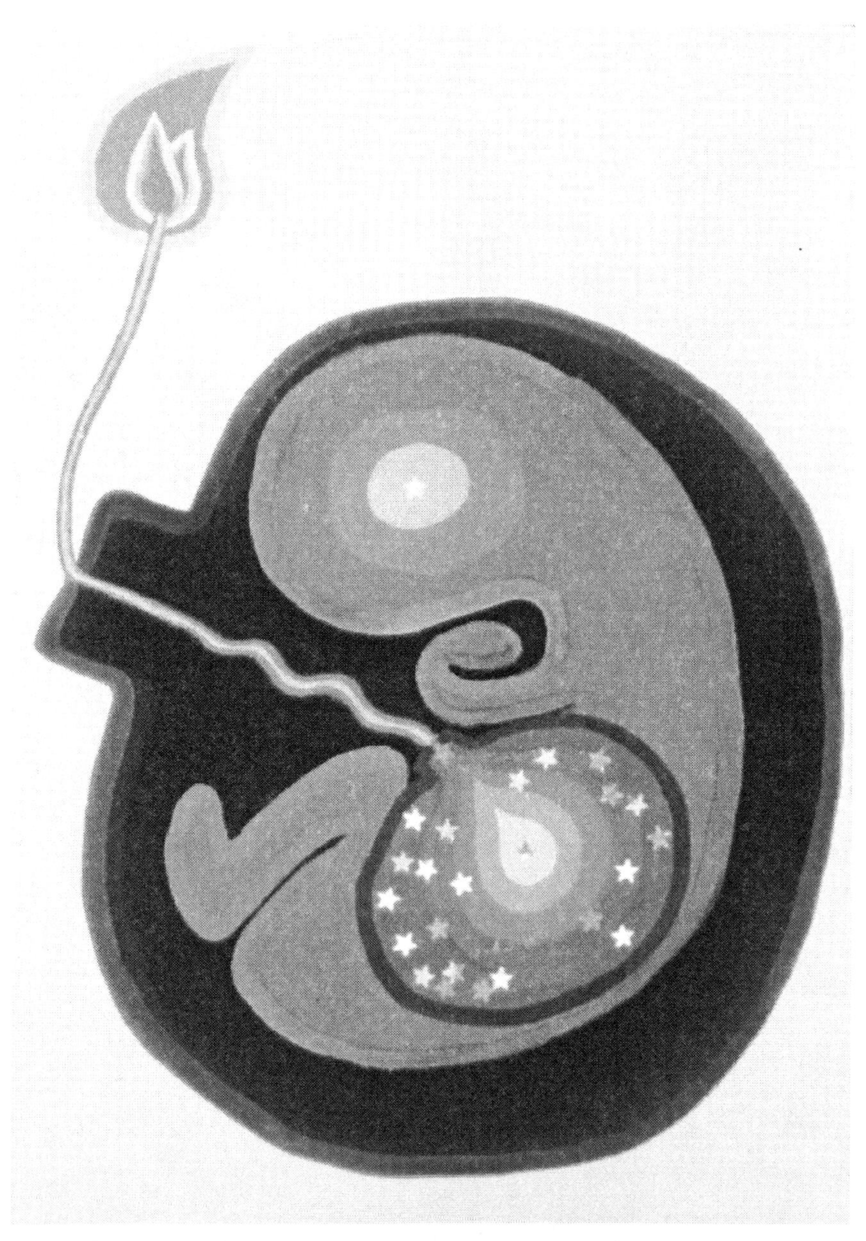

Identification with a fetus anticipating a major explosive event. This expectation is related not only to the forthcoming biological delivery, but also to the unleashing of creative power and potential for growth.

This is usually offered as a reason why biological birth is experientially irrelevant and why it is not recorded in memory.

The assumption of mainstream psychiatrists that the child is not conscious during this extremely painful and stressful ordeal and that the birth process does not leave any record in his or her brain seriously contradicts not only clinical observations, but common sense and elementary logic. It is certainly hard to reconcile with the fact that widely accepted psychological and physiological theories attribute great significance to the early relationship between the mother and the child, including such factors as bonding and nuances of nursing. The image of the newborn as an unconscious and unresponsive organism is also in sharp conflict with the growing body of literature describing the remarkable sensitivity of the fetus during the prenatal period (Verny and Kelly 1981, Tomatis 1991, Whitwell 1999).

The denial of the possibility of birth memory based on the fact that the cerebral cortex of the newborn is not fully myelinized is particularly absurd considering that the capacity for memory exists in many lower life forms that do not have a cerebral cortex at all. And it is well known that certain primitive forms of protoplasmatic memory exist even in unicellular organisms. Such blatant logical contradiction appearing in the context of rigorous scientific thinking is certainly surprising and is very likely the result of a profound emotional repression to which the memory of birth is subjected.

The amount of emotional and physical stress involved in childbirth clearly surpasses that of any postnatal trauma in infancy and childhood discussed in psychodynamic literature, with the possible exception of extreme forms of physical abuse. Various forms of experiential psychotherapy have amassed convincing evidence that biological birth is the most profound trauma of our life and an event of paramount psychospiritual importance. It is recorded in our memory in miniscule details down to the cellular level and it has profound effect on our psychological development.

Reliving of various aspects of biological birth can be very authentic and convincing and often replays this process in photographic detail. This can occur even in people who have no intellectual knowledge about their birth and lack elementary obstetric information. All these details can be confirmed if good birth records or reliable personal witnesses are available. For example, we can discover through direct experience that we had a breech birth, that a forceps was used during our delivery, or that we were born with the umbilical cord twisted around the neck. We can feel the anxiety, biological fury, physical pain, and suffocation that we experienced during birth and even accurately recognize the type of anesthesia used when we were born.

This is often accompanied by various postures and movements of the body, arms, and legs, as well as rotations, flections and deflections of the head that accurately recreate the mechanics of a particular type of delivery. When reliving birth, bruises, swellings, and other vascular changes can unexpectedly appear on the skin in the places where the forceps was applied or where the umbilical cord was constricting the throat. These observations suggest that the record of the trauma of birth reaches all the way down to the cellular level.

The intimate connection between birth and death in our unconscious psyche makes eminent sense. It reflects the fact that birth is a potential or actual life-threatening event. The delivery brutally terminates the intrauterine existence of the fetus. He or she "dies" as an aquatic organism and is born as an air-breathing, physiologically and even anatomically different form of life. And the passage through the birth canal is, in and of itself, a difficult and possibly life-threatening event.

Various complications of birth, such as serious discrepancy between the size of the child and the pelvic opening, transversal position of the fetus, breech birth, or placenta praevia can further increase the emotional and physical challenges associated with this process. The child and the mother can actually lose their lives during delivery, and children might be born severely blue from asphyxiation, or even dead and in need of resuscitation.

Conscious reliving and integration of the trauma of birth plays an important role in the process of experiential psychotherapy and self-exploration. The experiences originating on the perinatal level of the unconscious appear in four distinct experiential patterns, each of which is characterized by specific emotions, physical feelings, and symbolic imagery. These patterns are closely related to the experiences that the fetus has before the onset of birth and during the three consecutive stages of biological delivery. At each of these stages, the child experiences a specific and typical set of intense emotions and physical sensations. These experiences leave deep unconscious imprints in the psyche that later in life have an important influence on the life of the individual. I refer to these four dynamic constellations of the deep unconscious as *Basic Perinatal Matrices or BPMs.*

The spectrum of perinatal experiences is not limited to the elements that can be derived from the biological and psychological processes involved in childbirth. The perinatal domain of the psyche also represents an important gateway to the collective unconscious in the Jungian sense. Identification with the infant facing the ordeal of the passage through the birth canal seems to provide access to experiences involving people from other times and cultures, various animals, and even mythological figures. It is as if by connecting with the fetus struggling to be born, one reaches an intimate, almost mystical connection with other sentient beings who are in a similar difficult predicament.

The connections between the experiences of the consecutive stages of biological birth and various symbolic images associated with them are very specific and consistent. The reason why they emerge together is not understandable in terms of conventional logic. However, that does not mean that these associations are arbitrary and random. They have their own deep order that can best be described as "experiential logic." What this means is that the connection between the experiences characteristic for various stages of birth and the concomitant symbolic themes are not based on some formal external similarity, but on the fact that they share the same emotional feelings and physical sensations.

Perinatal matrices are rich and complex and have specific biological and psychological, as well as archetypal and spiritual dimensions. Experiential confrontation with birth and death seems to result automatically in a spiritual opening and discovery of the mystical dimensions of the psyche and of existence. It does not seem to make a difference whether this encounter takes a symbolic form, as in psychedelic and holotropic sessions and in the course of spontaneous psychospiritual crises ("spiritual emergencies") or whether it occurs in actual life situations, for example, in delivering women or in the context of near-death experiences (Ring 1982). The specific symbolism of these experiences comes from the collective unconscious, not from the individual memory banks. It can thus draw on any historical period, geographical area, and spiritual tradition of the world, quite independently from the subject's cultural or religious background.

Individual matrices have fixed connections with certain categories of postnatal experiences arranged in COEX systems. They have also associations with the archetypes of the Terrible Mother Goddess, the Great Mother Goddess, Hell, or Heaven, as well as racial, collective, and karmic memories, and phylogenetic experiences. I should also mention theoretically and practically important links between BPMs and specific aspects of physiological activities in the Freudian erogenous zones and to specific categories of emotional and psychosomatic disorders. All these interrelations are shown on the synoptic paradigm in table 2.1.

TABLE 2.1 **Basic Perinatal Matrices**

BPM I	BPM II	BPM III	BPM IV
Related Psychopathological Syndromes			
Schizophrenic psychoses (paranoid symptomatology, feelings of mystical union, encounter with metaphysical evil forces); hypochondriasis (based on strange and bizarre physical sensations); hysterical hallucinosis and confusing daydreams with reality	Schizophrenic psychoses (elements of hellish tortures, experience of meaningless "cardboard" world); severe inhibited "endogenous" depressions; irrational inferiority and guilt feelings; hypochondriasis (based on painful physical sensations); alcoholism and drug addiction, psoriasis; peptic ulcer	Schizophrenic psychoses (sadomasochistic and scatological elements, automutilation, abnormal sexual behavior); agitated depression, sexual deviations (sadomasochism, drinking of urine and eating of feces); obsessive-compulsive neurosis; psychogenic asthma, tics, and stammering; conversion and anxiety hysteria; frigidity and impotence; neurasthenia; traumatic neuroses; organ neuroses; migraine headache; enuresis and encopressis	Schizophrenic psychoses (death-rebirth experiences, messianic delusions, elements of destruction and recreation of the world, salvation and redemption, identification with Christ); manic symptomatology; exhibitionism
Corresponding Activities in Freudian Erogenous Zones			
Libidinal satisfaction in all erogenous zones; libidinal feelings during rocking and bathing; partial approximation to this condition after oral, anal, urethral, or genital satisfaction and after delivery of a child	Oral frustration (thirst, hunger, painful stimuli); retention of feces and/or urine; sexual frustration; experiences of cold, pain and other unpleasant sensations	Chewing and swallowing of food; oral aggression and destruction of an object; process of defecation and urination; anal and urethral aggression; sexual orgasm; phallic aggression; delivering of a child, statoacoustic eroticism (jolting, gymnastics, fancy diving, parachuting)	Satiation of thirst and hunger; pleasure of sucking; libidinal feelings after defecation, urination, sexual orgasm, or delivery of a child

TABLE 2.1 Basic Perinatal Matrices (*continued*)

BPM I	BPM II	BPM III	BPM IV
Associated Memories From Postnatal Life			
Situations from later life in which important needs are satisfied, such as happy moments from infancy and childhood (good mothering, play with peers, harmonious periods in the family, etc.), fulfilling love, romances; trips or vacations in beautiful natural settings; exposure to artistic creations of high aesthetic value; swimming in the ocean and clear lakes, etc.	Situations endangering survival and body integrity (war experiences, accidents, injuries, operations, painful diseases, near drowning, episodes of suffocation, imprisonment, brainwashing, and illegal interrogation, physical abuse, etc.); severe psychological traumatizations (emotional deprivation, rejection, threatening situations, oppressive family atmosphere, ridicule and humiliation, etc.)	Struggles, fights, and adventurous activities (active attacks in battles and revolutions, experiences in military service, rough airplane flights, cruises on stormy ocean, hazardous car driving, boxing); highly sensual memories (carnivals, amusement parks and nightclubs, wild parties, sexual orgies, etc.); childhood observations of adult sexual activities; experiences of seduction and rape; in females, delivering of their own children	Fortuitous escape from dangerous situations (end of war or revolution, survival of an accident or operation); overcoming of severe obstacles by active effort; episodes of strain and hard struggle resulting in a marked success; natural scenes (beginning of spring, end of an ocean storm, sunrise, rainbow, etc.)
Phenomenology in LSD Sessions			
Undisturbed intrauterine life: realistic recollections of "good womb" experiences; "oceanic" type of ecstasy, nature at its best ("Mother Nature"); experience of cosmic unity; visions of Heaven and Paradise; disturbances of intrauterine life: realistic recollections of "bad womb" experiences (fetal crises, diseases, and emotional upheavals	Cosmic engulfment; immense physical and psychological suffering; unbearable and inescapable situation that will never end; various images of hell; feelings of entrapment and engagement (no exit); agonizing guilt and inferiority feelings; apocalyptic view of the world (horrors of wars and concentration camps, terror of	Intensification of suffering to cosmic dimensions; borderline between pain and pleasure; "volcanic" type of ecstasy; brilliant colors; explosions and fireworks; sadomasochistic orgies; murders and bloody sacrifice, active engagement in fierce battles; atmosphere of wild adventure and dangerous explorations; intense sexual orgiastic feelings and scenes of harems and carnivals; experiences of	Enormous decompression; expansion of space; "illuminative" type of ecstasy, visions of gigantic halls; radiant light and beautiful colors (heavenly blue, golden, rainbow, peacock feathers); feelings of rebirth and redemption; appreciation of simple way of life; sensory enhancement; brotherly feelings; humanitarian and chari-

TABLE 2.1 Basic Perinatal Matrices (*continued*)

BPM I	BPM II	BPM III	BPM IV
of the mother, twin situation, attempted abortions), universal threat: paranoid ideation; unpleasant physical sensations ("hangover," chills and fine spasms, unpleasant tastes, disgust, feelings of being poisoned); encounter with demonic entities and other metaphysical evil forces	the Inquisition; dangerous epidemics; diseases; decrepitude and death. etc.): meaninglessness and absurdity of human existence; "cardboard world" or the atmosphere of artificiality and gadgets: ominous dark colors and unpleasant physical symptoms (feelings of oppression and compression, cardiac distress, hot flashes and chills, sweating, difficult breathing)	dying and being reborn, religions involving bloody sacrifice (Aztecs, Christ's suffering and death on the cross, Dionysus, etc.); intense physical manifestations (pressures and pains, suffocation, muscular tension and discharge in tremors and twitches, nausea and vomiting, hot flashes and chills, sweating, cardiac distress, problems of sphincter control, ringing in the ears)	table tendencies; occasionally manic activity and grandiose feelings, transition to elements of BPM 1; pleasant feelings can be interrupted by umbilical crisis: sharp pain in the navel, loss of breath, fear of death and castration, shifts in the body, but no external pressures

Stages of Delivery

0

1

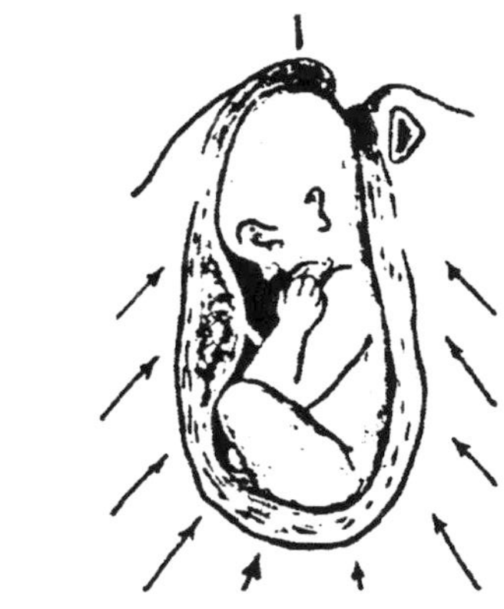
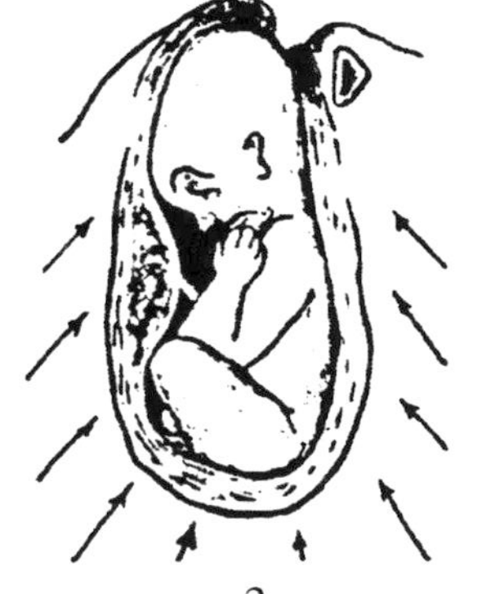

2

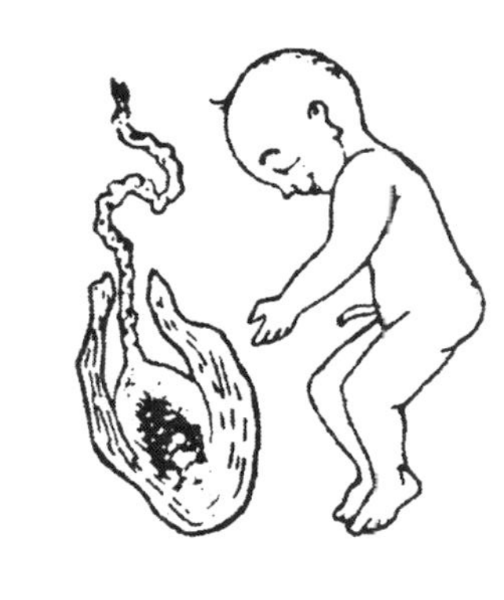

3

Reinforced by emotionally meaningful experiences from infancy, childhood, and later life arranged in COEX systems, perinatal matrices can shape our perception of the world, profoundly influence our everyday behavior, and contribute to the development of various emotional and psychosomatic disorders. On a collective scale, we can find echoes of perinatal matrices in religion, art, mythology, philosophy, and various forms of social and political psychology and psychopathology. Before exploring these broader implications of perinatal dynamics, I will describe the phenomenology of the individual BPMs.

First Basic Perinatal Matrix: BPM I (Primal Union with Mother)

This matrix is related to the intrauterine existence before the onset of the delivery. The experiential world of this period can be referred to as the "amniotic universe." The fetus does not have an awareness of boundaries and does not differentiate between the inner and the outer. This is reflected in the nature of the experiences associated with the reliving of the memory of the prenatal state. During episodes of undisturbed embryonal existence, we typically have experiences of vast regions with no boundaries or limits. We can identify with galaxies, interstellar space, or the entire cosmos.

A related experience is that of floating in the sea, identifying with various aquatic animals, such as fish, jelly fish, dolphins, or whales, or even becoming the ocean. This seems to reflect the fact that the fetus is essentially an aquatic creature. Positive intrauterine experiences can also be associated with archetypal visions of Mother Nature, safe, beautiful, and unconditionally nourishing like a good womb. We can envision fruit-bearing orchards, fields of ripe corn, agricultural terraces in the Andes, or unspoiled Polynesian islands. Mythological images from the collective unconscious that often appear in this context portray various celestial realms and paradises as they are described in mythologies of different cultures.

When we are reliving episodes of intrauterine disturbances, memories of the "bad womb," we have a sense of dark and ominous threat and often feel that we are being poisoned. We might see images that portray polluted waters and toxic dumps. This reflects the fact that many prenatal disturbances are caused by toxic changes in the body of the pregnant mother. Sequences of this kind can be associated with archetypal visions of frightening demonic entities or with a sense of insidious all-pervading evil. Those of us who relive episodes of more violent interference with prenatal existence, such as an imminent miscarriage or attempted abortion, usually

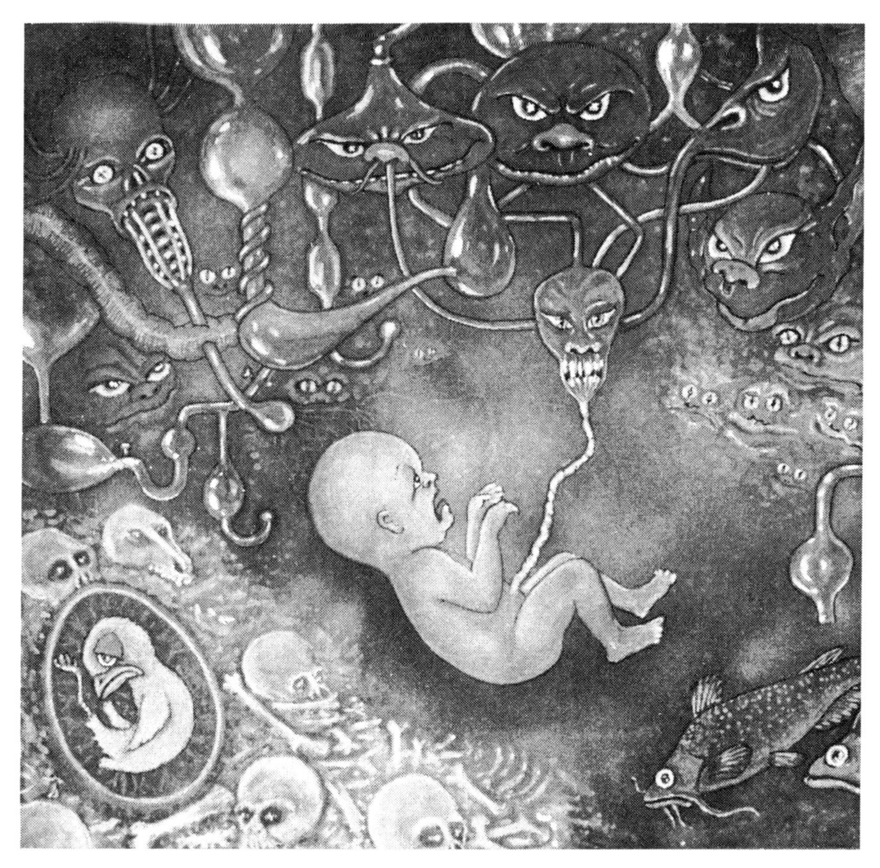

Painting representing a "bad womb" experience in a psychedelic session. Toxicity of the womb portrayed as a painful and frightening ordeal in a diabolical laboratory full of insidious demons. This experience is accompanied by identification with fish in polluted waters and with a chicken embryo in advanced stage of development when the inside of the egg is contaminated by metabolic side products (Robin Maynard-Dobbs).

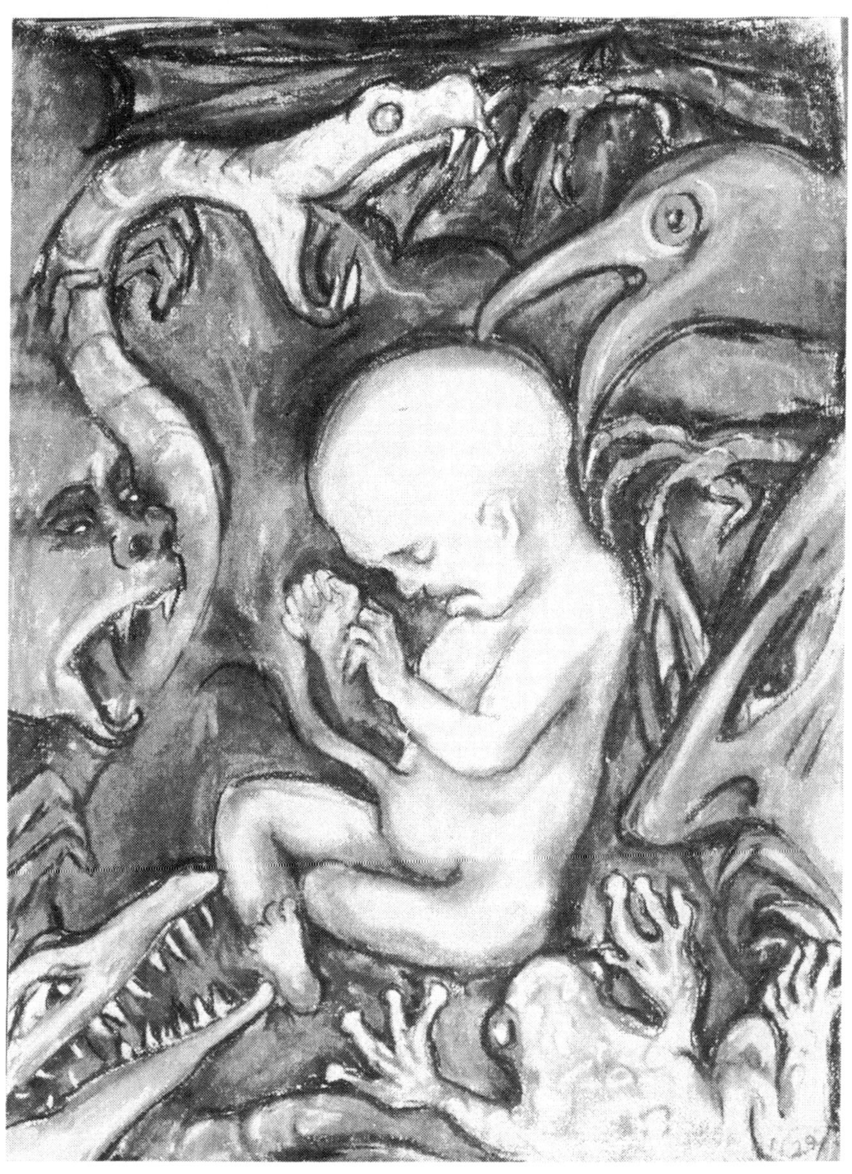

Painting representing a "bad womb" experience in a psychedelic session. Hostility of the womb experienced as attacks of vicious animals (Robin Maynard-Dobbs).

experience some form of universal threat or bloody apocalyptic visions of the end of the world. This again reflects the intimate interconnections between events in our biological history and the Jungian archetypes.

The following account of a high-dose psychedelic session can be used as a typical example of a BPM I experience, opening at times into the transpersonal realm.

> All that I was experiencing was an intense sense of malaise resembling a flu. I could not believe that a high dose of LSD, which in my previous sessions had produced dramatic psychological changes, could evoke such a minimal response. I decided to close my eyes and observe carefully what was happening. At this point, the experience seemed to deepen and I realized that what with my eyes open appeared to be an adult experience of a viral disease now changed into a realistic situation of a fetus suffering some strange toxic insults during its intrauterine existence.
>
> I was greatly reduced in size, and my head was considerably bigger than the rest of my body and my extremities. I was suspended in a liquid milieu and some harmful chemicals were being channeled into my body through the umbilical area. Using some unknown receptors, I was detecting these influences as noxious and hostile to my organism. While this was happening, I was aware that these toxic "attacks" had something to do with the condition and activity of the maternal organism. Occasionally, I could distinguish influences that appeared to be due to ingestion of alcohol, inappropriate food, or smoking. A different kind of discomfort seemed to be caused by chemical changes accompanying my mother's emotions—anxieties, nervousness, anger, and conflicting feelings about pregnancy.
>
> Then the feelings of sickness and indigestion disappeared, and I was experiencing an ever-increasing state of ecstasy. This was accompanied by a clearing and brightening of my visual field. It was as if multiple layers of thick, dirty cobwebs were being magically torn and dissolved, or a movie projection or television broadcast brought into focus by an invisible cosmic technician. The scenery opened up, and an incredible amount of light and energy enveloped me and streamed in subtle vibrations through my whole being.
>
> On one level, I was still a fetus experiencing the ultimate perfection and bliss of a good womb or a newborn fusing with a nourishing and life-giving breast. On another level, I became the entire universe. I was witnessing the spectacle of the macrocosm with countless pulsating and vibrating galaxies and was it at the same time. These radiant and breathtaking cosmic vistas were intertwined with experiences of the equally miraculous microcosm, from the dance of atoms and molecules to the origins of life and the biochemical world of individual cells. For the first time, I was experiencing the

universe for what it really is—an unfathomable mystery, a divine play of Absolute Consciousness.

For some time, I was oscillating between the state of a distressed, sickened fetus and a blissful and serene intrauterine existence. At times, the noxious influences took the form of insidious demons or malevolent creatures from the world of spiritual scriptures or fairy tales. During the undisturbed episodes of fetal existence, I experienced feelings of basic identity and oneness with the universe; it was the Tao, the Beyond that is Within, the "Tat tvam asi" (thou art That) of the Upanishads. I lost my sense of individuality; my ego dissolved, and I became all of existence.

Sometimes this experience was intangible and contentless, sometimes it was accompanied by many beautiful visions—archetypal images of Paradise, the ultimate cornucopia, golden age, or virginal nature. I became a dolphin playing in the ocean, a fish swimming in crystal-clear waters, a butterfly floating over mountain meadows, and a seagull gliding by the sea. I was the ocean, animals, plants, the clouds—sometimes all these at the same time.

Nothing concrete happened later in the afternoon and in the evening hours. I spent most of this time feeling one with nature and the universe, bathed in golden light that was slowly decreasing in intensity.

Second Perinatal Matrix: BPM II (Cosmic Engulfment and No Exit or Hell)

While reliving the onset of biological birth, we typically feel that we are being sucked into a gigantic whirlpool or swallowed by some mythic beast. We might also experience that the entire world or cosmos is being engulfed. This can be associated with images of devouring or entangling archetypal monsters, such as leviathans, dragons, whales, giant snakes, tarantulas, or octopuses. The sense of overwhelming vital threat can lead to intense anxiety and general mistrust bordering on paranoia. Another experiential variety of the beginning second matrix is the theme of descending into the depths of the underworld, the realm of death, or hell. As Joseph Campbell so eloquently described, this is a universal motif in the mythologies of the hero's journey (Campbell 1968).

In the fully developed first stage of biological birth, the uterine contractions periodically constrict the fetus, and the cervix is not yet open. Each contraction causes compression of the uterine arteries, and the fetus is threatened by lack of oxygen. Reliving this stage of birth is one of the worst experiences we can have during self-exploration that involves holotropic states. We feel caught in a monstrous claustrophobic nightmare, exposed to

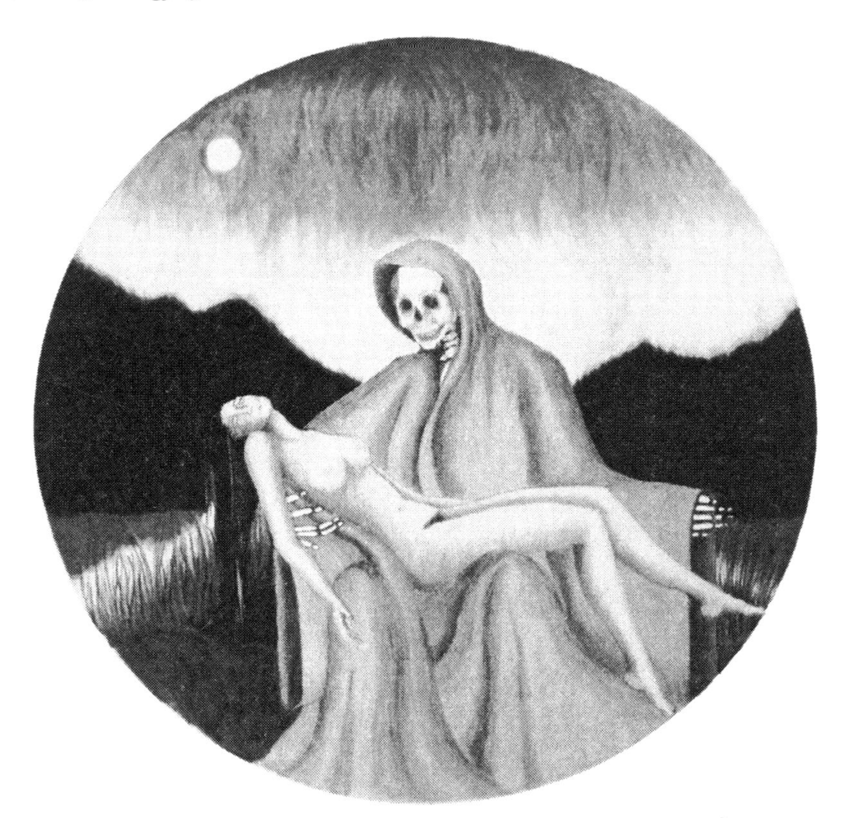

Painting from a holotropic breathwork session in which the artist experienced compassion for the suffering of humanity and herself. It represents Death, holding a human form. The accompanying text reads: "Melting of the boundaries of the physical body and of the mind frees the spirit and allows it to return once again to the splendor of divine light" (Kathleen Silver).

agonizing emotional and physical pain, and have a sense of utter helplessness and hopelessness. Feelings of loneliness, guilt, the absurdity of life, and existential despair reach metaphysical proportions. A person in this predicament often becomes convinced that this situation will never end and that there is absolutely no way out. An experiential triad characteristic for this state is a sense of dying, going crazy, and never coming back.

Reliving this stage of birth is typically accompanied by sequences that involve people, animals, and even mythological beings in a painful and hopeless predicament similar to that of the fetus caught in the clutches

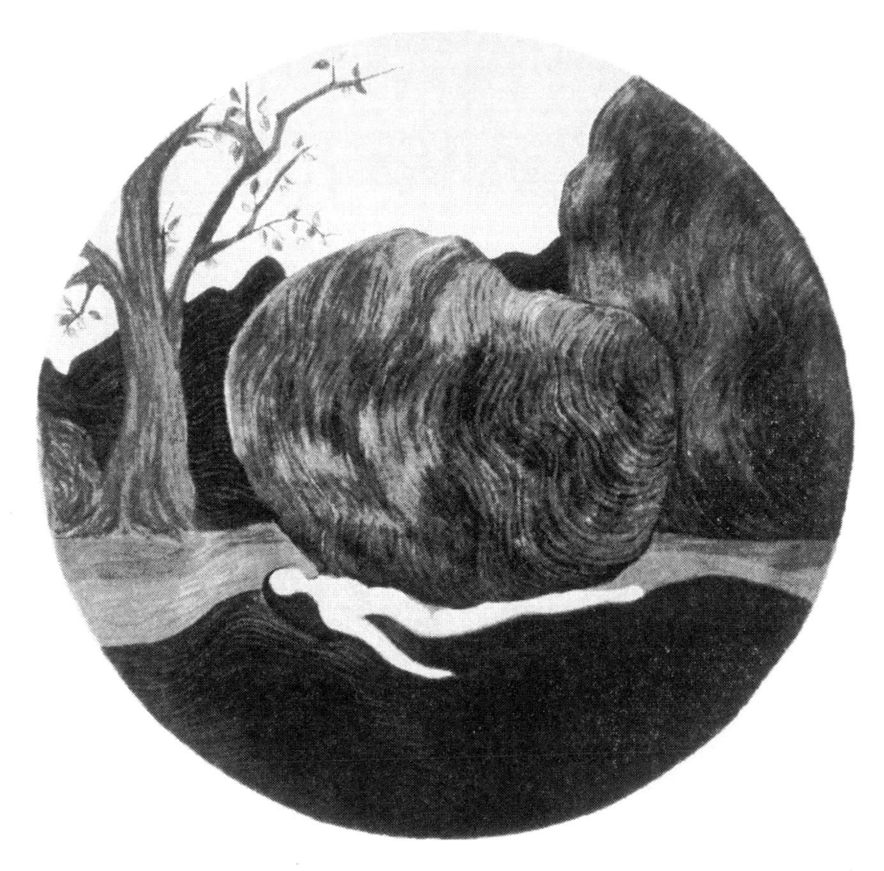

Painting from a holotropic breathwork session in which the artist reexperienced the lack of love and nurturance in her childhood combined with elements of BPM 11. It shows her being crushed by what should be the quintessential nurturing feminine principle—the Earth. The session resulted in feelings of immense compassion for herself and others, both victims and perpetrators. The persimmon tree on the left symbolizes new life, love, and hope (Kathleen Silver).

of the birth canal. We can experience identification with prisoners in dungeons, victims of the Inquisition, and inmates of concentration camps or insane asylums. Our suffering can take the form of pains of animals caught in traps or even reach dimensions that are archetypal.

We may feel the intolerable tortures of sinners in hell, the agony of Jesus Christ on the cross, or the excruciating torment of Sisyphus rolling his boulder up the mountain in the deepest pit of Hades. Other images that have appeared in sessions dominated by this matrix include the Greek archetypal symbols of endless suffering, Tantalus and Prometheus, and other figures representing eternal damnation, such as the Wandering Jew Ahasuerus or the Flying Dutchman.

While under the influence of this matrix, we are selectively blinded and are unable to see anything positive in our life and in human existence in general. The connection to the divine dimension seems to be irretrievably severed and lost. Through the prism of this matrix, life seems to be a meaningless Theater of the Absurd, a farce staging cardboard characters and mindless robots, or a cruel circus sideshow. In this state of mind, existential philosophy appears to be the only adequate and relevant description of existence. It is interesting in this regard that Jean Paul Sartre's work was deeply influenced by a badly managed and unresolved mescaline session dominated by BPM II (Riedlinger 1982). Samuel Beckett's preoccupation with death and birth and his search for Mother also reveal strong perinatal influences.

It is only natural that someone facing this aspect of the psyche would feel a great reluctance to confront it. Going deeper into this experience seems like meeting eternal damnation. Yet, the fastest way of terminating this unbearable state is surrendering to it completely and accepting it. This shattering experience of darkness and abysmal despair is known from the spiritual literature as the Dark Night of the Soul. It is an important stage of spiritual opening that can have an immensely purging and liberating effect.

The most characteristic features of BPM II can be illustrated by the following account.

> The atmosphere seemed increasingly ominous and fraught with hidden danger. It seemed that the entire room started to turn and I felt drawn into the very center of a threatening whirlpool. I had to think about Edgar Alan Poe's chilling description of a similar situation in "A Descent into the Maelstrom." As the objects in the room seemed to be flying around me in a rotating motion, another image from literature emerged in my mind—the cyclone that in Frank Baum's *Wonderful Wizard of Oz* sweeps Dorothy away from the monotony of her life in Kansas and sends her on a strange journey of adventure. My experience also had something to do with entering the rabbit hole in *Alice in Wonderland* and I awaited with great trepidation what world I would find on the other side of the looking glass. The entire universe seemed to be closing in on me and there was nothing I could do to stop this apocalyptic engulfment.

As I was sinking deeper and deeper into the labyrinth of my own unconscious, I felt an onslaught of anxiety, turning to panic. Everything became dark, oppressive, and terrifying. It was as if the weight of the whole world was encroaching on me exerting incredible hydraulic pressure that threatened to crack my skull and reduce my body to a tiny compact ball. A rapid fugue of memories from my past cascaded through my brain showing me the utter futility and meaninglessness of my life and existence in general. We are born naked, frightened, and in agony and we will leave the world the same way. The existentialist were right! Everything is impermanent, life is nothing else but waiting for Godot! Vanity of vanities, all is vanity!

The discomfort I felt turned to pain and the pain increased to agony. The torture intensified to the point where every cell in my body felt like it was being bored open with a diabolic dentist's drill. Visions of infernal landscapes and devils torturing their victims suddenly brought to me the awareness that I was in Hell. I thought of Dante's *Divine Comedy*: "Abandon all hope ye who enter!" There seemed to be no way out of this diabolical situation; I was forever doomed without the slightest hope for redemption.

Third Perinatal Matrix: BPM III (The Death-Rebirth Struggle)

Many aspects of this rich and colorful experience can be understood from its association with the second clinical stage of biological delivery, the propulsion through the birth canal after the cervix opens and the head descends into the pelvis. In this stage, the uterine contractions continue, but the cervix is now dilated and allows gradual propulsion of the fetus through the birth canal. This involves crushing mechanical pressures, pains, and often a high degree of anoxia and suffocation. A natural concomitant of this highly uncomfortable and life-threatening situation is an experience of intense anxiety.

Besides the interruption of blood circulation caused by uterine contractions and the ensuing compression of uterine arteries, the blood supply to the fetus can be further compromised by various complications. The umbilical cord can be squeezed between the head and the pelvic opening or be twisted around the neck. The placenta can detach during delivery or actually obstruct the way out (*placenta praevia*). In some instances, the fetus can inhale various forms of biological material that it encounters in the final stages of this process, which further intensifies the feelings of suffocation. The problems in this stage can be so extreme that they require instrumental intervention, such as the use of forceps or even an emergency Cesarean section.

BPM III is an extremely rich and complex experiential pattern. Besides the actual realistic reliving of different aspects of the struggle in the birth canal, it involves a wide variety of imagery drawn from history, nature, and archetypal realms. The most important of these are the atmosphere of titanic fight, aggressive and sadomasochistic sequences, experiences of deviant sexuality, demonic episodes, scatological involvement, and encounter with fire. Most of these aspects of BPM III can be meaningfully related to certain anatomical, physiological, and biochemical characteristics of the corresponding stage of birth.

The *titanic aspect* of BPM III is quite understandable in view of the enormity of the forces operating in the final stage of childbirth. When we encounter this facet of the third matrix, we experience streams of energy of overwhelming intensity, rushing through the body and building up to explosive discharges. At this point, we might identify with raging elements of nature, such as volcanoes, electric storms, earthquakes, tidal waves, or tornadoes.

The experience can also portray the world of technology involving enormous energies—tanks, rockets, spaceships, lasers, electric power plants, or even thermonuclear reactors and atomic bombs. The titanic experiences of BPM III can reach archetypal dimensions and portray battles of gigantic proportions, such as the cosmic battle between the forces of Light and Darkness, angels and devils, or the gods and the Titans.

Aggressive and sadomasochistic aspects of this matrix reflect the biological fury of the organism whose survival is threatened by suffocation, as well as the introjected destructive onslaught of the uterine contractions. Facing this aspect of BPM III, we might experience cruelties of astonishing proportions, manifesting in scenes of violent murder and suicide, mutilation and automutilation, massacres of various kinds, and bloody wars and revolutions. They often take the form of torture, execution, ritual sacrifice and self-sacrifice, bloody man-to-man combats, and sadomasochistic practices.

The experiential logic of the *sexual aspect* of the death-rebirth process is not as immediately obvious. It seems that the human organism has an inbuilt physiological mechanism that translates inhuman suffering, and particularly suffocation, into a strange kind of sexual arousal and eventually into ecstatic rapture. This can be illustrated by the experiences of the martyrs and of flagellants described in religious literature. Additional examples can be found in the material from concentration camps, from the reports of prisoners of war, and from the files of Amnesty International. It is also well known that men dying of suffocation on the gallows typically have an erection and even ejaculate.

Sexual experiences that occur in the context of BPM III are characterized by enormous intensity of the sexual drive, by their mechanical and unselective quality, and their exploitative, pornographic, or deviant nature. They depict scenes from red light districts and from the sexual underground, extravagant erotic practices, and sadomasochistic sequences. Equally frequent are episodes portraying incest and episodes of sexual abuse or rape. In rare instances, the BPM III imagery can involve the gory and repulsive extremes of criminal sexuality – erotically motivated murder, dismemberment, cannibalism, and necrophilia.

The fact that, on this level of the psyche, sexual arousal is inextricably connected with highly problematic elements—vital threat, extreme danger, anxiety, aggression, self-destructive impulses, physical pain, and various forms of biological material—forms a natural basis for the development of the most important types of sexual dysfunctions, variations, deviations, and perversions. This has important theoretical and practical implications that will be explored later in this book.

The *demonic aspect* of BPM III can present specific problems for the experiencers, as well as therapists and facilitators. The uncanny and eerie nature of the manifestations involved often leads to reluctance to face it. The most common themes observed in this context are scenes of the Sabbath of the Witches (*Walpurgi's Night*), satanic orgies and Black Mass rituals, and temptation by evil forces. The common denominator connecting this stage of childbirth with the themes of the Sabbath or with the Black Mass rituals is the peculiar experiential amalgam of death, deviant sexuality, pain, fear, aggression, scatology, and distorted spiritual impulse that they share. This observation seems to have great relevance for the recent epidemic of experiences of satanic cult abuse reported by clients in various forms of regressive therapy.

The *scatological aspect* of the death-rebirth process has its natural biological basis in the fact that, in the final phase of the delivery, the fetus can come into close contact with various forms of biological material—blood, vaginal secretions, urine, and even feces. However, the nature and content of these experiences by far exceed what the newborn might have actually experienced during birth. Experiences of this aspect of BPM III can involve such scenes as crawling in offal or through sewage systems, wallowing in piles of excrement, drinking blood or urine, or participating in repulsive images of putrefaction. It is an intimate and shattering encounter with the worst aspects of biological existence.

When the experience of BPM III comes closer to resolution, it becomes less violent and disturbing. The prevailing atmosphere is that of extreme passion and driving energy of intoxicating intensity. The imagery portrays exciting conquests of new territories, hunts of wild animals, challenging sports, and adventures in amusement parks. These experiences are clearly related to activities that involve "adrenaline rush" —car racing, bungie-cord jumping, dangerous circus performances, and acrobatic diving.

At this time, we can also encounter archetypal figures of deities, demigods, and legendary heroes representing death and rebirth. We can have visions of Jesus, his torment and humiliation, the Way of the Cross, and crucifixion, or even actually experience full identification with his suffering. Whether or not we know intellectually the corresponding mythologies, we can experience such mythological themes as resurrection of the Egyptian god Osiris, or death and rebirth of the Greek deities Dionysus, Attis, or Adonis. The experience can portray Persephone's abduction by Pluto, the descent into the underworld of the Sumerian goddess Inanna, or the ordeals of the Mayan Hero Twins of the Popol Vuh.

Just before the experience of psychospiritual rebirth, it is common to encounter the *element of fire*. The motif of fire can be experienced either in its ordinary everyday form or in the archetypal form of purgatorial fire (*pyrocatharsis*). We can have the feeling that our body is on fire, have visions of burning cities and forests, and identify with the victims of immolation. In the archetypal version, the burning seems to radically destroy whatever is corrupted in us and prepare us for spiritual rebirth. A classical symbol of the transition from BPM III to BPM IV is the legendary bird Phoenix who dies in fire and rises resurrected from the ashes.

The pyrocathartic experience is a somewhat puzzling aspect of BPM III, since its connection with biological birth is not as direct and obvious as is the case with the other symbolic elements. The biological counterpart of this experience might be the explosive liberation of previously blocked energies in the final stage of childbirth or the overstimulation of the fetus with indiscriminate "firing" of the peripheral neurons. It is interesting that this encounter with fire has its experiential parallel in the delivering mother who at this stage of delivery often feels that her vagina is on fire.

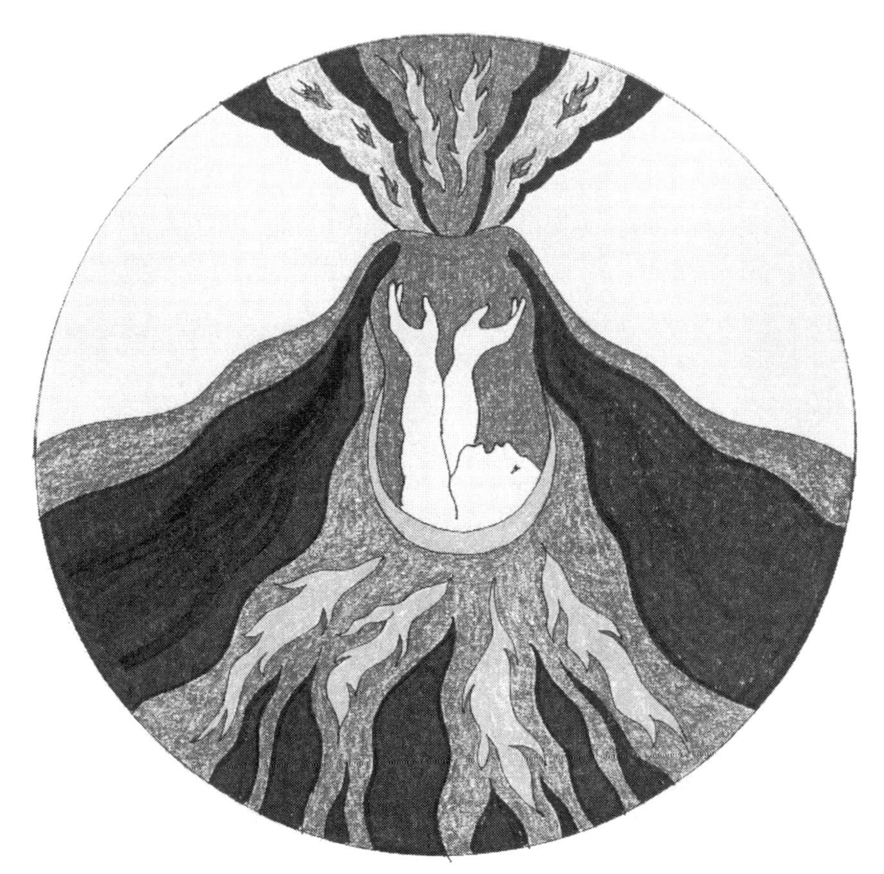

A painting representing psychospiritual rebirth in a holotropic session experienced as being born of fire at the center of the earth and emerging through a volcano (Tai Ingrid Hazard).

Several important characteristics of the third matrix distinguish it from the previously described no-exit constellation. The situation here is challenging and difficult, but it does not seem hopeless and we do not feel helpless. We are actively involved in a fierce struggle and have the feeling that the suffering has a definite direction, goal, and meaning. In religious terms, this situation relates to the concept of purgatory rather than hell.

In addition, we do not play exclusively the role of helpless victims. At this point, three different roles become available to us. Besides being observers of what is happening, we can also identify with both the aggressor and the victim. This can be so convincing that it might be difficult to distinguish and separate the roles. Also, while the no-exit situation involves sheer suffering, the experience of the death-rebirth struggle represents the borderline between agony and ecstasy and the fusion of both. It seems appropriate to refer to this type of experience as *Dionysian* or *volcanic ecstasy* in contrast to the *Apollonian* or *oceanic ecstasy* of the cosmic union associated with the first perinatal matrix.

The following account from a high-dose psychedelic session illustrates many of the typical themes associated with BPM III described above:

> Although I never really clearly saw the birth canal, I felt its crushing pressure on my head and all over, and I knew with every cell of my body that I was involved in the birth process. The tension was reaching dimensions that I had not imagined were humanly possible. I felt unrelenting pressure on my forehead, temples, and occiput, as if I were caught in the steel jaws of a vise. The tensions in my body had a brutally mechanical quality. I imagined myself passing through a monstrous meat grinder or a giant press full of cogs and cylinders. The image of Charlie Chaplin victimized by the world of technology in *Modern Times* briefly flashed through my mind.
>
> Incredible amounts of energy seemed to be flowing through my entire body, condensing and releasing in explosive discharges. I felt an amazing mixture of feelings; I was suffocated, frightened, and helpless, but also furious and strangely sexually aroused. Another important aspect of my experience was a sense of utter confusion. While I felt like an infant involved in a vicious struggle for survival and realized that what was about to happen was my birth, I was also experiencing myself as my delivering mother. I knew intellectually that being a man I could never give birth, yet I felt that I was somehow crossing that barrier and that the impossible was becoming a reality.
>
> There was no question that I was connecting with something primordial—an ancient feminine archetype, that of the delivering mother. My body image included a large pregnant belly and female genitals with all the nuances of biological sensations. I felt frustrated by not being able to surrender to this elemental process, to give birth and be born, to let go and to let the baby out. An enormous reservoir of murderous aggression emerged from the underworld of my psyche. It was as if an abscess of evil had suddenly been punctured by the cut of a cosmic surgeon. A werewolf or a berserk was taking me over; Dr. Jekyll was turning into Mr. Hyde. There were many images of the murderer and the victim as being one and the same person, just as earlier I could not distinguish between the child who was being born and the delivering mother.

I was a merciless tyrant, the dictator exposing the subordinates to unimaginable cruelties, and also a revolutionary, leading the furious mob to overthrow the tyrant. I became the mobster who murders in cold blood and the policeman who kills the criminal in the name of law. At one point, I experienced the horrors of the Nazi concentration camps. When I opened my eyes, I saw myself as an SS officer. I had a profound sense that he, the Nazi, and I, the Jew, were the same person. I could feel the Hitler and the Stalin in me and felt fully responsible for the atrocities in human history. I saw clearly that humanity's problem is not the existence of vicious dictators, but this Hidden Killer that we all harbor within our own psyches, if we look deep enough.

Then the nature of the experience changed and reached mythological proportions. Instead of the evil of human history, I now sensed the atmosphere of witchcraft and the presence of demonic elements. My teeth were transformed into long fangs filled with some mysterious poison, and I found myself flying on large bat wings through the night like an ominous vampire. This changed soon into wild, intoxicating scenes of a Witches' Sabbath. In this strange, sensuous ritual, all the usually forbidden and repressed impulses seemed to surface and were experienced and acted out. I was aware of participating in some mysterious sacrificial ceremony celebrating the Dark God.

As the demonic quality gradually disappeared from my experience, I still felt tremendously erotic and was engaged in endless sequences of the most fantastic orgies and sexual fantasies, in which I played all the roles. All through these experiences, I simultaneously continued being also the child struggling through the birth canal and the mother delivering it. It became very clear to me that sex and birth were deeply connected and that satanic forces had important links with the propulsion through the birth canal. I struggled and fought in many different roles and against many different enemies. Sometimes I wondered if there would ever be an end to my misery.

Then a new element entered my experience. My entire body was covered with some biological filth, which was slimy and slippery. I could not tell if it was the amniotic fluid, urine, mucus, blood, or vaginal secretions. The same stuff seemed to be in my mouth and even in my lungs. I was choking, gagging, making faces, and spitting, trying to get it out of my system and off my skin. At the same time, I was getting a message that I did not have to fight. The process had its own rhythm and all I had to do was surrender to it. I remembered many situations from my life, where I felt the need to fight and struggle and, in retrospect, that too felt unnecessary. It was as if I had been somehow programmed by my birth to see life as much more complicated and dangerous than it actually is. It seemed to me that this experience could open my eyes in this regard and make my life much easier and more playful than before.

Fourth Perinatal Matrix: BPM IV (The Death-Rebirth Experience)

This matrix is related to the third clinical stage of delivery, to the final expulsion from the birth canal and the severing of the umbilical cord. Experiencing this matrix, we complete the preceding difficult process of propulsion through the birth canal, achieve explosive liberation, and emerge into light. This can often be accompanied by concrete and realistic memories of various specific aspects of this stage of birth. These can include the experience of anesthesia, the pressures of the forceps, and the sensations associated with various obstetric maneuvers or postnatal interventions.

The reliving of biological birth is not experienced just as a simple mechanical replay of the original biological event, but also as psychospiritual death and rebirth. To understand this, one has to realize that what happens in this process includes some important additional elements. Because the fetus is completely confined during the birth process and has no way of expressing the extreme emotions and reacting to the intense physical sensations involved, the memory of this event remains psychologically undigested and unassimilated.

Our self-definition and our attitudes toward the world in our postnatal life are heavily contaminated by this constant reminder of the vulnerability, inadequacy, and weakness that we experienced at birth. In a sense, we were born anatomically but have not caught up with this fact emotionally. The "dying" and the agony during the struggle for rebirth reflect the actual pain and vital threat of the biological birth process. However, the ego death that precedes rebirth is the death of our old concepts of who we are and what the world is like, which were forged by the traumatic imprint of birth and are maintained by the memory of this situation that stays alive in our unconscious.

As we are clearing these old programs by letting them emerge into consciousness, they are losing their emotional charge and are, in a sense, dying. But we are so identified with them that approaching the moment of the ego death feels like the end of our existence, or even like the end of the world. As frightening as this process is, it is actually very healing and transforming. However, paradoxically, while only a small step separates us from an experience of radical liberation, we have a sense of all-pervading anxiety and impending catastrophe of enormous proportions.

What is actually dying in this process is the false ego that, up to this point in our life, we have mistaken for our true self. While we are losing all the reference points we know, we have no idea what is on the other side, or

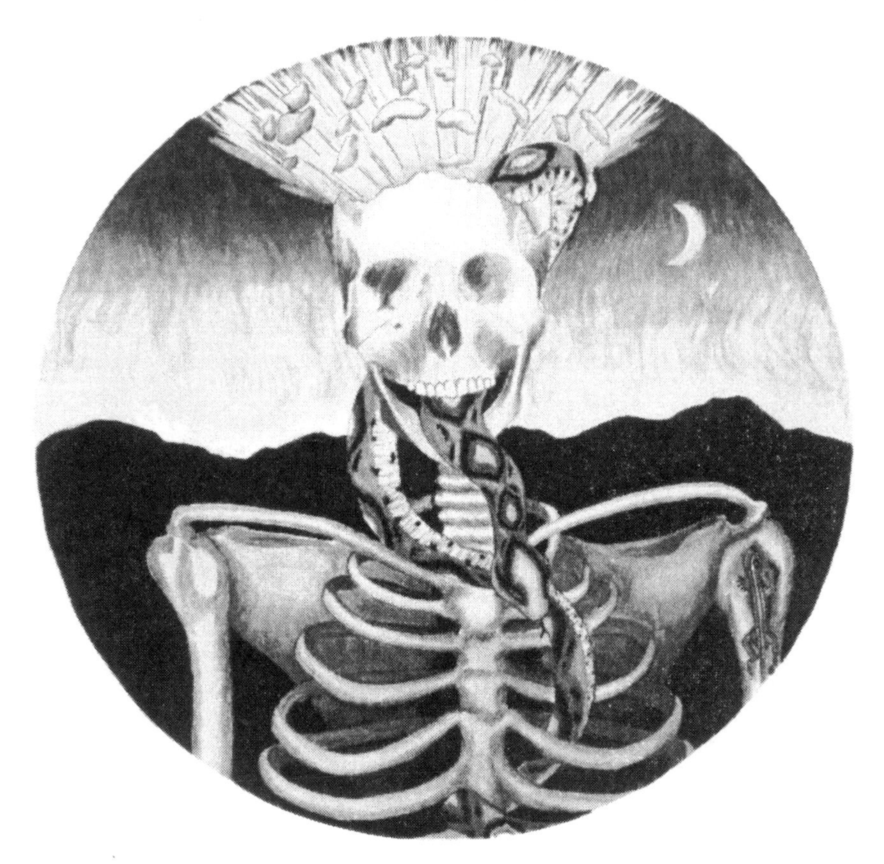

Experience of transcendence of death in an ayahuasca session. Vision of a skull and ribcage exploding into light of the Spirit and breaking the bondage of the mind and of the human form. This experience brought a sense of great freedom and joy (Kathleen Silver).

even if there is anything there at all. This fear tends to create enormous resistance to continue and complete the experience. As a result, without appropriate guidance many people can remain psychologically stuck in this problematic territory.

When we overcome the metaphysical fear encountered at this important juncture and decide to let things happen, we experience total annihilation on all imaginable levels—physical destruction, emotional disaster, intellectual and philosophical defeat, ultimate moral failure, and even spiritual damnation. During this experience, all reference points—everything

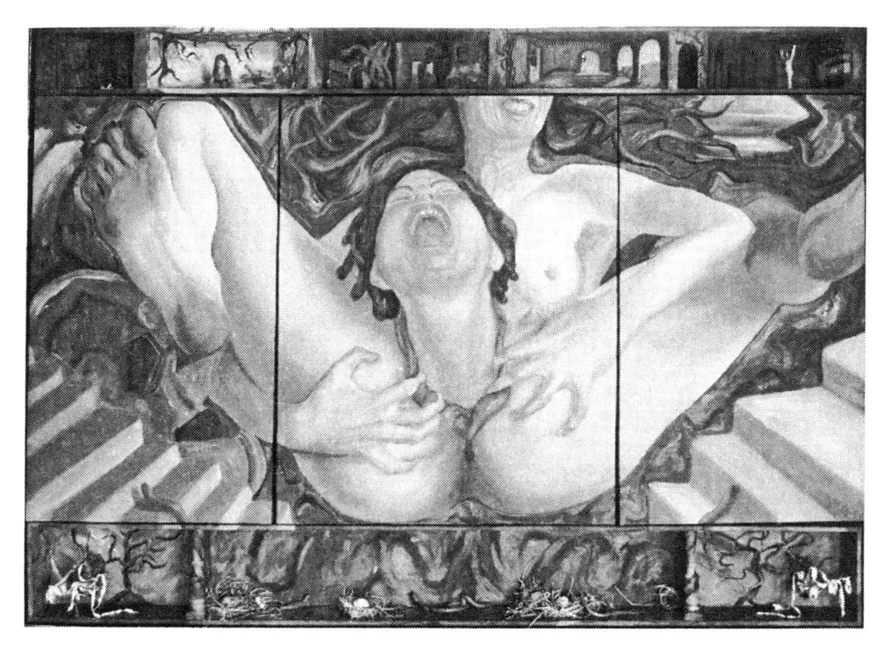

A painting representing the combined experience of giving birth and being born in a session of holotropic breathwork. Experiences of this kind can be very healing and transformative and result in a sense of giving birth to a new self. (Jean Perkins: "Coming Out of Darkness," 54"x74", 1999).

that is important and meaningful in our life—seem to be mercilessly destroyed. Immediately following the experience of total annihilation—hitting "cosmic bottom"—we are overwhelmed by visions of white or golden light of supernatural radiance and exquisite beauty that appears numinous and divine.

Having survived what seemed like an experience of total annihilation and apocalyptic end of everything, we are blessed only seconds later with fantastic displays of magnificent rainbow spectra, peacock designs, celestial scenes, and visions of archetypal beings bathed in divine light. Often, this is the time of a powerful encounter with the archetypal Great Mother Goddess, either in her universal form or in one of her culture-specific forms. Following the experience of psychospiritual death and rebirth, we feel redeemed and blessed, experience ecstatic rapture, and have a sense of reclaiming our divine nature and cosmic status. We are overcome by a surge of positive emotions toward ourselves, other people, nature, and existence in general.

It is important to emphasize that this kind of healing and life-changing experience occurs when birth was not too debilitating or confounded by heavy anesthesia. If that was the case, we do not have a sense of triumphant emergence into light and radical resolution. Instead, the postnatal period might feel like a slow recovering from a crippling disease or awakening from a hangover. As we will see later, anesthesia at birth can also have profound adverse psychological consequences for postnatal life.

The following account of a death-rebirth experience from a high-dose psychedelic session describes a typical sequence characteristic of BPM IV.

> However, the worst was yet to come. All of a sudden, I seemed to be losing all my connections to reality, as if some imaginary rug was pulled from under my feet. Everything was collapsing and I felt that my entire world was shattered to pieces. It was like puncturing a monstrous metaphysical balloon of my existence; a gigantic bubble of ludicrous self-deception had burst open and exposed the lie of my life. Everything that I ever believed in, everything that I did or pursued, everything that seemed to give my life meaning suddenly appeared utterly false. These were all pitiful crutches without any substance with which I tried to patch up the intolerable reality of existence. They were now blasted and blown away like the frail feathered seeds of a dandelion, exposing a frightening abyss of ultimate truth—the meaningless chaos of the existential Void.
>
> Filled with indescribable horror, I saw a gigantic figure of a deity towering over me in a threatening pose. I somehow instinctively recognized that this was the Hindu god Shiva in his destructive aspect. I felt the thunderous impact of his enormous foot that crushed me, shattered me to smithereens, and smeared me like an insignificant piece of excrement all over what I felt was the bottom of the cosmos. In the next moment, I was facing a terrifying giant figure of a dark Indian goddess whom I identified as Kali. My face was being pushed by an irresistible force toward her gaping vagina that was full of what seemed to be menstrual blood or repulsive afterbirth.
>
> I sensed that what was demanded of me was absolute surrender to the forces of existence and to the feminine principle represented by the goddess. I had no choice but to kiss and lick her vulva in utmost submission and humility. At this moment, which was the ultimate and final end of any feeling of male supremacy I had ever harbored, I connected with the memory of the moment of my biological birth. My head was emerging from the birth canal with my mouth in close contact with the bleeding vagina of my mother.
>
> I was flooded with divine light of supernatural radiance and indescribable beauty; its golden rays were exploding into thousands of exquisite peacock designs. From this brilliant golden light emerged a figure of the Great

Mother Goddess who seemed to embody love and protection of all ages. She spread her arms and reached toward me, enveloping me into her essence. I merged with this incredible energy field, feeling purged, healed, and nourished. What seemed to be some divine nectar and ambrosia, some archetypal essence of milk and honey, was pouring into me in absolute abundance.

Then the figure of the goddess gradually disappeared, absorbed by an even more brilliant light. It was abstract, yet endowed with definite personal characteristics and radiating infinite intelligence. It became clear to me that what I was experiencing was the merging with and absorption into the Universal Self, or Brahman, as I have read about it in books of Indian philosophy. This experience subsided after about ten minutes of clock-time; however, it transcended any concept of time and felt like eternity. The flow of the healing and nourishing energy and the visions of golden glow with peacock designs lasted through the night. The resulting sense of well-being stayed with me for many days. The memory of the experience has remained vivid for years and has profoundly changed my entire life philosophy.

The Transpersonal Domain of the Psyche

The second major domain that has to be added to mainstream psychiatry's cartography of the human psyche when we work with holotropic states is now known under the name *transpersonal.* This term means literally "reaching beyond the personal" or "transcending the personal." The experiences that originate on this level involve transcendence of our usual boundaries (our body and ego) and of the limitations of three-dimensional space and linear time that restrict our perception of the world in the ordinary state of consciousness. Transpersonal experiences can best be defined by comparison with the everyday experience of ourselves and of the world or, more specifically, with the way we have to experience ourselves and the environment to pass for "normal" according to the standards of our culture and of contemporary psychiatry.

In the ordinary, or normal, state of consciousness, we experience ourselves as Newtonian objects existing within the boundaries of our skin. The American writer and philosopher Alan Watts referred to this experience of oneself as identifying with the "skin-encapsulated ego." Our perception of the environment is restricted by the physiological limitations of our sensory organs and by the physical characteristics of the environment. We cannot see objects from which we are separated by a solid wall, ships that are beyond the horizon, or the other side of the moon. If we are in

Prague, we cannot hear what our friends are talking about in San Francisco. We cannot feel the softness of the lambskin unless the surface of our body is in direct contact with it.

In addition, we can experience vividly and with all our senses only the events that are happening in the present moment. We can recall the past and anticipate future events or fantasize about them; however, these are very different experiences from an immediate and direct experience of the present moment. In transpersonal states of consciousness, none of the above limitations are absolute; any of them can be transcended. There are no limits for the reach of our senses and we can experience with all the sensory qualities episodes that occurred in the past and occasionally even those that have not yet happened but will actually happen in the future.

The spectrum of transpersonal experiences is extremely rich and includes phenomena from several different levels of consciousness. Table 2.2 represents an attempt to list and categorize the various types of experiences that, in my opinion, belong to the transpersonal domain. I have personally experienced in my own psychedelic and holotropic sessions most of the phenomena that are listed in this synoptic table and I have also repeatedly observed them in my work with others. In the context of this book, I will not be able to provide definitions and descriptions of all these types of experiences and illustrate them with clinical examples. For this, I have to refer the interested readers to my previous publications (Grof 1975, 1985, 1988).

As the table shows, transpersonal experiences can be divided into three large categories. The first of these involves primarily transcendence of the usual spatial and temporal barriers. Experiential extension beyond the spatial limitations of the "skin-encapsulated ego" leads to experiences of merging with another person into a state that can be called "dual unity," assuming the identity of another person, or identifying with the consciousness of an entire group of people, such as all mothers of the world, the entire population of India, or all the inmates of concentration camps. Our consciousness can even expand to such an extent that it seems to encompass all of humanity. Experiences of this kind have been repeatedly described in the spiritual literature of the world.

In a similar way, we can transcend the limits of the specifically human experience and identify with the consciousness of various animals, plants, or even experience a form of consciousness that seems to be related to inorganic objects and processes. In the extremes, it is possible to experience consciousness of the biosphere, of our entire planet, or the whole material universe.

TABLE 2.2 **Transpersonal Experiences**

Experiential Extension within Space-Time and Consensus Reality

Transcendence of Spatial Boundaries

Experience of Dual Unity
Identification with Other Persons
Group Identification and Group Consciousness
Identification with Animals
Identification with Plants and Botanical Processes
Oneness with Life and All Creation
Experience of Inorganic Materials and Processes
Planetary Consciousness
Experiences of Extraterrestrial Beings and Worlds
Identification with the Entire Physical Universe
Psychic Phenomena Involving Transcendence of Space

Transcendence of Temporal Boundaries

Embryonal and Fetal Experiences
Ancestral Experiences
Racial and Collective Experiences
Past Incarnation Experiences
Phylogenetic Experiences
Experiences of Planetary Evolution
Cosmogenetic Experiences
Psychic Phenomena Involving Transcendence of Time

Experiential Exploration of the Microworld

Organ and Tissue Consciousness
Cellular Consciousness
Experience of the DNA
Experiences of the World of Atoms and Subatomic Particles

Experiential Extension beyond Space-Time and Consensus Reality

Spiritistic and Mediumistic Experiences
Energetic Phenomena of the Subtle Body
Experiences of Animal Spirits (Power Animals)
Encounters with Spirit Guides and Suprahuman Beings
Visits to Parallel Universes and Meetings with Their Inhabitants
Experiences of Mythological and Fairytale Sequences
Experiences of Specific Blissful and Wrathful Deities
Experiences of Universal Archetypes
Intuitive Understanding of Universal Symbols
Creative Inspiration and the Promethean Impulse
Experience of the Demiurg and Insights into Cosmic Creation
Experience of Cosmic Consciousness
The Supracosmic and Metacosmic Void

TABLE 2.2 **Transpersonal Experiences (*continued*)**

Transpersonal Experiences of Psychoid Nature
Synchronicities (Interplay between Intrapsychic Experiences and Consensus Reality)
Spontaneous Psychoid Events
Supernormal Physical Feats
Spiritistic Phenomena and Physical Mediumship
Recurrent Spontaneous Psychokinesis (Poltergeist)
UFOs and Alien Abduction Experiences
Intentional Psychokinesis
Ceremonial Magic
Healing and Hexing
Yogic Siddhis
Laboratory Psychokinesis

Incredible and absurd as it might seem to a Westerner committed to monistic materialism, these experiences suggest that everything we can experience in the everyday state of consciousness as an object, has in the holotropic state of consciousness a corresponding subjective representation. It is as if everything in the universe has its objective and subjective aspect, the way it is described in the great spiritual philosophies of the East. For example, the Hindus see all that exists as a manifestation of Brahman or the Taoists think about the universe in terms of transformations of the Tao.

Other transpersonal experiences in this first category are characterized primarily by overcoming of temporal rather than spatial boundaries, by transcendence of linear time. We have already talked about the possibility of vivid reliving of important memories from infancy and reexperiencing of the trauma of birth. This historical regression can continue farther and involve authentic fetal and embryonal memories from different periods of intrauterine life. It is not even unusual to experience, on the level of cellular consciousness, full identification with the sperm and the ovum at the time of conception.

But the process of experiential retracing of creation does not stop here. In holotropic states, we can experience episodes from the lives of our human or animal ancestors, or even those that seem to be coming from the racial and collective unconscious, as described by C. G. Jung. Quite frequently, experiences that seem to be happening in other cultures and historical periods are associated with a sense of personal remembering, a convinced feeling of *déjà vu* or *déjà vecu*. People then talk about reliving of memories from past lives, from previous incarnations.

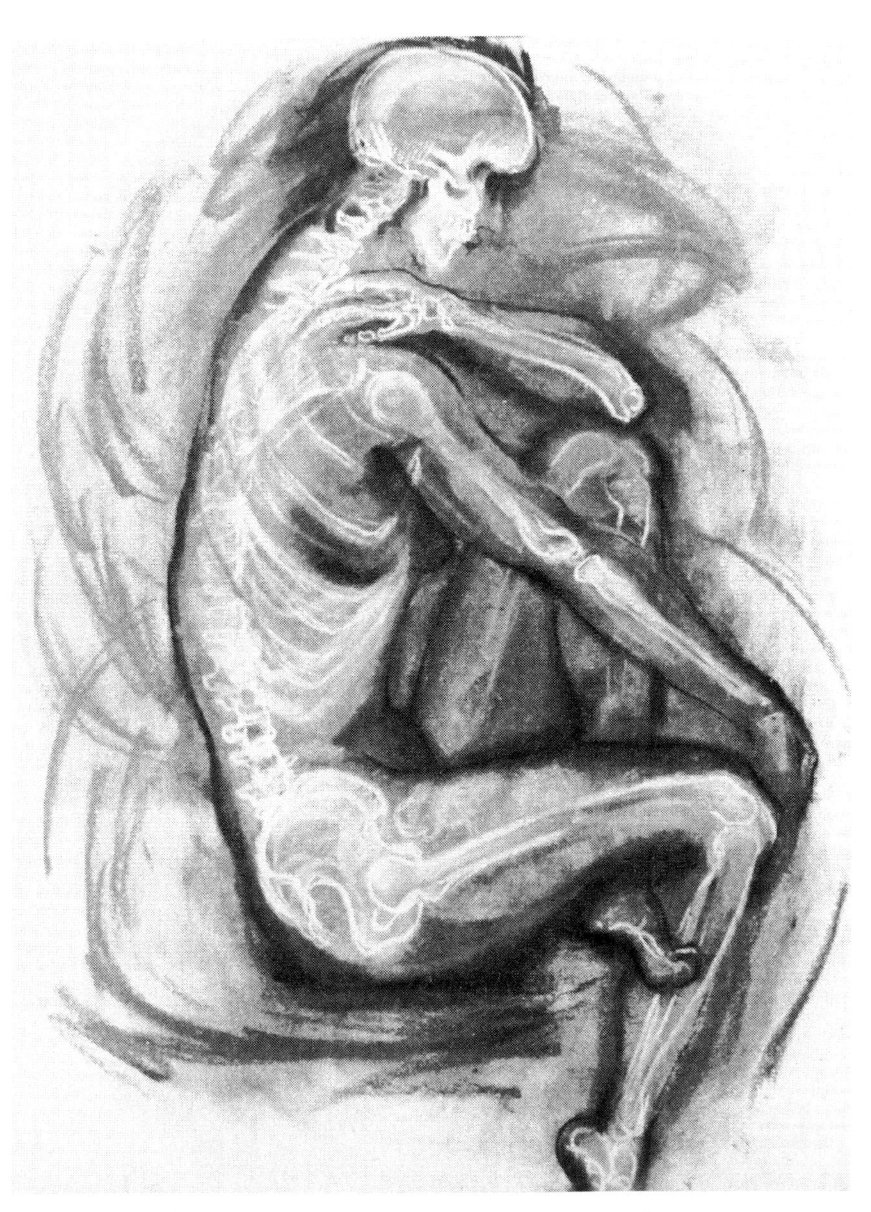

Inside I [above] and Inside II [right], two paintings reflecting experiences of the interior of the body in a psychedelic session. The capacity to experience one's skeleton and inner organs in holotropic states of consciousness throws interesting light on the 'X-ray art' of Siberian or Eskimo shamans and Australian Aborigines (Robin Maynard-Dobbs).

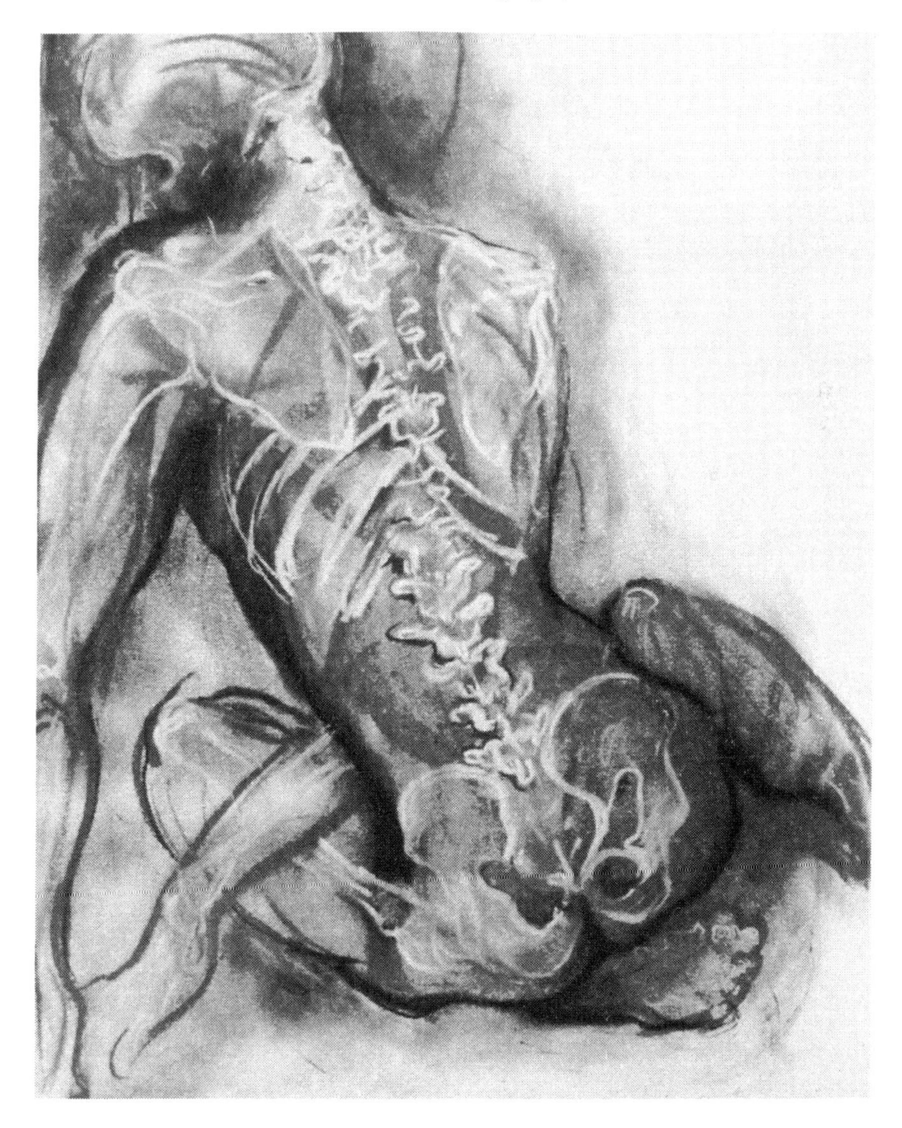

Experiences in holotropic states can also take us into the microworld, to structures and processes that are ordinarily not accessible to our unaided senses. Here belong sequences reminiscent of Isaac Asimov's film *Fantastic Voyage* that portray the world of our inner organs, tissues, and cells or even involve full experiential identification with them. Particularly fascinating are experiences of the DNA associated with insights into the ultimate mystery of life, reproduction, and heredity. Occasionally, this type of transpersonal experience can take us into the inorganic world of molecules, atoms, and subatomic particles.

The content of transpersonal experiences described so far consists of various phenomena existing in space-time. They involve elements of our everyday familiar reality—other people, animals, plants, materials, and events from the past. There is nothing that we would ordinarily consider unusual as far as these phenomena in and of themselves are concerned. They belong to a reality that we know; we accept their existence and take it for granted. What surprises us in regard to the two categories of transpersonal experiences described above is not their content, but the fact that we can witness or fully identify with something that is not ordinarily accessible to our senses.

We know that there are pregnant whales in the world, but we should not be able to have an authentic experience of being one. The fact that there once was the French revolution is readily acceptable to us, but we should not be able to have a vivid experience of being there and lying wounded on the barricades of Paris. We know that there are many things happening in the world in places where we are not present, but it is usually considered impossible to experience something that is happening in remote locations (without the mediation of the television and a satellite). We may also be surprised to find consciousness associated with lower animals, plants, and with inorganic nature.

The second category of transpersonal phenomena is even stranger. In holotropic states, our consciousness can extend into realms and dimensions that the Western industrial culture does not consider to be "real." Here belong numerous visions of or identification with archetypal beings, deities and demons of various cultures, and visits to fantastic mythological landscapes. In this context, we can attain intuitive understanding of universal symbols, such as the cross, the Nile cross or *ankh,* the swastika, the pentacle, the six-pointed star, or the yin-yang sign. We can also experience encounter and communication with discarnate and suprahuman entities, spirit guides, extraterrestrial beings, or inhabitants of parallel universes.

In its farthest reaches, our individual consciousness can transcend all boundaries and identify with Cosmic Consciousness or the Universal Mind known under many different names: Brahman, Buddha, the Cosmic Christ, Keter, Allah, the Tao, the Great Spirit, and many others. The ultimate of all experiences appears to be identification with the Supracosmic and Metacosmic Void, the mysterious and primordial emptiness and nothingness that is conscious of itself and is the ultimate cradle of all existence. It has no concrete content, yet it contains all there is in a germinal and potential form.

The third category of transpersonal experiences comprises phenomena that I call *psychoid,* using the term coined by the founder of vitalism Hans Driesch and adopted by C. G. Jung. This group includes situations in which intrapsychic experiences are associated with corresponding events in the external world (or, better, in consensus reality) that are meaningfully related to them. Psychoid experiences cover a wide range from synchronicities, spiritual healing, and ceremonial magic to psychokinesis and other mind-over-matter phenomena known from the yogic literature as *siddhis* (Grof 1988).

Transpersonal experiences have many strange characteristics that shatter the most fundamental metaphysical assumptions of the materialistic worldview and of the Newtonian-Cartesian paradigm. Researchers who have studied and/or personally experienced these fascinating phenomena realize that the attempts of mainstream science to dismiss them as irrelevant plays of human fantasy, or as erratic hallucinatory products of a diseased brain, are naïve and inadequate. Any unbiased study of the transpersonal domain of the psyche has to confirm that the phenomena encountered here represent a critical challenge not only for psychiatry and psychology, but for the entire philosophy of Western science.

Although transpersonal experiences occur in the process of deep individual self-exploration, it is not possible to interpret them simply as intrapsychic phenomena in the conventional sense. On the one hand, they appear on the same experiential continuum as the biographical and perinatal experiences and are thus coming from within the individual psyche. On the other hand, they seem to be tapping directly, without the mediation of the senses, into sources of information that are clearly far beyond the conventional reach of the individual.

Somewhere on the perinatal level of the psyche, a strange experiential switch seems to occur: what was up to that point deep intrapsychic probing becomes an extrasensory experience of various aspects of the universe at large. Some people who experienced this peculiar transition from the inner to the outer compared it with the graphic art of the Dutch painter Maurits Escher, others talked about a "multidimensional experiential Moebius strip." These observations confirm the basic tenet of some esoteric systems, such as Tantra, Cabala, or the Hermetic tradition, according to which each of us is a microcosm containing in a mysterious way the entire universe. In the mystical texts, this was expressed by such phrases as "as above so below" or "as without, so within."

These observations indicate that we can obtain information about the universe in two radically different ways. The conventional mode of learning is based on sensory perception and analysis and synthesis of the data by our brain. The radical alternative that becomes available in holotropic states is learning by direct experiential identification with various aspects of the world. In the context of old paradigm thinking, the claims of ancient esoteric systems that the microworld can reflect the macroworld, or the part can contain the whole, were utterly absurd, since they seemed to offend common sense and violate the elementary principles of Aristotelian logic. This has changed radically after the discovery of the laser and of optical holography, which opened new ways of understanding the relationship between the part and the whole. The holographic or holonomic thinking has provided for the first time a conceptual framework for a scientific approach to this extraordinary mechanism (Bohm 1980, Pribram 1981, Laszlo 1993).

The reports of subjects who have experienced episodes of embryonal existence, the moment of conception, and elements of cellular, tissue, and organ consciousness abound in medically accurate insights into the anatomical, physiological, and biochemical aspects of the processes involved. Similarly, ancestral, racial and collective memories and past-incarnation experiences often provide very specific details about architecture, costumes, weapons, art forms, social structure, and religious and ritual practices of the corresponding cultures and historical periods, or even concrete historical events.

People who experienced phylogenetic experiences or identification with existing life forms not only found them unusually authentic and convincing, but often acquired in the process extraordinary insights concerning animal psychology, ethology, specific habits, or unusual reproductive cycles. In some instances, this was accompanied by archaic muscular innervations not characteristic for humans, or even such complex behaviors as enactment of a courtship dance of a particular species.

The philosophical challenge associated with the already described observations, as formidable as it is, in and of itself, is further augmented by the fact that the transpersonal experiences correctly reflecting the material world of space-time often appear on the same continuum as, and intimately interwoven with, others that contain elements that the Western industrial world does not consider to be real. Here belong, for example, experiences involving deities and demons from various cultures, mythological realms such as heavens and paradises, and legendary or fairytale sequences.

For example, we can have an experience of Shiva's heaven, of the paradise of the Aztec rain god Tlaloc, of the Sumerian underworld, or of one of the Buddhist hot hells. It is also possible to communicate with Jesus, have a shattering encounter with the Hindu goddess Kali, or identify with the dancing Shiva. Even these episodes can impart accurate new information about religious symbolism and mythical motifs that were previously unknown to the person involved. Observations of this kind confirm C. G. Jung's idea that, besides the Freudian individual unconscious, we can also gain access to the collective unconscious that contains the cultural heritage of all humanity (Jung 1959).

My classification of transpersonal experiences is strictly phenomenological and not hierarchical; it does not specify the levels of consciousness on which they occur. It is, therefore, interesting to compare this scheme with Ken Wilber's description of the levels of spiritual evolution that, according to him, follow the full integration of the body and mind (postcentauric levels of consciousness evolution in his terminology) (Wilber 1980). It is not difficult to show the parallels between his developmental scheme and my cartography of transpersonal experiences.

Constructing his developmental map of psychospiritual development, Wilber used mostly material from ancient spiritual literature, particularly from Vedanta Hinduism and Theravada Buddhism. My own data are drawn from clinical observations in contemporary populations in Europe, North and South America, and Australia, complemented by some limited experience with Japanese and East Indian groups. My work thus provides empirical evidence for the existence of most of the experiences included in his scheme. It also shows that the descriptions in ancient spiritual sources are still to a great extent relevant for modern humanity. However, as we will see, the systems are not exactly identical and incorporating my material would require certain additions, modifications, and adjustments.

Wilber's scheme of the postcentauric spiritual domain includes the lower and higher subtle and lower and higher causal levels and the Ultimate or Absolute. According to him, the *low subtle,* or *astral-psychic, level of consciousness* is characterized by a degree of differentiation of consciousness from the mind and body that goes beyond that achieved on the level of the centaur. Consciousness is thus able to transcend the normal capacities of body/mind and operate in ways that appear impossible and fantastic to the ordinary mind.

In Wilber's own words, "the astral level includes, basically, out-of-body experiences, certain occult knowledge, the auras, true magic, 'astral travel,' and so on." Wilber's description of the psychic level includes various "psi" phenomena: ESP, precognition, clairvoyance, psychokinesis, and others. He also refers in this connection to Patanjali's *Yoga Sutras,* which include on the psychic level all the paranormal powers, mind-over-matter phenomena, or *siddhis.*

In the *higher subtle realm,* consciousness differentiates itself completely from the ordinary mind and becomes what can be called the "overself" or "overmind." Wilber places in this region high religious intuition and inspiration, visions of divine light, audible illuminations, and higher presences—spiritual guides, angelic beings, ishtadevas, Dhyani-Buddhas, and God's archetypes, which he sees as high archetypal forms of our own being.

Like the subtle level, the causal level can be subdivided into lower and higher. Wilber suggests that the *lower causal realm* is manifested in a state of consciousness known as *savikalpa samadhi,* the experience of final God, the ground, essence, and source of all the archetypal and lesser-god manifestations encountered in the subtle realms. The *higher causal realm* then involves a "total and utter transcendence and release into Formless Consciousness, Boundless Radiance." Wilber refers in this context to *nirvikalpa samadhi* of Hinduism, *nirodh* of Hinayana Buddhism, and to the eighth of the ten ox-herding pictures of Zen Buddhism.

On Wilber's last level, that of the *Absolute,* Consciousness awakens as its Original Condition and Suchness (*tathagata*), which is, at the same time, all that is, gross, subtle, or causal. The distinction between the witness and the witnessed disappears and the entire World Process then arises, moment to moment as one's own Being, outside of which and prior to which nothing exists.

As I mentioned earlier, my own experiences and observations bring supportive evidence for the experiential states included in Wilber's ontological and cosmological scheme. The subjects I have worked with over the years experienced and reported first-hand experiences of most of the phenomena included in his map. My own sessions were no exceptions in this regard; I have personally encountered and described in my writings most of these experiences. I consider this convergence to be very important, since my material represents actual direct observations in contemporary subjects.

In a hierarchical classification based on my own data, I would include in the *low subtle* or *astral-psychic level* experiences that involve elements of the material world, but provide information about them in a way that is radically different from our everyday perception. Here belong, above all, experiences that are traditionally studied by parapsychologists (and some of them also by thanatologists), such as out-of-body experiences, astral travel, ESP phenomena, precognition, and clairvoyance.

I would also add to this list experiences of phenomena that are closely connected to the material world, but reveal aspects or dimensions of reality not accessible to ordinary consciousness, such as direct experiential apprehension of the subtle or energy body and of its conduits (*nadis* or *meridians*) and fields (*auras*). The concept of crosspoints, bridges between the visible and invisible reality, found in Tantric literature seems to be particularly relevant in this context (Mookerjee and Khanna 1977).

I would include on the low subtle level also some important transpersonal experiences included in my map but not mentioned by Wilber. Here would belong experiential identification with various aspects of space-time—with other people, animals, plants, and organic materials and processes, as well as ancestral, racial, collective, phylogenetic, and karmic experiences. These are experiences that surprisingly receive close to no attention in Wilber's writings. I have shown in my previous publications that all these experiences provide access to accurate new information about the phenomena involved that is mediated by extrasensory channels. They play an important role in the process of spiritual opening (Grof 1975, 1980, 1985, 1988, 1998). Following Patanjali, I would also include here from my classification the yogic siddhis, as well as the entire group of phenomena that I call "psychoid."

The transpersonal experiences from my cartography that could be assigned to the *high subtle level* include visions of divine light, encounters with various blissful and wrathful archetypal deities, communication with spirit guides and superhuman entities, contact with shamanic power animals, direct apprehension of universal symbols, and episodes of religious and creative inspiration (the "Promethean epiphany"). The visions of archetypal beings, or experiential identification with these beings, can portray them in their universal form (e.g., the Great Mother Goddess) or in the form of their specific cultural manifestations (e.g., Virgin Mary, Isis, Cybele, Parvati, etc.).

Over the years, I have had the privilege of being in sessions of people whose psychedelic or holotropic experiences had the characteristics of those that are assigned in Wilber's scheme to the lower and higher causal realms and possibly even those of the Absolute. I have also had personal experiences that I believe qualified for these categories. In my classification these episodes are described under such titles as experiences of the Demiurg, of

Cosmic Consciousness, Absolute Consciousness, or Supracosmic and Metacosmic Void.

In the light of the above observations, I have no doubt that the phenomena that Wilber includes in his holoarchic scheme are not only experientially but also ontologically real and are not products of metaphysical speculation or pathological processes in the brain. I am also fully aware of the fact that having the experience of these levels does not necessarily mean moving permanently to higher levels of consciousness evolution. The problem of the critical factors that determine when transient experiences of higher states of consciousness lead to lasting changes in evolutionary structures of consciousness is an important issue. Ken and I have touched upon it in our past discussions and I hope we will explore it further at another place and time.

The general concept of the Great Chain of Being, according to which reality includes an entire hierarchy (or holarchy) of dimensions that are ordinarily hidden to our perception, is very important and well founded. It would be erroneous to dismiss this understanding of existence as primitive superstition or psychotic delusion, as has so frequently been done. Anybody attempting to do that would have to offer a plausible explanation for why the experiences that systematically support this elaborate and comprehensive vision of reality have in the past occurred so consistently in people of various races, cultures, and historical periods.

As I have tried to show in another context, anybody trying to defend in this respect the monistic-materialistic position of Western science would also have to account for the fact that these experiences continue to emerge in highly intelligent, sophisticated, and otherwise mentally healthy people of our era (Grof 1998). This happens not only under the influence of psychedelics, but also under such diverse circumstances as sessions of experiential psychotherapy, in the meditations of people involved in systematic spiritual practice, in near-death experiences, and in the course of spontaneous episodes of psychospiritual crisis.

It is not an easy task to summarize in a brief communication conclusions from daily observations amassed in the course of over forty years of research of holotropic states and make those statements believable. Although I myself had many personal experiences and the opportunity to observe closely a number of other people in these states and hear their accounts, it took me years to fully absorb the impact of this cognitive shock. Because of space considerations, I was not able to present detailed case histories that could help to illustrate the nature of transpersonal experiences and the insights they make available. However, I doubt that even that, in and of itself, would suffice to counteract the deeply ingrained programs that Western science instilled into our culture. The conceptual challenges that are involved are so formidable that nothing short of a deep personal experience will be adequate to the task.

The existence and nature of transpersonal experiences violates some of the most basic assumptions of mechanistic science. They imply such seemingly absurd notions as relativity and arbitrary nature of all physical boundaries, nonlocal connections in the universe, communication through unknown means and channels, memory without a material substrate, nonlinearity of time, or consciousness associated with all living organisms, and even inorganic matter. Many transpersonal experiences involve events from the microcosm and the macrocosm, realms that cannot normally be reached by unaided human senses, or from historical periods that precede the origin of the solar system, formation of planet earth, appearance of living organisms, development of the nervous system, and emergence of homo sapiens.

The research of holotropic states reveals a remarkable paradox concerning the nature of human beings. It clearly shows that, in a mysterious and yet unexplained way, each of us contains the information about the entire universe and all of existence, has potential experiential access to all of its parts, and in a sense *is* the whole cosmic network, to the same degree that he or she is just an infinitesimal part of it, a separate and insignificant biological entity. The new cartography reflects this fact and portrays the individual human psyche as being essentially commensurate with the entire cosmos and the totality of existence. As absurd and implausible as this idea might seem to a traditionally trained scientist and to our common sense, it can be relatively easily reconciled with new revolutionary developments in various scientific disciplines usually referred to as the new or emerging paradigm.

I firmly believe that the expanded cartography outlined above is of critical importance for any serious approach to such phenomena as shamanism, rites of passage, mysticism, religion, mythology, parapsychology, near-death experiences, and psychedelic states. This new model of the psyche is not just a matter of academic interest. As will be revealed in the following chapters of this book, it has deep and revolutionary implications for the understanding of emotional and psychosomatic disorders, including many conditions currently diagnosed as psychotic, and offers new revolutionary therapeutic possibilities.

CHAPTER THREE

Architecture of Emotional and Psychosomatic Disorders

Before we explore at some length the far-reaching implications of the study of holotropic states for the understanding of emotional and psychosomatic disorders, we will take a brief look at the conceptual frameworks that are currently accepted in academic circles and used in clinical work. The attempts to explain the nature and origins of these disorders fall into two broad categories. Some theoreticians and clinicians show a strong preference to see these disorders as resulting from causes that are primarily of a biological nature, others favor psychological explanations. In everyday clinical practice, psychiatrists also often choose an eclectic approach and assign different degrees of significance to elements from both categories, leaning to one or the other side of the argument.

The organically oriented psychiatrists believe that, since the psyche is a product of material processes in the brain, the final answers in psychiatry will come from neurophysiology, biochemistry, genetics, and molecular biology. According to them, these disciplines will one day be able to provide adequate explanations, as well as practical solutions for most of the problems in their field. This orientation is usually associated with rigid adherence to the medical model and with attempts to develop a fixed diagnostic classification for all emotional disorders, including those for which no organic basis has been found.

An alternative orientation in psychiatry emphasizes factors of a psychological nature, such as the role of traumatic influences in infancy, childhood, and later in life, pathogenic potential of conflict, the importance of family dynamics and interpersonal relationships, or the impact of social environment. In the extremes, this way of thinking is applied not only to neuroses and psychosomatic disorders, but also to those psychotic states for which medicine has no biological explanation.

A logical consequence of this approach is to seriously question the appropriateness of applying the medical model, including rigid diagnostic labels, to disorders that are not biologically determined and are thus clearly of a different order than the organic ones. From this perspective, psychogenic disorders reflect the complexity of developmental factors to which we have been exposed in the course of our lives (and from the perspective of transpersonal psychologists throughout our entire psychospiritual history). Since these influences differ widely from individual to individual, the efforts to squeeze the resulting disorders into the straitjacket of medical diagnosis makes little sense.

Although many professionals advocate an eclectic approach that acknowledges a complex interplay of nature and nurture, or biology and psychology, the biological approach dominates thinking in the academic circles and routine everyday psychiatric practice. As a result of its complex historical development, psychiatry has become established as a subspecialty of medicine, which gives it a strong biological bias. Mainstream conceptual thinking in psychiatry, the approach to individuals with emotional disorders and behavior problems, the strategy of research, basic education and training, and forensic measures, all these are dominated by the medical model.

This situation is a consequence of two important sets of circumstances. Medicine has been successful in establishing etiology and finding effective therapy for a specific, relatively small group of mental abnormalities of organic origin. It has also demonstrated its ability to control symptomatically many of those disorders for which specific organic etiology could not be found. The initial successes in unraveling the biological causes of mental disorders, however astonishing, were really isolated and limited to a small fraction of the problems that psychiatry deals with. The medical approach to psychiatry has failed to find specific organic etiology for problems vexing the absolute majority of its clients—psychoneuroses, psychosomatic disorders, manic-depressive disease, and functional psychoses.

The psychological orientation in psychiatry was inspired by the pioneering research of Sigmund Freud and his followers. Some of them, such as Carl Gustav Jung, Otto Rank, Wilhelm Reich, and Alfred Adler, left the psychoanalytic association or were expelled from it and started their own schools. Others stayed within the organization, but developed their own variations of psychoanalytic theory and technique. In the course of the twentieth century, this collective effort resulted in a large number of schools of "depth psychology," which differ significantly from each other in terms of their understanding of the human psyche and the nature of emotional disorders, as well as the therapeutic techniques they use.

Most of these individuals have had minimal or no influence on mainstream thinking in psychiatry and reference to their work appears in academic textbooks as a historical note or even footnote. Only Freud's early writings, the work of a few of his followers, and the modern developments in psychoanalysis known as "ego psychology" have had significant impact on the psychiatric field.

Freud and his colleagues formulated a dynamic classification of emotional and psychosomatic disorders that explains and ranks these conditions in terms of fixation on a specific stage of the libido development and the evolution of the ego. One of Freud's major contributions was the discovery that the libidinal interests of the infant gradually shift from the oral zone (at the time of nursing) to the anal and urethral zone (at the time of toilet training) and finally to the phallic zone (focus on the penis and clitoris at the time of the Oedipus and Electra complex). Traumatization or, conversely, overindulgence during these critical periods can cause specific fixation on one of these zones. This predisposes the individual to psychological regression to this area when in the future he or she encounters serious difficulties.

The understanding of psychopathology based on Freud's libido theory was summarized by the German psychoanalyst Karl Abraham (1927). In his famous scheme, Abraham defined major forms of psychopathology in terms of the primary fixation of the libido. According to him, fixation on the passive oral stage (before teething occurs) predisposes the individual to schizophrenia and fixation on the oral-sadistic or cannibalistic stage (after teething) can lead to manic-depressive disorders and suicidal behavior. Oral fixation plays also a critical role in the development of alcoholism and drug addiction.

The primary fixation for obsessive-compulsive neurosis and personality is on the anal level. Anal fixation also plays an important role in the genesis of so-called pregenital neuroses, such as stammering, psychogenic tics, and asthma. Urethral fixation is associated with shame and fear of blunder and a tendency to compensate for it by excessive ambition and perfectionism. Anxiety hysteria (various phobias) and conversion hysteria (paralysis, anesthesia, blindness, loss of voice, and hysterical attack) result from a fixation on the phallic stage.

Karl Abraham's scheme took into consideration not only the points of libidinal fixation, but also fixation on the stages of evolution of the ego from autoeroticism and primary narcissism to the establishment of object love. This aspect of psychopathology was elaborated in great detail in later development of psychoanalysis. Modern ego psychology inspired by the groundbreaking work of Anna Freud and Heinz Hartmann revised and refined classical psychoanalytic concepts and added some important new dimensions (Blanck and Blanck 1974, 1979).

Combining direct observations in infants and young children with deep knowledge of psychoanalytic theory, René Spitz and Margaret Mahler laid the foundations for a deeper understanding of the ego development and establishment of personal identity. Their work brought attention to the importance of the evolution of object relationships and the difficulties associated with them for the development of psychopathology. The description and definition of three phases in the evolution of the ego—the autistic, symbiotic, and separation-individuation phase—have important theoretical and clinical implications.

Margaret Mahler, Otto Kernberg, Heinz Kohut, and others expanded Karl Abraham's scheme by adding several disorders that, according to them, have their origin in the early disturbances of object relations—autistic and symbiotic infantile psychoses, narcissistic personality disturbance, and borderline personality disorders. This new understanding of the dynamics of ego evolution and its vicissitudes made it also possible to develop techniques of psychotherapy for psychiatric patients in these categories who cannot be reached by methods of classical psychoanalysis.

There is no doubt that ego psychologists improved, refined, and expanded the psychoanalytic understanding of psychopathology. However, they share with classical psychoanalysis the narrow understanding of the psyche limited to postnatal biography and the individual unconscious. The observations from the study of holotropic states of consciousness show that emotional and psychosomatic disorders, including many states currently diagnosed as psychotic, cannot be adequately understood solely from difficulties in postnatal development, such as problems in the development of the libido or vicissitudes involving formation of object relations.

According to the new insights, emotional and psychosomatic disorders have a multilevel, multidimensional structure with important additional roots on the perinatal and transpersonal levels. Bringing these elements into consideration provides a radically new, much fuller and more complete picture of psychopathology and opens exciting new perspectives for therapy. The recognition of perinatal and transpersonal roots of emotional disorders does not mean denying the significance of the biographical factors described by psychoanalysis and ego psychology. The events in infancy and childhood certainly continue to play an important role in the overall picture.

However, instead of being the primary causes of these disorders, the memories of traumatic events from postnatal biography function as important conditions for the emergence of elements from deeper levels of the psyche. What gives neurotic, psychosomatic, and psychotic symptoms their extraordinary dynamic power and specific content are complex COEX constellations not limited to biographical layers, but reaching deep into the perinatal and transpersonal domains. The pathogenic influences emphasized by Freudian analysis and ego psychology modify the content of the themes from deeper levels of the unconscious, add to their emotional charge, and mediate their access into conscious awareness.

The relationship between symptoms and the underlying multilayer COEX system comprising biographical, perinatal, and transpersonal elements can be illustrated by a typical example. It involves Norbert, a fifty-one-year-old psychologist and minister who participated in one of our five-day workshops at the Esalen Institute.

> During the group introduction preceding the first session of holotropic breathwork, Norbert complained about severe chronic pain in his shoulder and pectoral muscles that caused him great suffering and made his life miserable. Repeated medical examinations, including X-rays, had not detected any organic basis for his problem and all therapeutic attempts had remained unsuccessful. Serial Prokain injections had brought only brief transient relief for the time of the effect of the drug.
>
> At the beginning of the session of holotropic breathwork, Norbert made an impulsive attempt to leave the room, since he could not tolerate the music, which he felt was "killing" him. It took great effort to persuade him to stay with the process and to explore the reasons for his discomfort. He finally agreed and, for almost three hours, he experienced severe pains in his breast and shoulder, which intensified to the point of becoming unbearable. He struggled violently as if his life were seriously threatened, choked and coughed, and let out a variety of loud screams. Following this stormy episode, he quieted down and was relaxed and peaceful. With great surprise, he

realized that the experience had released the tension in his shoulder and muscles and that he was free from pain.

Retrospectively, Norbert reported that there were three different layers in his experience, all of them related to the pain in his shoulder and associated with choking. On the most superficial level he relived a frightening situation from his childhood in which he almost lost his life. When he was about seven years old, he and his friends were digging a tunnel on a sandy ocean beach. When the tunnel was finished, Norbert crawled inside to explore it. As the other children jumped around, the tunnel collapsed and buried him alive. He almost choked to death before he was rescued.

When the breathwork experience deepened, he relived a violent and frightening episode that took him back to the memory of biological birth. His delivery was very difficult, since his shoulder had been stuck for an extended period of time behind the pubic bone of his mother. This episode shared with the previous one the combination of choking and severe pain in the shoulder.

In the last part of the session, the experience changed dramatically. Norbert started seeing military uniforms and horses and recognized that he was involved in a battle. He was even able to identify it as one of the battles in Cromwell's England. At one point, he felt a sharp pain and realized that his shoulder had been pierced by a lance. He fell off the horse and experienced himself as being trampled by the horses running over his body and crushing his chest.

Norbert's consciousness separated from the dying body, soared high above the battlefield, and observed the scene from this perspective. Following the death of the soldier, whom he recognized as himself in a previous incarnation, his consciousness returned to the present and reconnected with his body that was now pain-free for the first time after many years of agony. The relief from pain brought about by these experiences turned out to be permanent. It has now been over twenty years since this memorable session and the symptoms have not returned.

The traumatic memory of certain aspects of birth seems to be an important component of psychogenic symptoms of all kinds. The unconscious record of the experiences associated with biological delivery represents a universal pool of difficult emotions and physical sensations that constitute a potential source of various forms of psychopathology. Whether emotional and psychosomatic disorders actually develop and which form they take then depends on the reinforcing influence of traumatic events in postnatal history or, conversely, on the mitigating effect of various favorable biographical factors.

As we have seen in Norbert's case, the roots of a problem can include not only the perinatal level, but reach deep into the transpersonal domain of the psyche. There they can take the form of various past-life experiences or of appropriate archetypal figures and motifs that are thematically connected with the symptoms. It is also not uncommon to discover that the symptoms are related on a deeper level to elements drawn from the animal or botanical kingdoms. The symptoms of emotional and psychosomatic disorders are thus the result of a complicated interplay involving biographical, perinatal, and transpersonal factors.

It is interesting to speculate what factors might be responsible for the origination of COEX constellations and the relationship between their biographical layers, perinatal matrices, and transpersonal components. The similarity of some the postnatal traumas with each other and their resemblance to certain aspects of the perinatal dynamics might be attributed to chance. The life of some individuals might accidentally bring at different times victimizing situations resembling BPM II, violent or sexual traumas with elements of BPM III, episodes involving pain and choking, and other insults similar to perinatal distress. When a COEX system is established, it has a self-replicating propensity and can unconsciously drive the individual to recreate situations of a similar kind and thus add new layers to the memory constellation, as we saw earlier in the case of Peter.

Many people involved in deep self-exploration reported also some interesting insights concerning the relationship between past-life experiences and the birth trauma. The reliving of birth often coincides or alternates with various karmic episodes that share with it the emotional quality or certain physical sensations. This connection suggests the possibility that the way in which we experience our birth is determined by our karma. This applies not only to the general nature of our birth experience, but also to specific details.

For example, being hanged or strangled in a past-life situation can translate into suffocation during birth caused by the umbilical cord twisted around the neck. Pains inflicted by sharp objects in karmic dramas can project into pains caused by uterine contractions and pressures. The experience of being in a medieval dungeon, torture chamber of the Inquisition, or a concentration camp can fuse with the no exit experience of BPM II, and so on. Karmic patterns can also underlie and shape traumatic events in postnatal biography.

After this general introduction, I will now show how our psychological understanding of the most important forms of psychopathology changes in the light of the observations from holotropic states of consciousness. The following discussion will focus exclusively on the role of psychological factors in the formation of symptoms. It thus does not include the disorders that are clearly organic in nature and belong in the realm of medicine.

Anxiety and Phobias

Most psychiatrists would agree that anxiety, whether in its free-floating variety, in the form of phobias involving specific persons, animals, and situations, or as a factor underlying various other symptoms, represents one of the most common and basic psychiatric problems. Since in nature anxiety is a response to situations that endanger survival or body integrity, it makes sense that one of the primary sources of clinical anxiety is the trauma of birth, which is an actually or potentially life-threatening situation.

Freud himself entertained briefly the possibility that the frightening experience of birth might be the prototype for all future anxieties. However, he did not elaborate this idea any further and when his colleague and follower Otto Rank later published the book *The Trauma of Birth* (1929), in which he made birth the center of a new psychology, he was expelled from the psychoanalytic movement.

The work with holotropic states shows that the perinatal level of the unconscious plays a critical role in the genesis of phobias. The relation to the birth trauma is most evident in *claustrophobia,* the fear of closed and narrow places. It manifests in confined situations, such as elevators, subways, and small rooms without windows. Individuals who are claustrophobic are under the selective influence of a COEX system that is associated with the beginning of BPM II, when the uterine contractions begin to close in on the fetus.

The biographical factors contributing to this disorder involve memories of uncomfortable confining situations in postnatal life. From the transpersonal level, the elements that are most significant for this phobia are karmic memories involving imprisonment, entrapment, and suffocation. While the general tendency of claustrophobic patients is to avoid situations that intensify symptoms, therapeutic change requires full experience of discomfort associated with the underlying memories.

Agoraphobia, the fear of open places or of the transition from an enclosed space to a wide open one, seems at first sight to be the opposite of claustrophobia. In actuality, agoraphobic patients are typically also claustrophobic, but the transition from an enclosed place to an open space has a stronger charge for them than the stay in the enclosed space itself. On the perinatal level, agoraphobia is associated with the very final stage of BPM III, when the sudden release after many hours of extreme confinement is accompanied by fear of losing all boundaries, being blown apart, and ceasing to exist. The experience of ego death and psychospiritual rebirth tends to bring significant relief from this condition.

Patients suffering from *thanatophobia,* or pathological fear of death, experience episodes of vital anxiety, which they interpret as the onset of a life-threatening heart attack, stroke, or suffocation. This phobia has its deep roots in the extreme physical discomfort and sense of impending catastrophe associated with the trauma of birth. The COEX systems involved are typically related to situations that endanger life, such as operations, diseases, and injuries, particularly those that interfere with breathing. Radical resolution of thanatophobia requires conscious reliving of the different layers of the underlying COEX system and experiential confrontation with death.

Nosophobia, pathological fear of having or contracting a disease, is closely related to thanatophobia and also to hypochondriasis, an unsubstantiated delusional conviction of already having a serious illness. Patients suffering from this disorder have a variety of strange body sensations that they cannot account for and they tend to interpret them in terms of actual somatic pathology. These symptoms involve pains, pressures, and cramps in different parts of the body, nausea, strange energy flows, paraesthesias, and other forms of unusual phenomena. They can also show signs of dysfunction of various organs, such as breathing difficulties, dyspepsia, nausea and vomiting, constipation and diarrhea, muscular tremors, general malaise, weakness, and fatigue.

Repeated medical examinations typically fail to detect any organic disorder that would explain the subjective complaints. The reason for this is the fact that the disturbing sensations and emotions are not related to a present physiological process, but to memories of past physical traumas. Patients with these problems often repeatedly demand various clinical and laboratory tests and can become a real nuisance in doctors' offices and hospitals. Many of them end up in the care of psychiatrists, where they often do not receive the compassionate acceptance they deserve.

Physical complaints that cannot be justified by appropriate laboratory findings are often dismissed as products of the clients' imagination. Nothing could be farther from truth. Despite the negative medical findings, the physical complaints of these patients are very real. However, they do not reflect any current medical problem but, rather, are caused by surfacing memories of serious physiological difficulties from the past. Their sources are various diseases, operations, injuries, and particularly the trauma of birth.

Three distinct varieties of nosophobia deserve special attention: cancerophobia, pathological fear of developing or having cancer, bacillophobia, fear of microorganisms and infection, and mysophobia, fear of dirt and contamination. All these problems have deep perinatal roots, although their specific forms are biographically codetermined. In *cancerophobia,* the important element is the similarity between cancer and pregnancy. It is well known from the psychonalytical literature that malignant growth of tumors is unconsciously identified with embryonic development. This similarity goes beyond the most obvious superficial parallel, a rapidly growing foreign object inside one's body. It can be actually supported by anatomical, physiological, and biochemical data. In many respects, the cancer cells actually resemble undifferentiated cells from early stages of embryonal development.

In *bacillophobia* and *mysophobia,* the pathological fear focuses on biological material, body odors, and uncleanness. The biographical determinants of these disorders usually involve memories from the time of toilet training, but their roots reach deeper, to the scatological aspect of the perinatal process. The key to the understanding of these phobias is the connection that exists within BPM III between death, aggression, sexual excitement, and various forms of biological material.

Patients suffering from these disorders are not only afraid that they themselves might get biologically contaminated, but they are also frequently preoccupied with the possibility of infecting others. Their fear of biological materials is thus closely associated with aggression that is oriented both inward and outward, which is precisely the situation characteristic of the final stages of birth.

On a more superficial level, the fear of infection and bacterial growth is also unconsciously related to sperm and conception and, thereby, again to pregnancy and birth. The most important COEX systems related to the above phobias involve relevant memories from the anal-sadistic stage of libidinal development and conflicts around toilet training and cleanliness. Additional biographical material is represented by memories that depict sex and pregnancy as dirty and dangerous. Like all emotional disorders, these phobias often have also transpersonal components.

Deep entanglement and identification with biological contaminants are also at the basis of a particular kind of low self-esteem that involves self-degradation and a sense of disgust with oneself, referred to colloquially as "shitty self-esteem." It is frequently associated with behaviors aimed at improving one's exterior that connect this problem with obsessive-compulsive neuroses. These involve rituals that, on a deeper level, represent an effort to avoid or neutralize the biological contamination. The most obvious of these rituals is *compulsive washing of hands or other parts of the body*. It can be so excessive that it results in serious wounding of the skin and bleeding.

A woman whose memory of perinatal events is close to the surface can suffer from a *phobia of pregnancy and delivery*. Being in touch with the memory of the birth agony makes it difficult for a woman to accept her femininity and her reproductive role, because motherhood means for her inflicting pain and suffering. The idea of becoming pregnant and having to face the ordeal of delivery can under these circumstances be associated with paralyzing terror.

A *phobia of mothering*, an emotionally tormenting condition that usually begins shortly after the child is born, is not a pure phobia, but involves obsessive-compulsive elements. It is a combination of violent impulses against the child with panic fear of actually hurting it. This is typically associated with overprotective behavior and unreasonable concerns that something might happen to the baby. Whatever the biographical determinants of this problem might be, the deeper source can be traced, in the last analysis, to the delivery of that child. This reflects the fact that the passive and active aspects of childbirth are intimately connected in the unconscious.

The states of biological symbiotic union between the mother and the child represent states of experiential unity. Women reliving their own birth typically experience themselves, simultaneously or alternately, as delivering. Similarly, memories of being a fetus in the womb are characteristically associated with an experience of being pregnant, and situations of being nursed, with those of nursing. The deep roots of the phobia of mothering lie in the first clinical stage of delivery (BPM II) when the mother and the child are in a state of biological antagonism, inflicting pain on each other and exchanging enormous amounts of destructive energy.

The experience of this situation tends to activate the mother's memory of her own birth, unleash the aggressive potential associated with it, and direct it toward the child. The fact that delivering a child opens experiential access to perinatal dynamics represents an important therapeutic opportunity. This is a very good time for women who just have delivered their babies to do some unusually deep psychological work.

On the negative side, the activation of the mother's perinatal unconscious can result in postpartum depressions, neuroses, or even psychoses. Postpartum psychopathology is usually explained by vague references to hormonal changes. This does not make much sense considering that women's response to delivery covers a very broad range from ecstasy to psychosis, while the hormonal changes follow a fairly standard pattern. In my experience, the perinatal memories play a crucial role in the phobias of pregnancy and mothering, as well as postpartum psychopathology. Experiential work on the trauma of birth and the early postnatal period seems to be a method of choice in these disorders.

Phobia of traveling by train and subway is based, among others, on certain similarities between the experience of birth and travel in these means of transportation. The most important common denominators of the two situations are the sense of entrapment and the experience of enormous forces and energies in motion without any control over the process. Additional elements are passing through tunnels and underground passages and the encounter with darkness. In the time of the old-fashioned steam engine, the elements of fire, the pressure of the steam, and the noisy siren, conveying a sense of emergency, seemed to be contributing factors. For these situations to trigger the phobia, the perinatal memories must be easily available to consciousness, due to their intensity and to the bridging effect of postnatal layers of the underlying COEX.

A phobia that is closely related to the above is *fear of traveling by airplanes.* It shares with the other situations the discomfort concerning entrapment, the fear of the powerful energy involved, and the inability to have any influence on the course of events. The lack of control seems to be an element of great importance in the phobias involving movement. This can be illustrated by *the phobia of traveling by car,* which is a means of transportation in which we can easily play both the role of the passenger and that of the driver. This phobia typically manifests only when we are passively driven and not when we are in the driver's seat and can deliberately change or stop the motion.

It is interesting to mention in this connection that *seasickness* and *airsickness* are also often related to perinatal dynamics and tend to disappear after the individual has completed the death-rebirth process. The essential element here seems to be the willingness to give up the need to be in control and the ability to surrender to the flow of events, no matter what they bring. Difficulties arise when the individual tries to impose his or her control on processes that have their own dynamic momentum. Excessive need for control of the situation is characteristic for individuals who are under a strong influence of BPM III and related COEX systems, while the capacity to surrender to the flow of events shows strong connection with positive aspects of BPM I and BPM IV.

Acrophobia, or *the fear of heights,* is not really a pure phobia. It is always associated with the compulsion to jump down or throw oneself from a high place—a tower, window, cliff, or bridge. The sense of falling with a simultaneous fear of destruction is a typical manifestation of the final stages of BPM III. The origin of this association is not clear, but it might involve a phylogenetic component. Some animals deliver standing and women in some native cultures deliver suspended on branches, squatting, or on all four. Another possibility is that this liaison reflects the first encounter with the phenomenon of gravity, including the possibility of being dropped or even an actual memory of such an event.

In any case, it is very common that people who in holotropic states are under the influence of this matrix have experiences of falling, acrobatic diving, or parachuting. A compulsive interest in sports and other activities that involve falling (parachuting, bungie-cord jumping, movie stunts, acrobatic flying) seems to reflect the need to exteriorize the feelings of impending disaster in situations that allow a certain degree of control (bungie-cord, string of a parachute) or involve some other forms of safeguards (termination of the fall in water). The COEX systems responsible for the manifestation of this particular facet of the birth trauma include childhood memories of being playfully tossed in the air by adults and accidents involving falling.

Because of the somewhat enigmatic relationship between the phobia of heights, experience of falling, and the final stages of birth, I will make an exception and illustrate this particular phobia with a specific example. It involves Ralph, a German emigrant to Canada, who many years ago attended our holotropic breathwork workshop in British Columbia. Case histories related to other types of phobias can be found in my other publications.

> In his holotropic session, Ralph experienced a powerful COEX system that he felt was the cause of his serious phobia of heights. The most superficial layer of this COEX contained a memory from prewar Germany. This

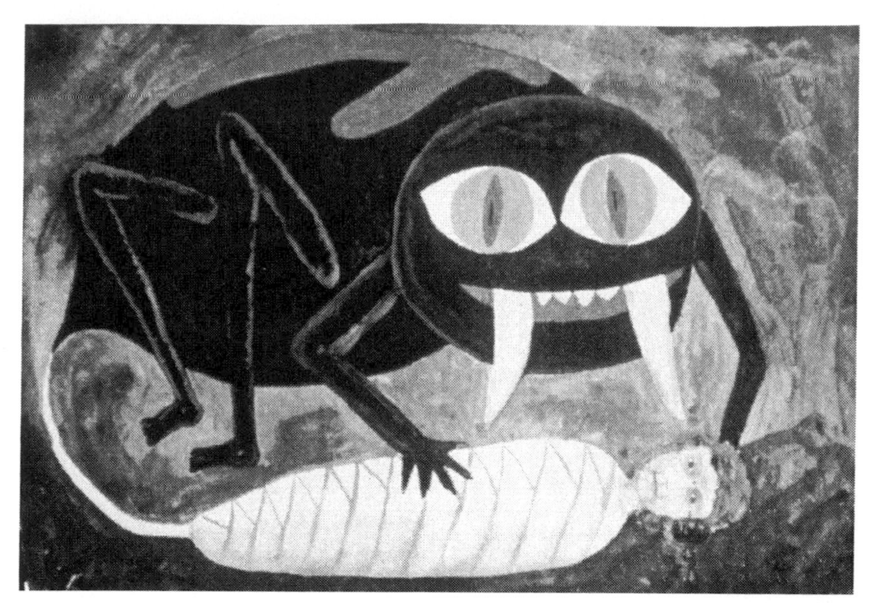

A series of paintings from the holotropic breathwork training of Jarina Moss, a young woman suffering from phobia of heights. They illustrate the psychodynamic connection that exists between this type of phobia and the experience of the final stage of birth.

Above: Experience from a session dominated by BPM II, in which Jarina is shown as a helpless victim of the Devouring Mother in the form of a giant tarantula.

Page 84. This painting shows Jarina in a later stage of her process, when she escaped what previously seemed to be an absolutely hopeless situation. She is now approaching the divine light (BPM III-IV), but the light is deep below her in an abyss and she has to face a fall to reach it.

Page 85. At this point, Jarina encounters a traumatic memory from infancy. She was born in Prague, Czechoslovakia, during WW2. Prague was liberated by the Red Army and immediately after the war, Soviet soldiers lived briefly in many private homes, including the house of Jarina's family. The picture shows the soldiers playing with Jarina insensitively by throwing her high into the air. This experience turned out to be part of a COEX underlying her phobia of heights.

Page 86. The image of the angel represents the promise of transcendence. However, reaching it requires letting go and the ego death. This is associated with great fear and Jarina is still holding on.

Page 87. The last picture of the series shows what happened when she finally let go. The old personality structure has split and disintegrated. Out of it emerges a new self (or Self) that has a spiritual connection. The title that Jarina chose for this picture is: LIBERATION.

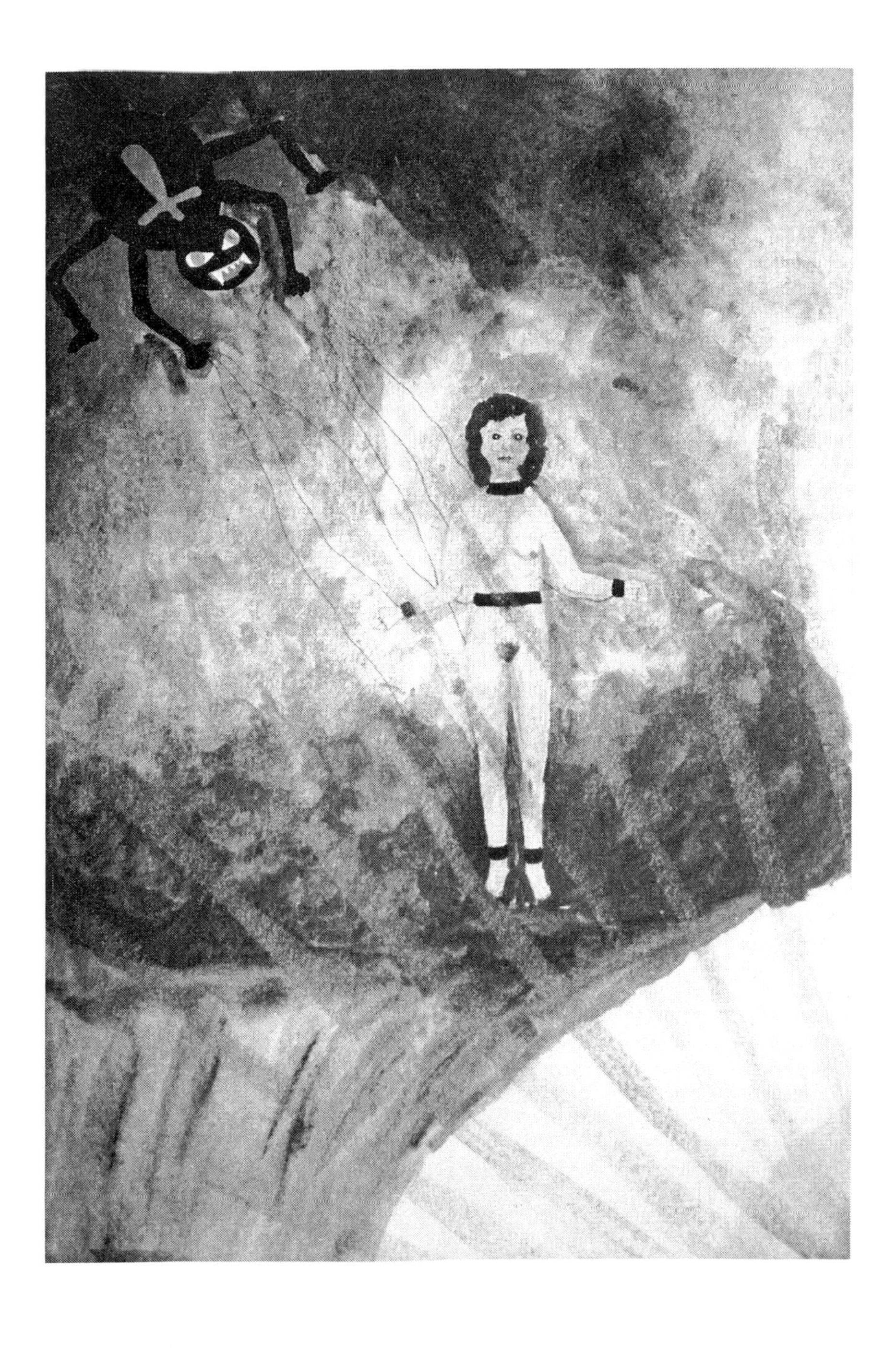

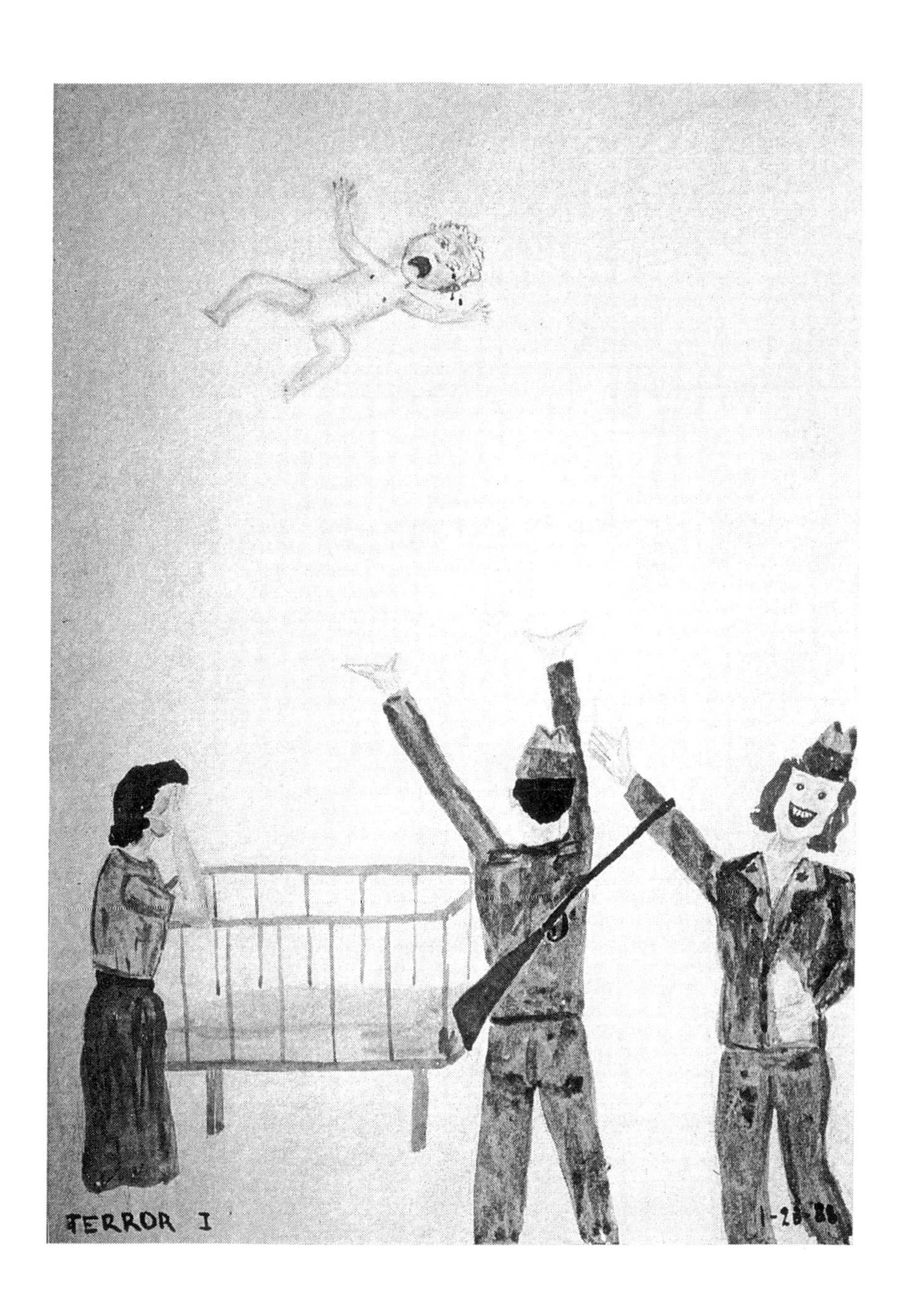
TERROR I

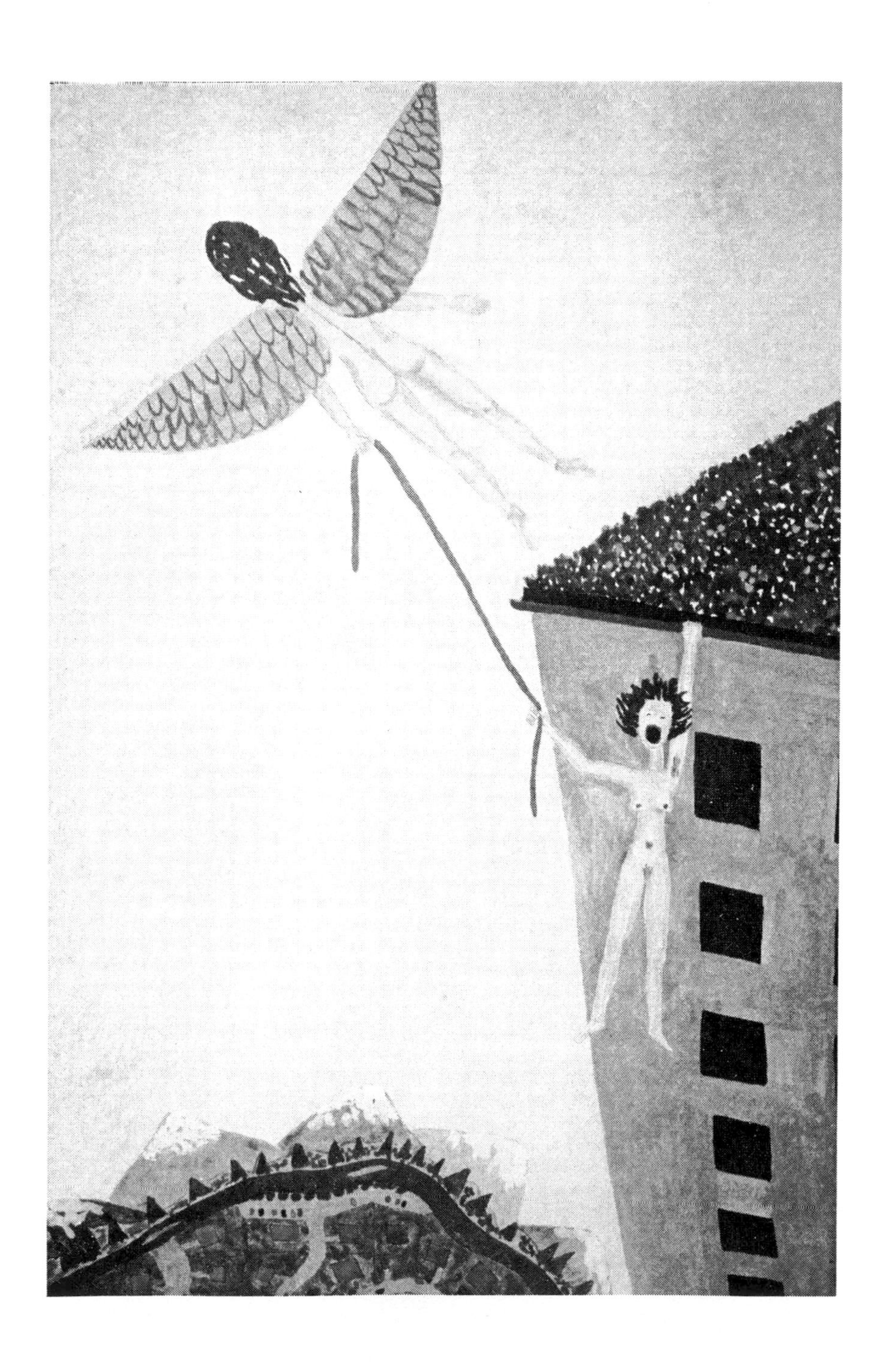

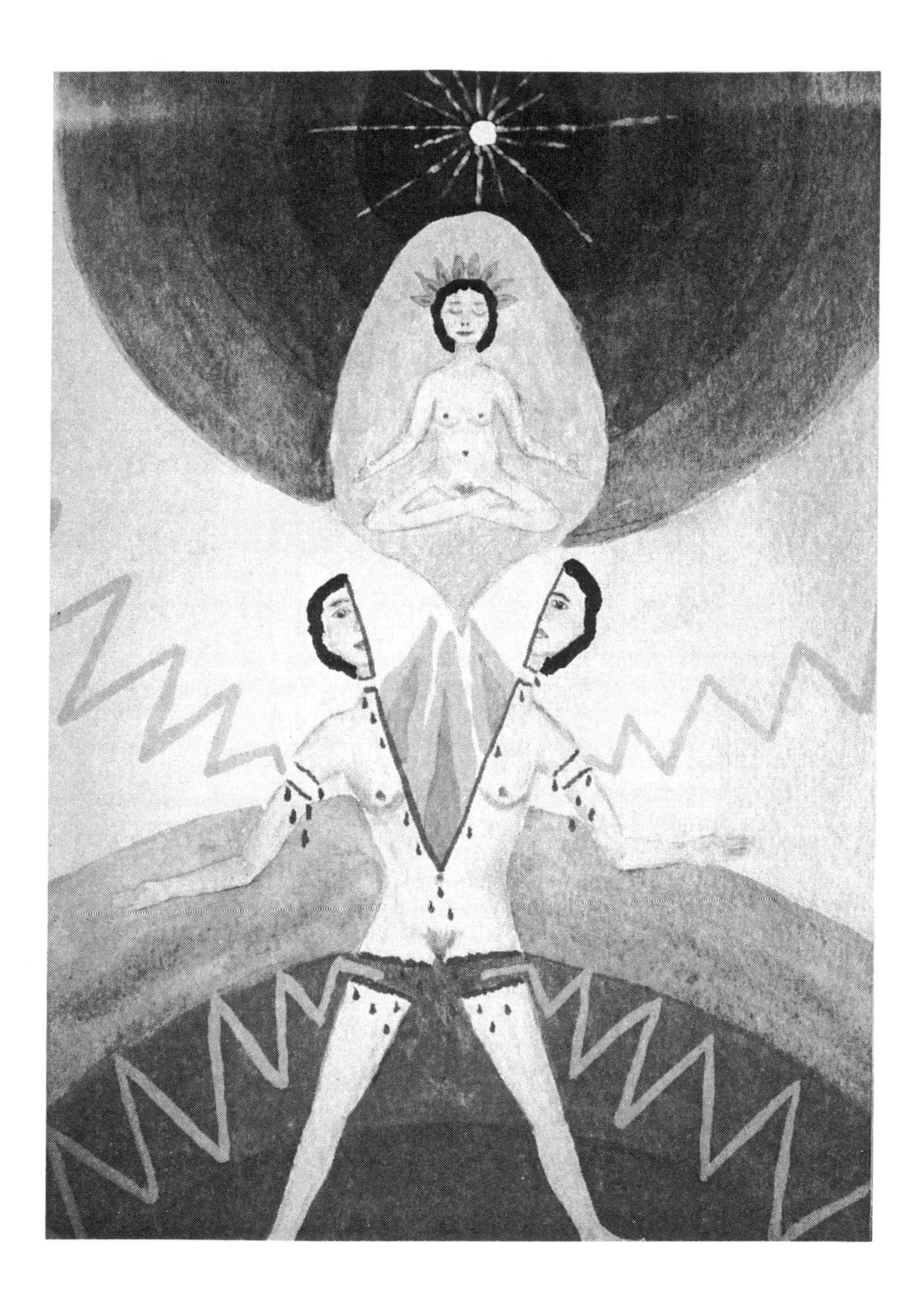

was the time of a hectic military build-up and of equally hectic preparations for the Olympic Games in Berlin, in which Hitler intended to demonstrate the superiority of the Nordic race.

Since the victory in the Olympics was for Hitler a matter of extreme political importance, many talented athletes were assigned to special camps for rigorous training. This was an alternative of being drafted into the Wehrmacht, the infamous German army. Ralph, a pacifist who hated the military, was selected for one of these camps, which was for him a welcome opportunity to avoid the draft.

The training involved a variety of sport disciplines and was incredibly competitive; all the performances were graded and those with least points were sent to the army. Ralph was lagging behind and had the last opportunity to improve his standing. The stakes and his motivation to succeed were very high, but the challenge was truly formidable. The task he was supposed to perform was something he had never done in his life, a head-first dive into a swimming pool from a sixty-foot-high tower.

The biographical layer of his COEX system consisted of reliving the enormous ambivalence and fear associated with the dive, as well as the sensations of the falling itself. The deeper layer of the same COEX that immediately followed this experience was the reliving of Ralph's struggle in the final stage of birth with all the emotions and physical sensations involved. The process then continued into what Ralph concluded must have been a past-life experience.

He became an adolescent boy in a native culture, who was involved with a group of peers in a dangerous rite of passage. One after the other, they climbed to the top of a tower made of wooden poles tied together with flexible vegetable tendrils. Once there, they attached to their ankles the end of a long liana and fixed its other end to the edge of the platform at the top of the tower. It was a status symbol and matter of great pride to have the longest liana and not to get killed.

When he experienced the feelings associated with the jump in this rite of passage, he realized that they were very similar both to the feelings associated with his dive in the Olympic camp and to those he encountered in the final stages of birth. All three situations were clearly integral parts of the same COEX.

Zoophobia, the fear of various animals, can involve many different forms of life, both large and dangerous beasts and small and harmless creatures. It is essentially unrelated to the actual danger that a particular animal represents for humans. In classical analysis, the feared animal was seen as a symbolic representation of the castrating father or the bad mother and always had a sexual connotation. The work with holotropic states has shown that such a biographical interpretation of zoophobias is inadequate and that these disorders have significant perinatal and transpersonal roots.

If the object of the phobia is a large animal, the most important elements seem to be either the theme of being swallowed and incorporated (wolf) or the relation to pregnancy and nursing (cow). It was mentioned earlier that the archetypal symbolism of the onset of BPM II is the experience of being swallowed and incorporated. This perinatal fear of engulfment can be projected on large animals, particularly predators.

In addition, certain animals have a special symbolic association with the birth process. Thus images of gigantic tarantulas frequently appear in the initial phase of BPM II as symbols of the devouring Feminine. This seems to reflect the fact that spiders catch free-flying insects in their webs, immobilize them, enwrap them, and kill them. It is not difficult to see a deep similarity between this sequence of events and the experiences of the child during biological delivery. This connection seems to be essential for the development of *arachnophobia.*

Another zoophobia that has an important perinatal component is *ophiophobia* or *serpentophobia, the fear of snakes.* Images of snakes that, on a more superficial level, have a phallic connotation are common symbols representing the birth agony and thus the destructive and devouring feminine. Poisonous vipers usually represent the threat of imminent death, while large boa constrictors symbolize the crushing and strangulation involved in birth. The fact that large constrictor snakes swallow their prey and appear pregnant further reinforces the perinatal connotation.

The serpentine symbolism typically extends deep into the transpersonal realm, where it can have many different culture-specific meanings (the snake from the Garden of Eden, Kundalini, the snake Muchalinda protecting the Buddha, Vishnu's Ananta, the Plumed Serpent Quetzalcoatl, the Rainbow Serpent of the Australian Aborigenes, and many others).

Phobias of small insects can frequently be traced to the dynamics of perinatal matrices. Thus bees seem to be related to reproduction and pregnancy because of their role in the transfer of pollen and fertilization of plants, as well as their capacity to cause swelling. Flies, as a result of their affinity for excrement and their propensity to spread infection, are associated with the scatological aspect of birth. As has already been pointed out, this has a close relation to phobias of dirt and microorganisms and the compulsive washing of hands.

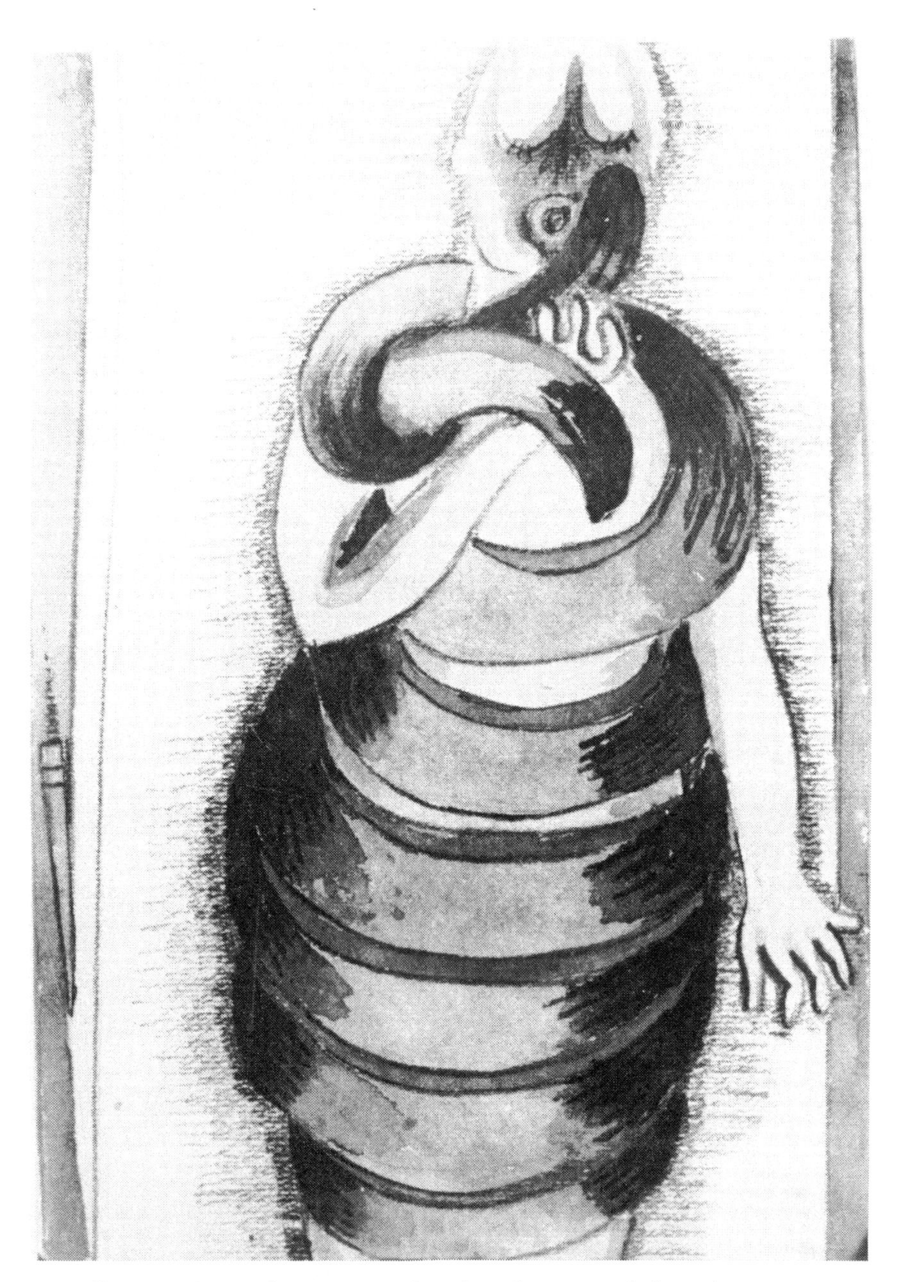

Freud's assumption that images of snakes always symbolize the penis was a gross oversimplification. Snakes also have a deep connection to the perinatal process, as indicated by these two paintings from therapeutic LSD sessions. Above: Uterine contractions experienced as an attack by a boa constrictor type of snake. Pythons swallow their prey without dismembering it,

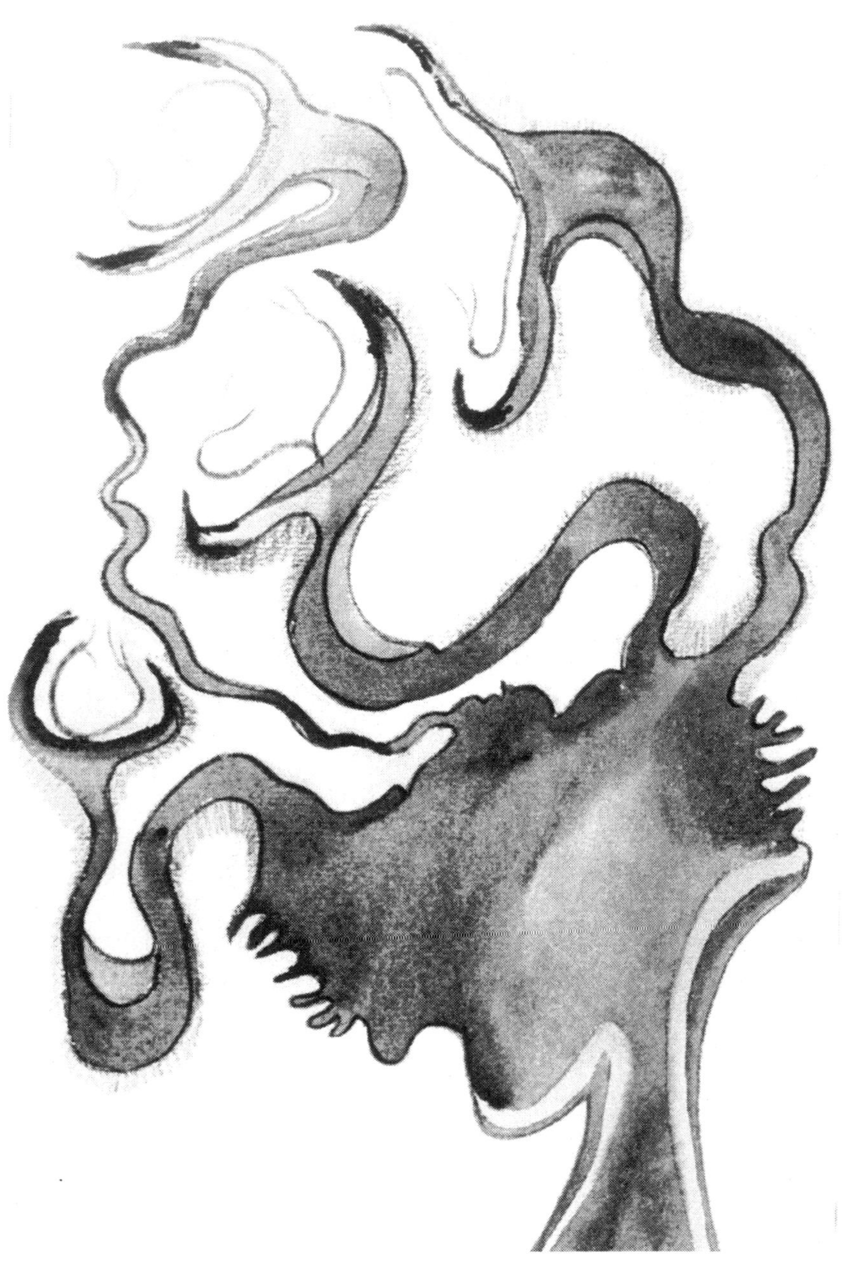

which makes them look pregnant. They also twist their bodies around the victims and crush. Both these characteristics make them ideal perinatal symbols. Above: The inside of the uterus experienced as a dangerous snake pit. Vipers symbolize imminence of death and because of their molting also rebirth.

Keraunophobia, or *pathological fear of thunderstorms,* is psychodynamically related to the transition between BPM III and BPM IV and thus to the ego death. Lightening represents an energetic connection between heaven and earth and electricity is a physical expression of divine energy. For this reason, an electric storm symbolizes the contact with the divine light that occurs at the culmination point of the death-rebirth process. During my work in Prague, I observed on several occasions patients who in their psychedelic sessions consciously relived electroshocks that had been administered to them earlier in their lives. They had these experiences at the time when their process of psychospiritual transformation reached the point of the ego death. The most famous person suffering from keraunophobia was Ludwig van Beethoven. He succeeded in confronting the subject of his fear when he included a magnificent musical representation of a thunderstorm in his Pastoral Symphony.

Pyrophobia, pathological fear of fire, also has deep psychological roots in the transition from BPM III to BPM IV. When we discussed the phenomenology of the perinatal matrices, we saw that individuals approaching the ego death typically have visions of fire. They also often experience that their body is burning and that they are passing through purifying flames. The motif of fire and purgatory is thus an important concomitant of the final stage of psychospiritual transformation. When this aspect of the unconscious dynamics reaches the threshold of consciousness, the liaison between the experience of fire and the impending ego death gives rise to pyrophobia.

In the individuals who are able to intuit the positive potential of this process, the fact that its final outcome would be psychospiritual rebirth, the effect can be exactly the opposite. They have the feeling that something fantastic would happen to them if they could experience the destructive force of fire. This expectation can be so strong that it results in an irresistible urge to actually start a fire. The observation of the resulting conflagration brings only transient excitement and tends to be disappointing. However, the feeling that the experience of fire should bring a phenomenal liberation is so convincing that these people try again and become arsonists. Pyrophobia is thus paradoxically closely related to pyromania.

Hydrophobia, pathological fear of water, also typically has a strong perinatal component. This reflects the fact that water plays an important role in connection to childbirth. If the pregnancy and delivery have a normal course, this connection is very positive. In that case, water represents for the child the comfort of the amniotic existence or of the postnatal period, when receiving a bath indicates that the danger of birth is over. However, various prenatal crises, inhalation of the amniotic fluid during birth, or postnatal bathing accidents can give water a distinctly negative charge. The COEX systems underlying hydrophobia also typically contain biographical elements (traumatic experiences with water in infancy and childhood) and transpersonal elements (shipwreck, flood, or drowning in a previous incarnation).

Conversion Hysteria

This psychoneurosis was much more prevalent in Freud's times than it is today and it played an important role in the history and development of psychoanalysis. Several of Freud's patients and many patients of his followers belonged to this diagnostic category. *Conversion hysteria* has rich and colorful symptomatology and is, according to the psychoanalytic psychogenetic scheme, closely related to the group of phobias, or anxiety hysteria.

This means that the major fixation for this disorder is on the phallic stage of libidinal development and that the psychosexual trauma which underlies it occurred at the time when the child was under a strong influence of the Electra or Oedipus complex. Of the several defense mechanisms involved in psychogenesis of conversion hysteria, the most characteristic one is conversion, which gave this form of hysteria its name. This term refers to symbolic transformation of unconscious conflicts and instinctual impulses into physical symptoms.

Examples of hysterical affliction of motor functions are *paralysis of arms or legs, loss of speech (aphonia),* and *vomiting.* Conversion focusing on sensory organs and functions can result in *temporary blindness, deafness,* or *psychogenic anesthesia.* Conversion hysteria can also produce a combination of symptoms that convincingly imitate pregnancy. This *false pregnancy* or *pseudokyesis* involves amenorrhea and a sizable extension of the abdominal cavity caused, at least partly, by retention of gases in the intestines. *Religious stigmata* simulating the wounds of Christ have also often been interpreted as hysterical conversions.

Freud suggested that, in hysterical conversions, repressed sexual thoughts and impulses find their vicarious expression in changes of physical functions and the affected organ is "sexualized," that is, it becomes a symbolic substitute for genitals. For example, the hyperemia and swelling of various organs might symbolize erection, or abnormal feelings in these organs might imitate genital sensations. In some instances, the emerging memory of the entire traumatic situation can be substituted by some physical sensations the individual was experiencing at that time.

The most complex and distinctive manifestation of hysteria is a specific form of psychosomatic attack, referred to as *major hysterical spell.* It is a condition associated with alternating crying and laughter, theatrical erotic movements, and extreme backward arching of the body (*arc de cercle*). According to Freud, hysterical spells are pantomimic expressions of memories of forgotten events from childhood and of fantasy stories constructed around these events. These spells represent disguised sexual themes related to the Oedipus and Electra complex and their derivatives. Freud pointed out that the behavior during hysterical spells clearly betrays their sexual nature. He compared the loss of consciousness at the height of the attack to the momentary loss of consciousness during sexual orgasm.

Observations from holotropic states show that conversion hysteria, in addition to the biographical determinants, has also significant perinatal and transpersonal roots. Underlying conversion phenomena, in general, and hysterical spells, in particular, are powerful bioenergetic blockages and conflicting innervations related to the dynamics of BPM III. The behavior of people experiencing the final stages of this perinatal matrix, especially the characteristic deflection of the head and extreme backward arching, often resembles a hysterical spell.

The nature and timing of the biographical material involved in the psychogenesis of conversion hysteria are in basic agreement with the Freudian theory. Experiential work typically reveals psychosexual traumas from the period of childhood when the patient reached the phallic stage of development and was under the influence of the Oedipus or Electra complex. The movements of the hysterical spell can be shown to represent, in addition to the mentioned perinatal elements, also symbolic allusions to certain specific aspects of the underlying childhood trauma.

The sexual content of the traumatic memories associated with conversion hysteria explains why they are part of a COEX system that also includes the sexual facet of BPM III. If we are not familiar with the fact that the memory of birth has a strong sexual element, it is easy to overlook the perinatal contribution to the genesis of conversion hysteria and attribute this disorder entirely to postnatal influences. It is interesting to mention in this context Freud's own observation and admission that the leading themes underlying hysterical spells often were not sexual seduction or intercourse, but pregnancy or childbirth.

The involvement of BPM III in the psychogenesis of conversion hysteria explains many important aspects of this disorder that have been often mentioned, but never adequately explained, in psychoanalytic literature. It is, above all, the fact that the analysis of hysterical symptoms reveals not only their connection to libidinal impulses and sexual orgasm, but also to "erection" generalized to the entire body (birth orgasm) and quite explicitly to childbirth and pregnancy. The same is true for strange links that exist in conversion hysteria between sexuality, aggression, and death.

The psychodynamic basis of conversion hysteria is quite similar to that of agitated depression. This becomes evident when we look at the fullest expression of this disorder, major hysterical spell. In general, agitated depression is a more serious disorder than conversion hysteria and it manifests in a much purer form the content and dynamics of BPM III. Observation of the facial expression and behavior of a patient with agitated depression leaves no doubt that there are reasons for grave concern. The high incidence of suicide and even suicide combined with murder found in these patients supports this impression.

A major hysterical spell shows a superficial resemblance to agitated depression. However, the overall picture is obviously far less severe and it lacks the depth of despair. It appears stylized and contrived and has definite theatrical features with unmistakable sexual overtones. In general, a hysterical attack has many basic characteristics of BPM III—excessive tension, psychomotor excitement and agitation, a mixture of depression and aggression, loud screaming, disturbances of breathing, and dramatic arching. However, the experiential template appears here in a considerably more mitigated form than in agitated depression and is substantially modified and colored by later traumatic events.

The dynamic connection between conversion hysteria, agitated depression, and BPM III becomes very evident in the course of deep experiential therapy. At first, the holotropic states tend to trigger or amplify hysterical symptoms and the client discovers their source in specific psychosexual traumas from childhood. Later sessions typically increasingly resemble agitated depression and eventually reveal the underlying elements of BPM III. The reliving of birth and connection to BPM IV then brings alleviation, or even disappearance of the symptoms. The deepest roots of hysterical conversions can reach to the transpersonal level and take the form of karmic memories or archetypal motifs.

Hysterical paralysis of the hands and arms, inability to stand (*abasia*), loss of speech (*aphonia*) and other conversion symptoms also have strong perinatal components. These conditions are not caused by lack of motor impulses, but by a dynamic conflict of antagonistic motor impulses that cancel each other. The source of this situation is the painful and stressful experience during childbirth to which the organism of the child responds by excessive chaotic generation of neuronal impulses for which there is no adequate discharge.

A similar interpretation of hysterical conversion symptoms was first suggested by Otto Rank, in his pioneering book, *The Trauma of Birth* (1929). While Freud saw conversions as expressions of a psychological conflict expressed in body language, Rank believed that their real basis was physiological, reflecting the original situation that existed during birth. The problem for Freud was how a primarily psychological problem could be translated into a physical symptom. Rank had to face the opposite problem—to explain how a primarily somatic phenomenon could acquire, through a secondary elaboration, psychological content and symbolic meaning.

Some serious manifestations of hysteria that border on psychosis, such as *psychogenic stupor, uncontrolled daydreaming,* and *mistaking fantasy for reality (pseudologia fantastica),* seem to be dynamically related to BPM I. They reflect a deep need to reinstitute the blissful emotional condition characteristic of undisturbed intrauterine existence and the symbiotic union with the mother. While the component of emotional and physical satisfaction involved in these states can easily be detected as surrogates of the desired good womb and good breast situation, the concrete content of daydreaming and fantasies uses themes and elements related to the individual's childhood, adolescence, and adult life.

Obsessive-Compulsive Neurosis

Patients suffering from *obsessive-compulsive disorders* are tormented by intrusive irrational thoughts that they cannot get rid of and they feel compelled to perform certain absurd and meaningless repetitive rituals. If they refuse to comply with these strange urges, they are overwhelmed by free-floating anxiety. There is a general agreement in psychoanalytical literature that conflicts related to homosexuality, aggression, and biological material form the psychodynamic basis of this disorder, together with an inhibition of genitality and a strong emphasis on pregenital drives, particularly those that are anal in nature. These aspects of obsessive-compulsive neurosis point to a strong perinatal component in this disorder, particularly to the scatological aspect of BPM III.

Another characteristic feature of this neurosis is strong ambivalence and conflict concerning religion and God. Many obsessive-compulsive patients live in constant severe conflict about God and religious faith and experience strong rebellious and blasphemous thoughts, feelings, and impulses. For example, they associate the image of God with masturbation or defecation or have an irresistible temptation to laugh aloud, scream obscenities, and pass gas in church or at a funeral. This alternates with desperate tendencies to repent, expiate, and punish themselves to undo their transgressions and sins.

As we saw earlier in the discussion of the phenomenology of perinatal matrices, this close association of sexual and aggressive impulses with the numinous and divine element is characteristic for the transition between BPM III and BPM IV. Similarly, a strong conflict between the revolt against an overwhelming force and a wish to surrender to it is characteristic of the final stages of the death-rebirth process. In holotropic states, this unrelenting authoritative force can be experienced in an archetypal figurative form.

We can envision it as a strict, punishing, and cruel God comparable to Yahweh of the Old Testament, or even a fierce pre-Columbian deity demanding bloody sacrifice. The biological correlate of this punishing deity is the restricting influence of the birth canal that inflicts extreme, life-threatening suffering on the individual and, in turn, prevents any external expression of the instinctual energies of sexual and aggressive nature activated by the ordeal of biological birth.

The restricting force of the birth canal represents the biological basis for the part of the superego that Freud called "savage." It is a primitive and barbaric element of the psyche that can drive an individual to self-mutilation or even bloody suicide. Freud saw this part of the superego as being instinctual in nature and thus a derivative of the id. Postnatally, the restrictive and coercive influence takes far more subtle forms of injunctions and prohibitions coming from parental authorities, penal institutions, and religious commandments. Yet another aspect of the superego, Freud's "ideal ego," reflects our tendency to identify with and emulate the person whom we admire.

An important perinatal source of obsessive-compulsive neurosis is the unpleasant or even life-threatening encounter with various forms of biological material in the final stages of birth. The COEX systems that are psychogenetically associated with this disorder involve traumatic experiences related to the anal zone and to biological material, such as a history of strict toilet training, painful enemas, anal rape, and gastrointestinal diseases. Another important category of related biographical material includes memories of various situations representing a threat to genital organization. Quite regularly, transpersonal elements with similar themes play an important role in the genesis of this difficult condition.

Depression, Mania, and Suicidal Behavior

In psychoanalysis, *depression* and *mania* are seen as disorders that are related to serious problems in the active (sadistic or cannibalistic) oral period, such as interference with nursing, emotional rejection and deprivation, and difficulties in the early mother-child relation. Suicidal tendencies are then interpreted as acts of hostility against the introjected object, the image of the "bad mother," primarily her breast. In view of the observations from holotropic states, this picture has to be revised and substantially extended. In its present form, it is implausible and unconvincing and does not explain some very fundamental clinical observations regarding depressions.

For example, why do we have two radically different forms of depression, the inhibited and the agitated variety? Why are depressed people typically bioenergetically blocked, as exemplified by high incidence of headaches, pressure on the chest, psychosomatic pains, and retention of water? Why are they physiologically inhibited and show loss of appetite, gastrointestinal dysfunction, constipation, and amenorrhea? Why do individuals who are depressed, including those who have an inhibited depression, show high levels of biochemical stress? Why do they feel hopeless and refer to themselves often as "feeling stuck"?

These questions cannot be answered by psychotherapeutic schools that are conceptually limited to postnatal biography and the Freudian individual unconscious. Even less successful in this regard are theories that try to explain depressive disorders simply as results of chemical aberrations in the organism. It is highly unlikely that a chemical change could, in and of itself, account for the complexity of the clinical picture of depression, including its close link with mania and suicide. This situation changes dramatically once we realize that these disorders have significant perinatal and transpersonal components. We start seeing the problems related to depression in an entirely new light and many of the manifestations of depression suddenly appear logical.

Inhibited depressions have typically important roots in the second perinatal matrix. The phenomenology of the sessions governed by BPM II, as well as the periods immediately following poorly resolved experiences dominated by this matrix, show all the essential features of deep depression. The person who is under the influence of BPM II, experiences agonizing mental and emotional pain—hopelessness, despair, overwhelming feelings of guilt, and a sense of inadequacy. He or she feels deep anxiety, lack of initiative, loss of interest in anything, and an inability to enjoy existence. In this state, life appears to be utterly meaningless, emotionally empty, and absurd.

The world and one's own life are seen as if through a negative stencil, with selective awareness of the painful, bad, and tragic aspects of life and blindness for anything positive. This situation appears to be utterly unbearable, inescapable, and hopeless. Sometimes this is accompanied by the loss of the ability to see colors; when that happens, the entire world is perceived as a black and white film. In spite of the extreme suffering involved, this condition is not associated with crying or any other dramatic external manifestations; it is characterized by a general motor inhibition.

As I mentioned earlier, inhibited depression is associated with bioenergetic blockages in various parts of the body and severe inhibition of major physiological functions. Typical physical concomitants of this form of depression are feelings of oppression, constriction and confinement, a sense of suffocation, tensions and pressures in different parts of the body, and headaches. Very common is also retention of water and urine, constipation, cardiac distress, loss of interest in food and sex, and a tendency to hypochondriacal interpretation of various physical symptoms.

All these symptoms are consistent with the understanding of this type of depression as a manifestation of BPM II. This is further supported by paradoxical biochemical findings. People suffering from inhibited depression typically show a high degree of stress, as indicated by the elevation of catecholamines and steroid hormones in the blood and urine. This biochemical picture fits well the fact that BPM II represents a highly stressful inner situation with no possibility of external action or manifestation ("sitting on the outside, running on the inside").

The theory of psychoanalysis links depression to early oral problems and emotional deprivation. Although this connection is obviously correct, it does not account for important aspects of depression—the sense of being stuck, hopelessness with feelings of no exit, and bioenergetic blockage, as well as the physical manifestations, including the biochemical findings. The present model shows the Freudian explanation as essentially correct but partial. While the COEX systems associated with inhibited depression include biographical elements emphasized by psychoanalysis, a fuller and more comprehensive understanding has to include the dynamics of BPM II.

The early deprivation and oral frustration has much in common with BPM II and the inclusion of both of these situations in the same COEX system reflects deep experiential logic. BPM II involves interruption of the symbiotic connection between the fetus and the maternal organism, which is caused by uterine contractions and the resulting compression of the arteries. This severing and loss of biologically and emotionally meaningful contact with the mother terminates the supply of oxygen, nourishment, and warmth to the fetus. Additional consequences of the uterine contractions are temporary accumulation of toxic products in the body of the fetus and exposure to an unpleasant and potentially dangerous situation.

It thus makes good sense that the typical constituents of COEX systems dynamically related to inhibited depression (and to BPM II) involve separation from and absence of the mother during infancy and early childhood and the ensuing feelings of loneliness, cold, hunger, and fear. They represent, in a sense, a "higher octave" of the more acute and disturbing deprivation caused during the delivery by the uterine contractions. More superficial layers of the relevant COEX systems reflect family situations that are oppressive and punishing for the child and permit no rebellion or escape. They also often include memories of playing the role of scapegoat in various peer groups, having abusive employers, and suffering political or social oppression. All these situations reinforce and perpetuate the role of victim in a no-exit predicament characteristic of BPM II.

An important category of COEX systems instrumental in the dynamics of depression involves memories of events that constituted a threat to survival or body integrity and in which the individual played the role of a helpless victim. This observation is an entirely new contribution of holotropic research to the understanding of depressions. Psychoanalysts and psychodynamically oriented academic psychiatrists emphasize the role of psychological factors in the pathogenesis of depression and do not take into consideration psychotraumas resulting from physical insults.

The psychotraumatic effects of serious diseases, injuries, operations, and episodes of near drowning have been overlooked and grossly underestimated by mainstream psychiatrists, which is surprising in view of their general emphasis on biological factors. For theoreticians and clinicians who see depression as a result of fixation on the oral period of libidinal development, the finding that physical traumas play an important role in the development of this disorder represents a serious conceptual challenge. However, it seems perfectly logical in the context of the presented model, which attributes pathogenic significance to COEX systems that include the combined emotional-physical trauma of birth.

In contrast to the inhibited depression, the phenomenology of *agitated depression* is psychodynamically associated with BPM III. Its basic elements can be seen in experiential sessions and postsession intervals governed by the third matrix. The pent-up energies from birth are not completely blocked, as it is the case in inhibited depression related to BPM II. Here the previously completely jammed energies find a partial outlet and discharge in the form of various destructive and self-destructive tendencies. It is important to emphasize that agitated depression reflects a dynamic compromise between energetic block and discharge. A full discharge of these energies would terminate this condition and result in healing.

Characteristic features of this type of depression are a high degree of tension, anxiety, psychomotor excitement, and restlessness. People experiencing agitated depression are very active. They tend to roll on the floor, flail around, and beat their heads against the wall. Their emotional pain finds expression in loud crying and screaming and they might scratch their faces and tear their hair and clothes. Physical symptoms that are often associated with this condition are muscular tensions, tremors, painful cramps, and uterine and intestinal spasms. Intense headaches, nausea, and breathing problems complete the clinical picture.

The COEX systems associated with this matrix deal with aggression and violence, cruelties of various kinds, sexual abuse and assaults, painful medical interventions, and diseases involving choking and a struggle for breath. In contrast with the COEX systems related to BPM II, the subjects involved in these situations are not passive victims; they are actively engaged in attempts to fight back, defend themselves, remove the obstacles, or escape. Memories of violent encounters with parental figures or siblings, fist fights with peers, scenes of sexual abuse and rape, and episodes from military battles are typical examples of this kind.

The psychoanalytic interpretation of *mania* is even less satisfactory and convincing than that of depression, as many analysts themselves admit (Fenichel 1945). However, most authors seem to agree that mania represents a means of avoiding the awareness of underlying depression, and that it includes a denial of painful inner reality and flight into the external world. It reflects the victory of ego and id over superego, a drastic reduction of inhibitions, an increase of self-esteem, and an abundance of sensual and aggressive impulses.

In spite of all this, mania does not give the impression of genuine freedom. Psychological theories of manic-depressive disorders emphasize the intensive ambivalence of manic patients and the fact that simultaneous feelings of love and hate interfere with their ability to relate to others. The typical manic hunger for objects is usually seen as a manifestation of strong oral fixation, and the periodicity of mania and depression is considered an indication of its relation to the cycle of satiety and hunger.

Many of the otherwise puzzling features of manic episodes become easily understandable when seen in their relation to the dynamics of the perinatal matrices. Mania is psychogenetically linked to the experiential transition from BPM III to BPM IV. It indicates that the individual is partially in touch with the fourth perinatal matrix, but nevertheless still under the influence of the third. Since the manic person is regressed all the way to the level of biological birth, the oral impulses are progressive and not regressive in nature. They point to the state the manic individual is craving and aiming for and has not yet consciously achieved, rather than representing regression to the oral level. Relaxation and oral satisfaction are characteristic of the state following biological birth. To be peaceful, to sleep, and to eat—the typical triad of wishes found in mania—are the natural goals of an organism flooded by the impulses associated with the final stage of birth.

In experiential psychotherapy one can occasionally observe transient manic episodes *in statu nascendi* as phenomena suggesting incomplete rebirth. This usually happens when the individuals involved in the transformation process have reached the final stage of the experience of the death-rebirth struggle and have gotten a taste of the feelings of release from the birth agony. However, at the same time, they are unwilling and unable to face the remaining unresolved material related to BPM III. As a result of anxious clinging to this uncertain and tenuous victory, the new positive feelings become accentuated to the point of a caricature. The image of "whistling in the dark" seems to fit this condition particularly well. The exaggerated and forceful nature of manic emotions and behavior clearly betrays that they are not expressions of genuine joy and freedom, but reaction formations to fear and aggression.

LSD subjects whose sessions terminate in a state of incomplete rebirth show all the typical signs of mania. They are hyperactive, move around at a hectic pace, try to socialize and fraternize with everybody in their environment, and talk incessantly about their sense of triumph and well-being, wonderful feelings, and the great experience they have just had. They tend to extol the wonders of LSD treatment and spin messianic and grandiose plans to transform the world by making it possible for every human being to have the same experience. The breakdown of the superego restraints results in seductiveness, promiscuous tendencies, and obscene talk. Extreme hunger for stimuli and social contact is associated with increased zest, self-love, and self-esteem, as well as indulgence in various aspects of life.

The need for excitement and the search for drama and action that are characteristic of manic patients serve a dual purpose. On the one hand, they provide outlet for the impulses and tensions that are part of the activated BPM III. On the other hand, engaging in external turbulent situations that match the intensity and quality of the inner turmoil helps to reduce the intolerable "emotional-cognitive dissonance" that threatens manic persons – the terrifying realization that their inner experiences do not correspond to external circumstances. And, naturally, serious discrepancy between the inner and the outer implies insanity.

Otto Fenichel (1945) pointed out that many important aspects of mania link it to the psychology of carnivals, events that provide opportunity for socially sanctioned unleashing of otherwise forbidden impulses. This further confirms the deep connection of mania with the dynamic shift from BPM III to BPM IV. In the final stages of the death-rebirth process, many people spontaneously experience visions of colorful carnival scenes. Like in the real life mardi gras pageants, this can include images of skulls, skeletons, and other death-related symbols and motifs appearing in the context of exuberant celebration. In holotropic states, this occurs in the culmination of BPM III, when we start feeling that we might prevail and survive our confrontation with death.

When individuals experiencing this state can be convinced to turn inward, face the difficult emotions that remained unresolved, and complete the (re)birth process, the manic quality disappears from their mood and behavior. The experience of BPM IV in its pure form is characterized by radiant joy, increased zest, deep relaxation, tranquility, and serenity. In this state of mind, people have a sense of inner peace and total satisfaction. Their joy and euphoria are not exaggerated to the point of grotesque caricature and their behavior does not have the driven and flamboyant quality characteristic of manic states.

The COEX systems psychogenetically related to mania comprise memories of situations in which satisfaction was experienced under circumstances of insecurity and uncertainty about the genuineness and continuation of the gratification. Similarly, expectation or demand of overtly happy behavior in situations that do not justify it seems to feed into the manic pattern. In addition, one frequently finds in the history of manic patients contrary influences on their self-esteem, such as hypercritical and undermining attitudes of one parental figure alternating with overestimation, psychological inflation, and a building up of unrealistic expectations coming from the other one. I have also observed in several of my European patients that the alternating experience of total constraint and complete freedom that characterized the custom of swaddling infants seemed to be psychogenetically related to mania.

All the above observations from experiential work seem to suggest that biological birth, with its sudden shift from agony to a sense of dramatic relief, represents the natural basis for the alternating patterns of manic-depressive disorders. This, of course, does not exclude the participation of biochemical factors in the clinical picture. For example, it is conceivable that positive and negative COEX systems have their specific biochemical correlates or can even be selectively activated by certain chemical changes in the organism. However, even if research could demonstrate that depression and mania have consistent biochemical concomitants, the chemical factors, in and of themselves, would not be able to explain the complex nature and specific psychological features of these emotional disorders.

It would be hard to imagine a situation more clearly chemically defined than a clinical LSD session. And yet, our knowledge of the exact chemical composition of the trigger and of the administered dosage is of little help in explaining the psychological content of the experience. Depending on circumstances, the LSD subject can experience an ecstatic rapture or a depressive, manic, or paranoid state. Similarly, naturally occurring depression or mania in all the complexity of their clinical picture cannot be accounted for by some simple chemical equation. There is also always the question whether biological factors play a causal role in the disorder or are its symptomatic concomitants. For example, it is conceivable that the physiological and biochemical changes in manic-depressive disorders represent a replay of the conditions in the organism of a child who is being born.

The new understanding of depression that includes the dynamics of basic perinatal matrices offers fascinating new insights into the psychology of *suicide,* a phenomenon which in the past represented a serious theoretical challenge for psychoanalytically oriented interpretations. Any theory that tries to explain the phenomenon of suicide has to answer two important questions. The first is why a particular individual wants to commit suicide, an act that obviously violates the otherwise mandatory dictate of the self-preservation drive, a powerful force that propels the evolution of life in nature. The second, equally puzzling question is the specificity in the choice of the means of suicide. There seems to be a close connection between the state of mind the depressed person is in and the type of suicide he or she contemplates or attempts.

The suicidal drive thus is not simply an impulse to terminate one's life but to do it in a particular way. It might seem natural that a person who takes an overdose of tranquilizers or barbiturates would not jump off the cliff or under a train. However, the selectivity of choice also works the other way round: a person who chooses bloody suicide would not use drugs, even if they were easily available. The material from psychedelic research and other forms of deep experiential work with holotropic states throw new light on both the deep motives for suicide and the intriguing question of the choice of methods.

Suicidal ideation and tendencies can occasionally be observed in any stage of work with holotropic states. However, they are particularly frequent and urgent at the time when subjects are confronting the unconscious material related to the negative perinatal matrices. Observations from psychedelic and holotropic sessions and from episodes of spiritual emergency reveal that suicidal tendencies fall into two distinct categories that have very specific relations to the perinatal process. We have seen that the experience of inhibited depression is dynamically related to BPM II and that agitated depression is a derivative of BPM III. Various forms of suicidal fantasies, tendencies, and actions can then be understood as unconsciously motivated attempts to escape these unbearable psychological states, using two routes. Each of these reflects a specific aspect of the individual's early biological history.

Suicide I, or *nonviolent suicide,* is based on the unconscious memory that the no-exit situation of BPM II was preceded by the experience of intrauterine existence. An individual suffering from inhibited depression tries to escape the intolerable experience of the second perinatal matrix by choosing a way that is most easily available in this state, that of regression into the original undifferentiated unity of the prenatal condition (BPM I). The level of the unconscious involved in this process is usually not accessible, unless the individual has the opportunity for deep experiential self-exploration. Lacking the necessary insight, he or she is attracted to situations and means in everyday life that seem to share certain elements with the prenatal situation.

The basic unconscious intention underlying this form of suicidal tendencies and behavior is to reduce the intensity of painful stimuli associated with BPM II and eventually eliminate them. The final goal is to reach the undifferentiated state of "oceanic consciousness" that characterizes embryonic existence. Mild forms of suicidal ideas of this type are manifested as a wish not to exist, or to fall into a deep sleep, forget everything, and not to awaken ever again. Actual suicidal plans and attempts in this group involve the use of large doses of hypnotics or tranquilizers, drowning, and inhalation of carbon monoxide or domestic gas.

In winter, this unconscious drive to return to the womb can take the form of walking in nature, lying down, and being covered by a layer of snow. The fantasy behind this situation is that the initial discomfort of freezing disappears and is replaced by feelings of coziness and warmth, like being in a good womb. Suicide by cutting one's wrists in a bathtub full of warm water also belongs to this category. Ending one's life in this way was fashionable in ancient Rome and was used by such illustrious men as Petronius and Seneca. This form of suicide might appear on the surface to be different from others in this category, since it involves blood. However, the psychological focus is on dissolution of boundaries and merging with the aquatic environment, not on violation of the body.

Suicide II, or *violent suicide,* follows unconsciously the pattern once experienced during biological birth. It is closely associated with the agitated form of depression and is related to BPM III. For a person who is under the influence of this matrix, regression into the oceanic state of the womb is not a feasible option, because it would lead through the hellish no-exit stage of BPM II. This would be psychologically far worse than BPM III, since it involves a sense of total despair and hopelessness.

However, what is available as a psychological escape route is the memory that once a similar state was terminated by the explosive release and liberation at the moment of biological birth. To understand this form of suicide, it is important to realize that during our biological birth we were born anatomically, but did not emotionally and physically integrate this overwhelming event. The individual contemplating violent suicide is using the memory of his or her biological birth as a recipe for coping with the "second birth," the emergence of the unassimilated emotions and physical sensations for conscious processing.

As is the case with nonviolent suicide, the individuals involved in this process typically do not have experiential access to the perinatal level of the unconscious. They thus lack the insight that the ideal strategy in their situation would be to complete the process internally—relive the memory of their birth and connect experientially with the postnatal situation. Unaware of this option, they exteriorize the process and tend to enact a situation in the external world that involves the same elements and has similar experiential components. The basic strategy of violent suicide follows the pattern experienced during delivery – intensification of the tension and emotional suffering to a critical point and reaching explosive resolution amidst various forms of biological material.

This description applies equally to biological birth and to violent suicide. Both involve abrupt termination of excessive emotional and physical tension, instant discharge of enormous destructive and self-destructive energies, extensive tissue damage, and the presence of organic material, such as blood, feces, and entrails. The juxtaposition of photographs showing biological birth and those depicting victims of violent suicide clearly demonstrate the deep formal parallels between the two situations. It is thus easy for the unconscious to confuse one with the other. The connection between the type of birth trauma and the choice of suicide has been confirmed by clinical research (Jacobson et al. 1987).

The suicidal fantasies and acts that belong to this category involve death under the wheels of a train, in the turbine of a hydroelectric plant, or in suicidal car accidents. Additional examples involve cutting one's throat, blowing one's brains out, stabbing oneself with a knife, or throwing oneself from a window, tower, or cliff. Suicide by hanging seems to belong to an earlier phase of BPM III, characterized by feelings of strangulation, suffocation, and strong sexual arousal. The category of violent suicide also includes some culture-bound forms of suicide such as harakiri, kamikaze, and running amok.

The last three were in the past seen as exotic forms of suicidal behavior occurring exclusively in Oriental cultures. In recent decades, episodes similar to running amok, involving indiscriminate killing and ending with the death of the aggressor, have become increasingly frequent in the United States and other Western countries. A very disturbing aspect of these episodes has been their growing incidence among adolescents and even school children. Kamikaze type of behavior has been repeatedly observed in the Middle Eastern Arab countries as a form of sabotage.

The work with holotropic states has also provided fascinating insights into the intriguing problem of the choice of a particular type and specific form of suicide that has been poorly understood in the past. Nonviolent suicide reflects a general tendency to reduce the intensity of painful emotional and physical stimuli. The specific choice of means for this type of suicide seems to be determined by biographical or transpersonal elements. Violent suicide involves a mechanism of an entirely different kind. Here I have repeatedly observed that the individuals who were contemplating a particular form of suicide were often already experiencing in their everyday life the physical sensations and emotions that would be involved in its actual enactment. Experiential work typically intensified these feelings and sensations and brought them to a very sharp relief.

Thus, those persons whose self-destructive fantasies and tendencies focus on trains or hydroelectric turbines already suffer from intense feelings of being crushed and torn to pieces. Individuals, who have a tendency to cut or stab themselves, often complain about unbearable pains exactly in those parts of their bodies that they intend to injure, or experience pains in those locations during experiential psychotherapy. Similarly, the tendency to hang oneself is based on strong and deep preexisting feelings of strangulation and choking. Both the pains and choking sensations are easily recognizable as elements of BPM III. If the intensification of symptoms would happen in a therapeutic situation and with adequate guidance, it could result in resolution of those uncomfortable sensations and have therapeutic results. The above self-destructive tendencies can thus be seen as unconscious, misguided, and truncated efforts at self-healing.

The mechanism of violent suicide requires a relatively clear memory of the sudden transition from the struggle in the birth canal to the external world and of the ensuing explosive liberation. If this transition was blurred by heavy anaesthesia, the individual would be programmed for the future, almost on a cellular level, to escape from severe stress and discomfort into a drugged state. This would create a disposition to alcoholism and drug abuse in a person otherwise dominated by BPM III. Under extreme circumstances, this could lead to a suicide involving drugs. In the study of individual cases of suicidal behavior, detailed examination of the birth process must be complemented with biographical analysis, since postnatal events can significantly codetermine and color the pattern of suicide.

When suicidal individuals undergo psychedelic or holotropic therapy and complete the death-rebirth process, they see suicide retrospectively as a tragic mistake based on lack of self-understanding. The average person does not know that one can safely experience liberation from unbearable emotional and physical tension through a symbolic death and rebirth or through reconnecting to the state of prenatal existence. As a result, he or she might be driven by the intensity of discomfort and suffering to seek a situation in the material world that involves similar elements. The extreme outcome is often tragic and irreversible.

The discussion of suicide would not be complete without mentioning the relationship between self-destructive behavior and transcendence. As we have seen earlier, the experiences of BPM I and BPM IV do not represent only regression to symbiotic biological states, but have also very distinct spiritual dimensions. For BPM I it is the experience of oceanic ecstasy and cosmic union, for BPM IV that of psychospiritual rebirth and divine epiphany. From this perspective, suicidal tendencies of both types appear to be distorted and unrecognized craving for transcendence. They represent a fundamental confusion between suicide and egocide. The best remedy for self-destructive tendencies and the suicidal urge is, then, the experience of ego death and rebirth and the ensuing feelings of cosmic unity.

Not only are the aggressive and self-destructive impulses consumed in the process of psychospiritual death and rebirth, but the individual connects experientially with the transpersonal context in which suicide no longer seems to be a solution. This sense of the futility of suicide is connected with the insight that the transformations of consciousness and the cycles of death and rebirth will continue after one's biological demise. More specifically, this results from the recognition of the impossibility of escaping one's karmic patterns.

Alcoholism and Drug Addiction

The observations from holotropic states are in general agreement with psychoanalytic theory that sees *alcoholism and narcotic drug addiction* as being closely related to manic-depressive disorders and suicide. But they differ considerably in regard to the nature of the psychological mechanisms involved and the level of the psyche on which they operate. Like suicidal individuals, addicts experience a great amount of emotional pain, such as depression, general tension, anxiety, guilt, and low self-esteem, and they have a strong need to escape these unbearable feelings. We saw earlier that the psychology of depression and suicide cannot be adequately accounted for by oral fixation, which is the interpretation offered by Freudian psychoanalysis. The same is certainly true for alcoholism and drug addiction.

The most basic psychological characteristic of alcoholics and addicts and their deepest motive for taking intoxicant drugs is not only the need to regress to the breast, but also a much deeper craving for the experience of blissful undifferentiated unity of the undisturbed intrauterine life. As we saw earlier, regressive experiences of both of these symbiotic states have intrinsic numinous dimensions. The deepest force behind alcoholism and addiction is thus unrecognized and misguided craving for transcendence. Like suicide, these disorders involve a tragic error based on inadequate understanding of one's own unconscious dynamics.

In our psychedelic and holotropic research, alcoholics and drug addicts who had the opportunity and good fortune to reach experientially positive BPM IV or BPM I told us repeatedly that these were the states they craved and not the alcoholic or narcotic intoxication. But until they experienced prenatal and perinatal satisfaction, they did not really know what they were looking for and their yearning had a very vague form.

Excessive consumption of alcohol or narcotic drugs seems to be a mitigated analogue of suicidal behavior. Alcoholism and addiction have frequently been described as prolonged and slow forms of suicide. The principal mechanism characteristic for these two groups of patients is the same as for the nonviolent variety of suicide. It reflects an unconscious need to undo the birth process and return to the womb, to the state that existed prior to the onset of delivery. Alcohol and narcotics tend to inhibit various painful emotions and sensations and produce a state of diffused consciousness and indifference toward one's past and present problems. This state bears some superficial similarity to fetal consciousness and the experience of cosmic unity.

However, resemblance is not identity, and there are also some fundamental differences between alcoholic or narcotic intoxications and transcendental states. Alcohol and narcotics dull the senses, obnubilate consciousness, interfere with intellectual functions, and produce emotional anesthesia. Transcendental states are characterized by a great enhancement of sensory perception, serenity, clarity of thinking, abundance of philosophical and spiritual insights, and unusual richness of emotions. In spite of some shared features, the intoxication with alcohol and hard drugs represents just a pitiful caricature of the mystical state. Yet, the similarity, however tenuous, seems to be sufficient to seduce the addicts into self-destructive abuse.

The tendency to escape painful emotions associated with BPM II and related COEX systems by an attempt to recreate the situation in the womb appears to be the most common psychodynamic mechanism underlying alcoholism and drug abuse. However, I have also worked with alcoholics and addicts whose symptoms indicated that they were under the influence of BPM III and yet sought the pharmacological solution for their problems. Clearly, these instances involved an alternative mechanism and required a different explanation. All these people happened to be been born under heavy anesthesia and several of them independently had convincing insights that linked this fact to their addiction.

This explanation certainly makes a lot of sense. Birth is typically the first significant challenge we encounter in our life and the first major painful and stressful situation. A possible exception to this rule could be situations where severe crises occurred already during embryonal existence. The extraordinary influence of early events in life on subsequent behavior has been repeatedly documented in experiments by ethologists, researchers studying animal instinctual behavior, and is known as "imprinting" (Lorenz 1963, Tinbergen 1965).

The nature of our delivery and the way it was handled has a powerful impact on our future life. When our delivery is of average duration and severity and we emerge into the world after having successfully negotiated it, it leaves us with a feeling of optimism and confidence in regard to challenges that we encounter in the future. Conversely, a prolonged and debilitating delivery creates in us a sense of pessimism and defeatism. It forges an impression of the world as being too difficult to cope with successfully and of ourselves as being helpless and ineffective.

If the pain and discomfort associated with our delivery is alleviated or terminated by anesthesia, it leaves a very deep and convincing imprint in our psyche that the way to deal with difficulties in life is to escape into a drug state. It might not be just a meaningless coincidence that today's epidemic of drug abuse involves individuals who have been born since the time when obstetricians started routinely using anesthesia during childbirth, often against the will of the delivering mothers. Since the founding of the Association of Pre- and Perinatal Psychology and Health (APPPAH), a discipline that applies the findings of experiential therapies and fetal research to birth practices, obstetricians are becoming increasingly aware of the fact that birthing involves more than body mechanics.

The way delivery and the postnatal period are handled has a profound influence on the emotional and social life of the individual and has important implications for the future of our society. It lays the foundations for a loving and altruistic relationship with fellow humans or, conversely for a mistrusting and aggressive attitude toward society (Odent 1995). And it might also be a critical factor determining whether the individual will be able to cope with the vicissitudes of life in a constructive way or will tend to escape the challenges of existence by opting for alcohol or narcotics.

The fact that alcoholism and narcotic drug abuse represent a misguided search for transcendence can also help us understand the healing and transformative effect of profound crises that are usually referred to as "hitting bottom." In many instances, reaching a state of total emotional bankrupcy and annihilation becomes a turning point in the life of the alcoholic or drug addict. In the context of our discussion, this would mean that the individual experienced ego death as part of the transition from BPM III to BPM IV. At this point, alcohol or narcotics are not any more able to protect him or her from the onslaught of the deep unconscious material. The eruption of the perinatal dynamics then results in a psychosomatic death-rebirth experience that often represents a positive turning point in the life of the alcoholic or addict. The implications of this observation for therapy will be discussed later in this book.

Like all emotional problems, alcoholism and addiction have not only biographical and perinatal, but also transpersonal roots. Most important among these are influences from the archetypal domain. This aspect of addiction has been explored particularly by therapists with Jungian orientation. Among archetypes that show important connection with addiction, that of *puer aeternus* with its varieties of Icarus and Dionysus, seems to play an important role (Lavin 1987). Many people with whom I have worked also discovered karmic material that seemed to be meaningfully related to their addiction.

Sexual Disorders and Deviations

In classical psychoanalysis, the interpretation of sexual problems rests on several fundamental concepts formulated by Freud. The first of these is the notion of *infantile sexuality.* One of the basic cornerstones of the psychoanalytic theory is that sexuality does not manifest in puberty, but already in early infancy. As the libido develops through several evolutionary stages—oral, anal, urethral, and phallic—frustration or overindulgence in any of them can lead to fixation. In mature sexuality, the primary focus is genital and the pregenital components play a secondary role, mostly as part of the foreplay. Specific psychological stress in later life can cause regression to earlier developmental stages of libidinal development where fixation occurred. Depending on the strength of the defense mechanisms that oppose these impulses, this can result in perversions or psychoneuroses (Freud 1953).

Another important concept in the psychoanalytic approach to sexual problems is the *castration complex.* "Freud believed that both sexes attribute extreme value to the penis and he considered this to be an issue of paramount importance for psychology. According to him, boys experience excessive fear that they might lose this highly valued organ. Girls believe that they once had a penis and lost it, which makes them more prone to masochism and guilt. Freud's critics repeatedly argued that this point of view represents a serious distortion and misunderstanding of female sexuality, since it portrays women as castrated males.

The discussion of Freud's understanding of sexuality would not be complete without mentioning another important concept, his famous *vagina dentata,* the observation that children see the female genitals as a dangerous organ equipped with teeth, one that can kill or castrate. Together with the Oedipal and Electra complexes and the castration complex, the fantasy of the ominous female genitals plays a crucial role in the psychoanalytic interpretation of sexual deviations and psychoneurosis.

Freud suggested two reasons for which the sight of female genitals may arouse anxiety in boys. First, the recognition that there are human beings without a penis leads to the conclusion that one might become one, which lends power to the castration fears. And second, the perception of the female genitals as a castrating instrument capable of biting is due to an association with old oral anxieties (Fenichel 1945). None of these two reasons is particularly compelling and convincing.

The observations from holotropic states radically expand and deepen the Freudian understanding of sexuality by adding to the individual unconscious the perinatal domain. They suggest that we do not experience our first sexual feelings on the breast, but already in the birth canal. As I have discussed earlier, the suffocation and agony during BPM III seems to generate a sexual arousal of extreme intensity. This means that our first encounter with sexual feelings occurs under very precarious circumstances.

Birth is a situation in which our life is threatened and we experience suffocation and other forms of extreme physical and emotional discomfort. We inflict pain on another organism and another organism inflicts pain on us. In addition, we are in contact with various forms of biological material—blood, vaginal secretions, amniotic fluid, and possibly even feces and urine. The typical response to this predicament is a mixture of vital anxiety and rage. These problematic associations form a natural basis for the understanding of the basic sexual dysfunctions, deviations, and perversions.

The recognition of the profound influence of perinatal dynamics on sexuality also clears some serious theoretical problems associated with Freud's concept of the castration complex. Several important characteristics of this complex do not make any sense as long as we relate it to the penis. According to Freud, the intensity of castration fear is so excessive that it equals the fear of death. He also saw castration as psychologically equivalent to loss of an important human relationship and suggested that it could actually be activated by such a loss. Among the free associations that often emerge in connection with the castration complex are those dealing with situations involving suffocation and loss of breath. And, as I mentioned earlier, the castration complex is found in both men and women.

None of the above connections could be adequately accounted for if the castration complex reflected only concerns about the loss of the penis. Observations from holotropic states show that the experiences, which Freud considered to be the source of the castration complex, actually represent the surface layer of a COEX system superimposed over the traumatic memory of the severing of the umbilical cord. All the inconsistencies that I discussed earlier disappear when we realize that many puzzling characteristics of Freud's castration complex actually refer to the separation from the mother at the time when the umbilical cord was cut and not to the loss of the penis.

Unlike facetious verbal threats of castration by adults, spontaneous castration fantasies, and even surgical interventions on the penis, such as circumcision or correction of the adhesion of the foreskin (*fimosis*), cutting of the cord is associated with a situation that is potentially or actually life threatening. Since it severs the vital connection with the maternal organism, it is the prototypical loss of an important relationship. The association of the cutting of the umbilical cord with suffocation also makes eminent sense, since the cord is the source of oxygen for the fetus. And, last but not least, it is an experience that is shared by both sexes.

Similarly, the image of the vagina dentata that Freud saw as a primitive infantile fantasy appears in a new light once we accept that the newborn is a conscious being or, at least, that the trauma of birth is recorded in the memory. Rather than being an absurd and silly fabrication of the child's immature psyche, the image of the vagina as a perilous organ reflects correctly the dangers associated with female genitals in one particular situation, namely during childbirth. Far from being a mere fantasy that does not have any basis in reality, it represents a generalization of one's experience in a life-threatening situation to other contexts in which it is not appropriate.

The link between sexuality and the potentially life-threatening trauma of birth creates a general disposition to sexual disturbances of various kinds. Specific disorders then develop when these perinatal elements are reinforced by postnatal traumas in infancy and childhood. As it is the case with emotional and psychosomatic disorders in general, the traumatic experiences that psychoanalysts see as primary causes of these problems actually reinforce certain aspects of the birth trauma and facilitate their emergence into consciousness. And like other psychogenic disorders, sexual problems also typically have deeper roots in the transpersonal domain linking them to various karmic, archetypal, and phylogenetic elements. After this general introduction, I will now briefly review the insights from holotropic states concerning various specific forms of human sexual experience and behavior.

Homosexuality has many different types and subtypes and undoubtedly many different determinants. In the early developmental stages, the human embryo is anatomically and physiologically bisexual. Homoerotic experimentation in adolescence is extremely common, even for boys and girls who in adulthood become distinctly heterosexual. In situations where heterosexual choice is impossible, such as prisons, military service, or long stay at sea, it is not unusual for heterosexual persons to resort to homosexual activities. Some native American tribes recognize and honor not two or four, but six sexes (Tafoya 1994).

Sexual preference and behavior can be influenced by genetic predisposition and by hormones, as well as cultural, social, and psychological factors. The research using holotropic states provides access to deep unconscious dynamics and renders interesting psychological insights that cannot be obtained in any other way. This work reveals the existence of perinatal and transpersonal determinants of sexual behavior. It thus contributes an interesting piece to the complex mosaic of our knowledge concerning sexual preferences, which has been amassed by various other disciplines. The following discussion should be seen from this perspective.

My clinical experience with homosexuality was rather biased, since it was limited to a great extent to individuals who came into treatment because they considered their homosexuality a problem and had serious conflicts about it. My patients who were homosexual typically had other clinical problems, such as depression, suicidal tendencies, neurotic symptoms, or psychosomatic manifestations. These considerations are important in drawing any general conclusions from my observations.

In addition, I have also had the opportunity to conduct psychedelic and holotropic sessions with a number of gay and lesbian individuals who participated in our psychedelic program for professionals and in our holotropic breathwork training. Their primary motivation was not therapy but professional training or personal growth. For many of them, homosexuality was clearly a preference and they enjoyed their way of life. Their major problem was a conflict with intolerant society rather than an intrapsychic conflict and struggle.

Most of the male homosexual patients I have worked with were able to form good social relations with women, but were incapable of relating to them sexually. They often resorted to homosexual activities after repeated frustrating experiences with women. During treatment, this problem could be traced back to the Freudian castration fears and vagina dentata. As we have already discussed, these concepts had to be radically reinterpreted and given perinatal and often transpersonal meaning.

Some of these patients also traced their predisposition to the passive homosexual role to deep unconscious identification with the delivering mother. This involved a specific combination of sensations characteristic of BPM III—the feeling of a biological object inside one's body, a mixture of pleasure and pain, and a combination of sexual arousal with anal pressure. They realized that this was the experience that they sought in the homosexual act. The fact that anal intercourse tends to have a strong sadomasochistic component suggests connection between this form of male homosexuality and the dynamics of BPM III.

On a more superficial level, there were often biographical factors that seemed to contribute to my patients' sexual choice. Particularly frequent was either the absence or emotional distance of the father figure and resulting deep craving for affection from a male figure. In an adult male, a strong need for an intimate, loving, and affectionate relationship with a male figure can be satisfied only in a homosexual relationship. Another common factor was a strong fixation on the mother, associated with boundary problems, and incest taboo.

As I mentioned before, some gay men who participated in our LSD training program for professionals and in our holotropic breathwork program did not show significant inner conflict about their sexual orientation. In their sessions, they traced their sexual orientation to transpersonal sources. For some of them, it was the influence of a particular archetypal figure, such as a culture-specific form of *puer aeternus*. Others traced their preference to a past-life experience as a person of the opposite gender or as an individual living in a culture that accepted or even extolled homosexuality; for example, ancient Greece. A few simply understood and accepted their orientation as an experiment of cosmic consciousness, a variation in the universal design reflecting the curiosity of the creative principle.

My comments concerning the *lesbian orientation* must be presented with reservations similar to those on male homosexuality, since my sample was equally limited and biased. One important factor in my lesbian patients was certainly an unsatisfied need for intimate contact with the female body, reflecting a period of emotional deprivation in infancy. If the anaclitic needs are not satisfied in infancy, they tend to persist throughout the entire life. In adulthood, the only way to resolve this unfulfilled craving is in the nonsexual context of regressive therapy. The alternative—giving this longing an expression in everyday life—naturally results in a sexual lesbian situation.

Another important component of the lesbian orientation seems to be a tendency to return psychologically to the memory of release at the time of birth, which occurred in close contact with female genitals. This would be essentially similar to the psychodynamics of male heterosexual preference for oral-genital practices. An additional perinatal element related to the memory of birth is the fear of being dominated, overpowered, and violated, which is more likely to occur in a sexual situation with a male partner. Very frequently negative experiences with a father figure in childhood are contributing factors for seeking women and avoiding men.

In general, female homosexuality seems to be less connected with negative perinatal matrices and with issues of life and death relevance than it is the case with its male counterpart. Lesbian tendencies reflect a positive perinatal component of attraction toward the maternal organism (BPM I and IV), while male homosexuality is associated with the memory of the life-threatening vagina dentata. Erotic contact between women also appears more natural, because intimate contact with the female body is something both sexes experience in their early history. Society's greater tolerance of lesbianism than of male homosexuality seems to be consistent with this view. Like homosexual men, some lesbians show an unequivocal preference for the same sex and do not seem to have intrapsychic conflicts about it. The determining factors here seem to be either biological or transpersonal in nature.

Erectile dysfunction (*impotence*), the inability to develop or maintain an erection, and *orgastic incompetence* (*frigidity*), the inability to attain an orgasm, have a similar psychodynamic basis. The conventional approach to these problems sees impotence as an expression of sexual weakness, lack of masculine power or prowess. Orgastic incompetence in women, as its old name "frigidity" indicates, is usually interpreted as sexual coldness and lack of erotic responsivity. According to my experience, the opposite seems to be true; in both conditions, it is actually excess of sexualized perinatal energy that is the problem.

Individuals suffering from these disorders are under strong influence of the sexual aspect of BPM III. This makes it impossible for them to experience sexual arousal without simultaneously activating all the other elements of this matrix. The intensity of the energy, the aggressive impulses, vital anxiety, and fear of loss of control associated with BPM III then inhibit the sexual act. In both instances, the sexual problems are connected with COEX systems that, besides this perinatal component, have also biographical layers and transpersonal roots – individual and karmic memories of sexual abuse, rape, association between sex and pain or danger, and similar themes.

The empirical support for the involvement of perinatal dynamics in "impotence" and "frigidity" comes from experiential psychotherapy. When we create a nonsexual situation in which the elements of BPM III can be brought into consciousness and the energy associated with them discharged, impotence can be temporarily replaced by a condition called *satyriasis*—an excessive sexual drive and appetite. This is due to the fact that a connection has been established between the penis and the sexual energy generated by the trauma of birth. It is now this perinatal energy and not the ordinary libido that is being used in the sexual act.

Because of the excessive amount of energy available on the perinatal level, this situation can result in an insatiable appetite and ability to perform sexually. The men who previously were not able to maintain erection at all are now capable of having intercourse several times in a single night. The release is usually not fully satisfactory and, as soon as they reach orgasm and ejaculate, the sexual energy starts to build up again. More nonsexual experiential work is necessary to bring this energy to a niveau that can be comfortably handled in a sexual situation.

In a similar way, women who were previously unable to let go and attain an orgasm can become orgastic when they discharge in a nonsexual situation some of the excessive energy associated with BPM III. When this happens, the initial orgasms tend to be overwhelming. They are often accompanied by loud intense involuntary screams and followed by several minutes of violent shaking. There might be a tendency to briefly lose control and bruise or scratch the partner. Under these circumstances, it is not uncommon for the woman to experience multiple orgasms. This initial liberation can also lead to an increase of sexual appetite to such a degree that it appears insatiable. We thus can see a temporary transformation of "frigidity" into a condition known as *nymphomania.* And again, as in the case of impotent men, additional inner work in a nonsexual situation is necessary to bring the energy to a level that can be comfortably handled in a sexual context.

The understanding of perinatal dimensions of sexuality throws an interesting new light on *sadomasochism,* a condition that represented a formidable challenge for Freud's theoretical speculations. He struggled with it until the end of his life and never really found a satisfactory solution. Active seeking of pain exhibited by sadomasochistic individuals contradicted one of the cornerstones of Freud's early model, the "pleasure principle." According to this concept, the deepest motivating force in the psyche was pursuit of pleasure and avoidance of discomfort. Freud was also baffled by the strange fusion of two basic instincts, sexuality and aggression, that is an essential feature of sadomasochism.

It was the existence of sadomasochism and other conditions "beyond the pleasure principle" that forced Freud to abandon his early theories and to create an entirely new system of psychoanalysis that included the controversial Thanatos, or death instinct (Freud 1955, 1964). Although he never made the link between death and birth, these late speculations clearly reflected his intuitive insight that sadomasochism borders on matters of life and death. They also reflected Freud's belief that a viable psychological theory had to incorporate the problem of death. Clearly, his thinking in this regard was far ahead of his followers, some of whom formulated theories of sadomasochism that focused on relatively trivial biographical situations.

Kučera's (1959) theory linking sadomasochism to the experience of teething, when active efforts of the child to bite become painful, is an example of such efforts. Explanations of this kind do not even begin to account for the depth of sadomasochistic impulses.

Sadomasochism and the bondage syndrome can be naturally understood from the connections that exists in the context of BPM III between sexual arousal, physical confinement, pain, and suffocation. This accounts for the fusion between sexuality and aggression, as well as the link between sexuality and inflicted or experienced pain that characterize these two conditions. The individuals who need to combine sex with such elements as physical restriction, dominance and submission, inflicting and experiencing pain, and strangling or choking, simply repeat a combination of sensations and emotions that they experienced during their birth. The primary focus of these activities is perinatal, not sexual. Sadomasochistic experiences and visions are a frequent occurrence in sessions dominated by BPM III.

The need to create a sadomasochistic situation and exteriorize the above unconscious experiential complex is not only symptomatic behavior but also a truncated attempt of the psyche to expurgate and integrate the original traumatic imprint. The reason why this effort is unsuccessful and does not result in self-healing is the fact that it does not reach deep enough into the unconscious and lacks the element of introspection, insight, and understanding of the nature of the process. The experiential complex is acted out without the recognition and awareness of its unconscious sources.

The same is true for *coprophilia, coprophagia,* and *urolagnia,* sexual deviations characterized by a strong need to bring into the sexual situation feces and urine. Individuals showing these aberrations seek intimate contact with biological materials that are usually considered repulsive, they become sexually aroused by them, and tend to incorporate them into their sexual life. In the extremes, such activities as being urinated or defecated on, smeared with feces, eating excrements, and drinking urine can be a necessary condition for reaching sexual satisfaction.

A combination of sexual excitement and scatological elements is a rather common experience during the final stages of the death-rebirth process. This seems to reflect the fact that, in the deliveries where no catheterization or enemas are used, many children experience intimate contact not only with blood, mucus, and amniotic fluid, but also with feces and urine. The natural basis of this seemingly extreme and bizarre deviation is oral contact with feces and urine at the moment when, after many hours of agony and vital threat, the head is released from the firm grip of the birth canal. Intimate contact with such material thus becomes the symbol of a total orgastic release, as well as its necessary prerequisite.

According to psychoanalytical literature, the infant—because of his or her essentially animal nature—is originally attracted to various forms of biological material and only secondarily develops aversion toward them as a result of parental and societal repressive measures. Observations from psychedelic research suggest that this is not necessarily so. The attitude toward biological material is significantly codetermined by the nature of the encounter with this material during the birth experience. Depending on the specific circumstances, this attitude can be extremely positive or negative.

In some deliveries, the child simply encounters vaginal secretions, urine, or feces as part of the ambience of physical and emotional liberation. In others, this material is inhaled, obstructs the respiratory pathways, and causes terrifying suffocation. In extreme situations of this kind, the life of the newborn has to be saved by intubation and suction that clears the trachea and bronchi. These are two radically different forms of encounter with biological material at birth, one of them positive, the other frightening and traumatic. A situation, in which breathing is triggered prematurely and the inhaled biological material threatens the life of the child can generate intense fear and become the basis for future obsessive-compulsive disorder, as we discussed earlier.

A rich source of fascinating information about sexual deviations is *A Sexual Profile of Men in Power,* by Janus, Bess, and Saltus (1977). Their study is based on more than seven hundred hours of interviews with high-class call-girls from the East Coast of the United States. Unlike many other researchers, the authors were less interested in the personalities of the prostitutes than in the preferences and habits of their customers. Among these were many prominent representatives of American politics, business, law, and justice.

The interviews revealed that only an absolute minority of the clients sought simply sexual intercourse. Most of them were interested in various devious erotic practices that would qualify as "heavy kinky sex." Very common were requests for bondage, whipping, and other forms of torture. Some of these clients were willing to pay high prices for psychodramatic staging of complex sadomasochistic scenes. One of the clients, for example, requested a realistic enactment of a situation in which he played the role of an American pilot shot down and captured in Nazi Germany during World War II. The prostitutes were asked to dress as bestial Gestapo women wearing high boots and military helmets. Their task was to subject the client to various ingenious tortures.

Among the frequently requested and highly priced practices were the "golden shower" and "brown shower," being urinated and defecated on in a sexual context. According to the accounts of the call-girls, after the sadomasochistic and scatological experience culminated and their clients reached sexual orgasm, many of these extremely ambitious and influential men regressed to an infantile state. They wanted to be held, suck on the prostitutes' nipples, and be treated like little babies. This behavior was in sharp contrast with the public image these men had been trying to project in their everyday life.

The interpretations of these findings offered in the book are strictly biographical and Freudian in nature. The authors link tortures to parental punishments, the golden shower and brown shower to problems related to toilet training, the need for sucking the breast to frustrated nursing needs and mother fixation, and the like. However, closer inspection reveals that the clients actually enacted classical perinatal themes rather than postnatal childhood events. The combination of physical restraint, pain and torture, sexual arousal, scatological involvement, and subsequent regressive oral behavior are unmistakable indications of the activation of BPM III and IV.

I will briefly mention here another illustration of the connection between similar sexual practices and the perinatal process. An Australian friend of mine, who was seeing in therapy a prostitute from a large city and was well informed about the situation in this city's sexual underworld, described to me what was the most popular and most frequently requested attraction offered by local call-girls. The client could lock himself in a special room with three teenage girls, all dressed as nuns. As he chased them and attacked them sexually, they faked panic and either resisted him or feigned attempts at escape. All this was happening while several loudspeakers played sacred music, such as Gounod's Saint Cecilia Mass or Mozart's Requiem. This combination of sex, aggression, and spiritual elements is very typical for the transition between BPM III and IV.

The conclusions of Janus, Bess, and Saltus deserve special notice. The authors appealed to the American public not to expect their politicians and other prominent figures to be models of sexual behavior. In the light of their research, this expectation would be highly unrealistic. Their findings indicated that excessive sexual drive and inclination to deviant sexuality are inextricably linked with the high degree of ambition that it takes in today's society to become a successful public figure. We thus should not be surprised by the scandals in the highest social and political circles—the Profumo affair that shook the British parliament, escapades of Ted Kennedy that destroyed his chances as presidential candidate, John Kennedy's peccadillos that threatened national security, and Bill Clinton's sexual extravaganzas that for many months paralyzed the U.S. government.

The realization of the perinatal roots of human behavior offers an unexpected solution to the old argument between Freud and Adler, whether the sexual drive or will to power is the dominant element in the human psyche. According to Freud, the strongest force driving our thoughts, emotions, and behavior is pursuit of sexual satisfaction. And we want power, because it makes us more desirable and increases our sexual opportunities. For Adler, the decisive motivating element in the psyche was the feeling of inferiority and a determined drive to overcompensate for it—striving for power or the "masculine protest" as he called it. What we want most is power and we use sex to get it and improve our position in the world.

Janus, Bess, and Saltus suggest that strong sexual drive and intense ambition are not in conflict, but are actually two sides of the same coin. This suggestion is in perfect agreement with the perinatal model; in the context of BPM III, the two forces are inextricably linked. As we have seen, choking and pain experienced in the birth canal generate an extraordinarily intense sexual drive that seeks discharge. And the confrontation with the elemental forces of the uterine contractions and with the resistance of the birth canal makes the fetus feel helpless and inadequate. At the same time, the extreme discomfort and vital threat of birth mobilizes the survival instinct and results in desperate efforts to deal with the challenge and overcome it. Events in postnatal life then constitute COEX systems that can reinforce one or the other element in this complementary dyad.

Some extreme forms of criminal sexual pathology, such as *rapes, sadistic murder,* and *necrophilia,* clearly betray definite perinatal roots. Individuals experiencing the sexual aspects of BPM III frequently talk about the fact that this stage of the birth process has many characteristics in common with rape. This comparison makes a lot of sense if one considers some of the essential experiential features of rape. For the victim, it involves the element of serious danger, vital anxiety, extreme pain, physical restraint, a struggle to free oneself, choking, and imposed sexual arousal. The experience of the rapist, in turn, involves the active counterparts of these elements—endangering, threatening, hurting, restricting, choking, and enforcing sexual arousal. The experience of the victim has many elements in common with that of the child suffering in the clutches of the birth canal, while the rapist exteriorizes and acts out the introjected forces of the uterine contractions, while simultaneously taking revenge on a mother surrogate.

If the memory of BPM III is close to consciousness, it can create a strong psychological pressure on the individual to enact its elements in everyday life—to engage in violent consensual sex or even unconsciously invite dangerous sexual situations. While this mechanism certainly does not apply to all victims of sexual crimes, in some instances it can play an important role. While clearly self-destructive, such behavior contains an unconscious healing impulse. Similar experiences generated by the subject's own psyche in the context of experiential therapy and with insights into their unconscious sources would lead to healing and psychospiritual transformation.

Because of this similarity between the experience of rape and the birth experience, the rape victim suffers a psychological trauma that reflects not only the painful impact of the recent situation but also the breakdown of the defenses protecting her or him against the memory of biological birth. The frequent long-term emotional problems following rapes are very probably caused by the emergence into consciousness of perinatal emotions and psychosomatic manifestations. Therapeutic resolution will have to include work on the trauma of birth.

The influence of the third perinatal matrix is even more obvious in the case of *sadistic murders,* which are closely related to rapes. In addition to a combined discharge of the sexual and aggressive impulses, these acts involve the elements of death, mutilation, dismemberment, and scatological indulgence in blood and intestines. This is clearly a combination characteristic of the reliving of the final stages of birth.

The dynamics of sadistic murder is closely related to that of bloody suicide. The only difference is that, in the former, the individual overtly assumes the role of the aggressor; whereas, in the latter, also that of the victim. In the last analysis, both roles represent separate aspects of the same personality: that of the aggressor reflects the introjection of the oppressive and destructive forces of the birth canal, that of the victim the memory of the emotions and sensations of the child during delivery.

A similar combination of elements, but in somewhat different proportions seems to underlie the clinical picture of *necrophilia.* Necrophilia

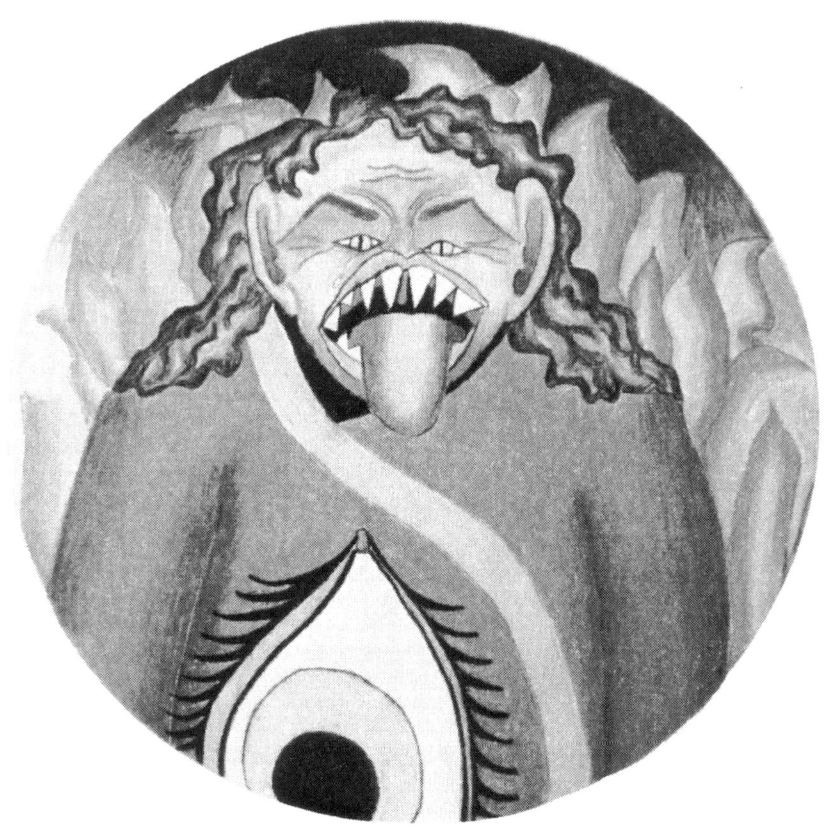

Painting from a holotropic breathwork session in which the artist had an experience of a little man trapped in her stomach. She felt that this figure was involved in the psychodynamics of her nausea and bulimia. The man's green stretched out tongue seemed to be of special importance; it was a very apt and graphic representation of sickness and revulsion (Kathleen Silver).

occurs in many different forms and degrees, from fairly innocuous to manifestly criminal. Its most superficial varieties involve sexual excitement produced by the sight of corpses or attraction to cemeteries, graves, or objects connected with them. More serious forms of necrophilia are characterized by a strong craving to touch corpses, smell or taste them, and indulge in putrefaction and decay. The next step is actual manipulation of corpses with a sexual emphasis, culminating in actual intercourse with the dead bodies in morgues, funeral homes, and cemeteries.

Extreme cases of this sexual perversion combine sexual abuse of corpses with acts of mutilation, dismemberment of the bodies, and cannibalism. Analysis of necrophilia reveals that same strange amalgam of sexuality, death, aggression, and scatology which is so characteristic of the third perinatal matrix. The deepest roots of this serious disorder seem to involve phylogenetic regression into the animal kingdom and identification with the consciousness of carnivorous scavenger species.

Psychosomatic Manifestations of Emotional Disorders

Many emotional disorders, such as psychoneuroses, depressions, and functional psychoses, have distinct physical manifestations. Most common among these are headaches, heart palpitations, excessive sweating, tics and tremors, psychosomatic pains, and various skin afflictions. Equally frequent are gastrointestinal disturbances, such as nausea, loss of appetite, constipation, and diarrhea. Among typical concomitants of emotional problems are also various sexual dysfunctions, for example, amenorrhea, irregularities of the cycle, menstrual cramps, or painful vaginal spasms during intercourse. We have already discussed earlier the erectile dysfunction and the inability to achieve an orgasm. These conditions can either accompany other neurotic problems or occur as independent primary symptoms.

In some psychoneuroses, such as conversion hysteria, the physical symptoms are very distinct and characteristic and can represent the predominant feature of the disorder. This is also true for a category of disorders that classical psychoanalysts called *pregenital neuroses;* it includes various tics, stammering, and psychogenic asthma. These conditions represent hybrids between obsessive-compulsive neurosis and conversion hysteria. The personality structure underlying them is obsessive-compulsive, but the main mechanism of defense and symptom formation is conversion, like in hysteria. There also exists a group of medical disorders, in which the role of psychological factors is so significant that even traditional medicine refers to them as *psychosomatic diseases.*

This category includes *migraine headaches, functional hypertension, colitis* and *peptic ulcers, psychogenic asthma, psoriasis, various eczemas,* and, according to some, even certain forms of *arthritis.* Mainstream physicians and psychiatrists accept the psychogenic nature of these disorders, but do not offer plausible explanation of the psychogenetic mechanisms involved. Much of the clinical work, theoretical speculation, and research until this day has been based on the ideas of psychoanalyst Franz Alexander, considered to be the founder of psychosomatic medicine. In 1935, Alexander proposed a theoretical model explaining the mechanism of psychosomatic disorders. His key contribution was the recognition that psychosomatic symptoms result from the physiological concomitants of psychological conflict and trauma. According to him, emotional arousal during acute anxiety, grief, or rage gives rise to intense physiological reactions, which lead to the development of psychosomatic symptoms and diseases (Alexander 1950).

Alexander made a distinction between conversion reactions and psychosomatic disorders. In the former, the symptoms have a symbolic significance and serve as a defense against anxiety; this is an important characteristic of psychoneuroses. In psychosomatic disorders, the source of the underlying emotional state can be traced to psychological trauma, neurotic conflicts, and pathological interpersonal relationships, but the symptoms do not serve a useful function. They actually represent a failure of psychological mechanisms to protect the individual against excessive affective arousal. Alexander emphasized that this somatization of emotions occurs only in those individuals who are predisposed and not in healthy ones; however, neither he nor his successors have been able to define the nature of this disposition.

More than six decades later, the situation in the field of psychosomatic medicine is generally very disappointing. It is characterized by a fundamental lack of agreement about the mechanisms involved in the psychogenesis of somatic symptoms and no conceptual framework is considered entirely satisfactory (Kaplan and Kaplan 1967). The lack of clear answers is responsible for the fact that many authors subscribe to the idea of multicausality. According to this view, psychological factors play a significant role in psychosomatic disorders, but one has to take into consideration also a variety of other factors, such as constitution, heredity, organ pathology, nutritional status, environment, and social and cultural determinants. These, of course, cannot be adequately specified, which leaves the question of etiology of psychosomatic disorders very vague and fuzzy.

As we have seen earlier, psychedelic therapy and holotropic breathwork have brought clear evidence that postnatal psychological traumas, in and of themselves, are not sufficient to account for the development of emotional disorders. This is also true, even to a much greater extent, for psychosomatic symptoms and disorders. Psychological conflict, loss of an important relationship, excessive dependency, the child's observation of parental intercourse, and other similar factors, which psychoanalysts see as causal factors, simply cannot account for the nature and intensity of the physiological disturbances involved in psychosomatic disorders.

In the light of deep experiential work, any of the psychoanalytically oriented theories of psychosomatic diseases that try to explain them as based solely on psychological traumas in postnatal biography are superficial and unconvincing. Equally implausible is the assumption that these disorders can be effectively treated by verbal therapy. Holotropic research has contributed important insights to the theory and therapy of psychosomatic disorders. Probably the most important of these findings was the discovery of enormous amounts of blocked emotional and physical energy underlying psychosomatic symptoms.

While there can be justifiable doubts that purely psychological biographical traumas could cause deep functional disturbances or even gross anatomical damage to the organs, this is more than a reasonable possibility in the case of the primordial and elemental destructive energies that manifest in holotropic states. In the most general sense, this observation confirmed the concepts of the brilliant and controversial renegade pioneer of psychoanalysis, Wilhelm Reich. On the basis of his observations from therapeutic sessions, Reich concluded that the main factor underlying emotional and psychosomatic disorders is jamming and blockage of significant amounts of bioenergy in the muscles and viscera, constituting what he referred to as *character armor* (Reich 1949, 1961).

But here the parallel between Reichian psychology and the observations from holotropic research ends. According to Reich, this jammed energy is sexual in nature and the reason for its blockage is a fundamental conflict between our biological needs and repressive influence of society, which interferes with full orgastic release and satisfactory sexual life. Residual sexual energy that remains unexpressed then jams and finds deviant expression in the form of perversions and neurotic or psychosomatic symptoms. The work with holotropic states offers a radically different explanation. It shows that the pent-up energy we carry in our organism is not accumulated, unexpressed libido, but emotional and physical charge bound in COEX systems.

Part of this energy belongs to biographical layers of these systems that contain memories of psychological and physical traumas from infancy and childhood. A considerable proportion of this energetic charge is perinatal in origin and reflects the fact that the memory of birth has not been adequately processed and continues to exist in the unconscious as an emotionally and physically incomplete gestalt of major importance. During delivery, extraordinary amounts of energy are generated by excessive stimulation of the neurons and cannot be discharged, because of the confinement of the birth canal. The reason Reich mistook this energy for jammed libido was probably the strong sexual arousal associated with BPM III.

In some instances, prenatal traumas can significantly contribute to the overall negative charge of the COEX systems and participate in the genesis of psychosomatic symptoms. Some people have a very difficult prenatal history that involves such factors as extreme emotional and physical stress of the pregnant mother, impending miscarriage, attempted abortion, toxic womb, or Rh incompatibility. The deepest sources of the energy underlying psychosomatic disorders can typically be traced to the transpersonal domain, particularly to karmic and archetypal elements (see the story of Norbert on pp. 74–75).

Of particular interest and importance is the observation from deep experiential work that the primary driving forces behind all psychosomatic manifestations are not psychological traumas. What plays the crucial role in their genesis are unassimilated and unintegrated physical traumas, such as memories of the discomfort associated with childhood diseases, operations, injuries, or near drowning. On a deeper level, the symptoms are related to the trauma of birth and even to physical traumas associated with past-life memories. For example, the material underlying psychosomatic pains can include memories of accidents, operations, or diseases from infancy, childhood, and later life, the pain experienced during the birth process, and physical suffering connected with injuries or death in a previous incarnation.

This is in sharp contrast with the views of most psychodynamic schools that tend to attribute the primary role in the genesis of psychosomatic symptoms to psychological conflicts and traumas. According to them, symptoms originate in such a way that these psychological issues are expressed in symbolic body language, or "somatized." For example, emotional holding on and riddance are seen as psychological factors underlying constipation and diarrhea. Severe pain in the neck muscles is a symbolic expression of the fact that the client "carries too much responsibility on his or her shoulders."

Similarly, stomach problems develop in people who are unable to "swallow" or "stomach" something. Hysterical paralysis reflects a defense against an objectionable infantile sexual action. Breathing difficulties are caused by a mother who is "smothering" the client, asthma is a "cry for the mother," and oppressive feelings on the chest result from "heavy grief." In the same vein, stammering is seen as resulting from suppression of verbal aggression and an urge to utter obscenities and severe skin disorders serve as protection against sexual temptation.

A psychological system that, unlike most others, recognizes the paramount psychotraumatic impact of physical traumas, is Ron Hubbard's scientology (Hubbard 1950). Scientologists discovered the great psychological significance of physical insults by *auditing*, a process of exploration and therapy that is objectively guided by galvanometers measuring the skin resistance and indicating the emotional charge of the material that is discussed in the sessions. This feedback then becomes the guideline for the auditor in directing the exploratory interview and is an invaluable tool in detecting material that is truly emotionally relevant. In holotropic states, this guidance is provided automatically by the "inner radar" that we discussed earlier.

The theoretical system of scientology recognizes not only physical traumas in postanatal life, but also the trauma of birth and somatic traumas in past lives. Hubbard referred to imprints of physical traumatizations as *engrams* and saw them as primary sources of emotional problems. In his terminology, the usual psychological traumas are called *secondaries;* they borrow their emotional power from their associations with engrams. To a certain extent, the more practical and down-to-earth aspects of Hubbard's conceptual framework show a certain similarity with the material discussed in this book (Gormsen and Lumbye 1979). Unfortunately, the reckless abuse of scientology for pursuit of power and money and Hubbard's wild speculations about extraterrestrial influences have discredited his interesting theoretical contributions.

The work with holotropic states provides rich opportunities for insights into the dynamics of psychosomatic disorders. It is actually not uncommon to see transient occurrence of asthmatic attacks, migraine headaches, various eczemas, and even psoriatic skin eruptions *in statu nascendi,* that is as they emerge into manifestation in psychedelic and holotropic therapy. This is usually associated with insights concerning their psychodynamic roots. On the positive side, dramatic and lasting improvements of various psychosomatic disorders have been reported by therapists and facilitators who use deep experiential techniques in their work. These reports typically describe reliving of physical traumas, in particular the birth trauma, and various transpersonal experiences as the most effective therapeutic mechanisms.

Space considerations do not allow me to describe in more detail the new insights into the psychodynamics of the specific psychosomatic disorders and offer illustrative case histories. In this regard, I have to refer the interested readers to my earlier publications (Grof 1980, 1985).

Autistic and Symbiotic Infantile Psychoses, Narcissistic Personality, and Borderline States

Pioneers of ego psychology, Margaret Mahler, Otto Kernberg, Heinz Kohut, and others, contributed to the classical psychoanalytic classification several new diagnostic categories that, according to them, have their origin in the early disturbances of object relations. A healthy psychological development proceeds from the autistic and symbiotic stage of primary narcissism through the process of separation and individuation to the attainment of constant object relations. Severe interference with this process and lack of gratification of basic needs at these early stages can result in serious disorders. According to the degree of these adversities and their timing, these disturbances can lead to *autistic and symbiotic infantile psychoses, narcissistic personality disturbance,* or *borderline personality disorders.*

The analysis of the disturbances of object relationships underlying these disorders, found in the literature on ego psychology, is unusually detailed and refined. However, like classical psychoanalysts, ego psychologists fail to recognize that postnatal biographical events, in and of themselves, cannot adequately account for the symptomatology of emotional disorders. Observations from holotropic states suggest that early traumas in infancy have a profound impact on the psychological life of the individual not only because they happen to a very immature organism and affect the very foundations of personality, but also because they interfere with the recovery from the birth trauma. They leave the access to the perinatal unconscious wide open.

The terms used in ego psychology for describing the postnatal dynamics of these disorders betray their underlying prenatal and perinatal dimensions. The symbiotic gratification, to which ego psychologists attribute great significance, applies not only to the quality of breast feeding and anaclitic satisfaction in infancy, but also to the quality of the prenatal state. The same is true for the detrimental effects of symbiotic deprivation. I will use here as an illustration Margaret Mahler's description of the symbiotic phase: "During the symbiotic phase the infant behaves and functions as though he and his mother were an omnipotent system (a dual unity) within one common boundary—a symbiotic membrane as it were" (Mahler 1961). Similarly, the regression to autism and to an objectless state has distinct characteristics of a psychological return to the womb, not just to the early postnatal state.

Other important aspects of the disorders caused by disturbances in the development of object relations clearly point to perinatal dynamics. Thus splitting of the object world into good and bad, characteristic of borderline patients, reflects not just inconsistency of mothering ("good" and "bad mother") emphasized by ego psychologists. On a deeper level, its source is the fundamental ambiguity of the role that the mother plays in the life of the child, even under the best of circumstances. Prenatally and postnatally, she represents the life-giving and life-sustaining principle, while during delivery she turns into a life-threatening element.

The experiences of children suffering from infantile symbiotic psychosis, who are caught between the fear of separation and fear of engulfment, also clearly have their source in the trauma of birth, rather than just the transition from primary narcissism to object relations. Similarly the intensity of rage characterizing this category of patients betrays perinatal origins.

Psychodynamics of Adult Psychotic States

In spite of enormous investment of time, energy, and money into psychiatric research, the nature of the psychotic process has remained a mystery. Extensive systematic studies have revealed and explored important variables related to constitutional and genetic factors, hormonal and biochemical changes, biological correlates, psychological and social determinants, environmental precipitating influences, and many others. None of these has so far proved to be sufficiently consistent to provide a convincing explanation of the etiology of functional psychoses.

However, even if biological and biochemical research were able to detect processes that would show consistent correlation with the occurrence of psychotic states, that, in and of itself, would not help in understanding the nature and content of psychotic experiences. I have already touched upon this problem in an earlier chapter, while discussing laboratory research with psychedelic substances. In the states induced by chemically pure psychedelics, the biochemical trigger and its dosage are precisely known. And yet, all this gives no clues whatsoever for understanding the nature and content of the experiences involved and their interindividual and intraindividual variability. It only explains the emergence of deep unconscious material into consciousness.

The same dose given under the same circumstances to various people can induce a broad spectrum of experiences ranging from recollective-analytical self-exploration through manic and paranoid states to profound mystical revelations. This shows that the prospect of finding a simple biological solution for the complex problem of psychoses (and mystical states) is very meager indeed. In view of all these facts, it is difficult to accept speculations of this kind as serious scientific propositions. The potential to create these experiences is clearly an inherent property of the human psyche per se. The phenomenology of functional psychoses combines in various ways perinatal and transpersonal phenomena, with occasional admixture of postnatal biographical elements.

The experiences characteristic of BPM I are represented in the symptomatology of psychotic states both in their positive and negative form. Many patients experience episodes of symbiotic union with the Great Mother Goddess and a sense of being nourished in her womb or on her breast. This is also often experienced as an ecstatic union with Mother Nature, with the entire universe, and with God. When such experiences are supported, they can provide a powerful corrective experience for the lack of symbiotic satisfaction in the patient's own early history.

Conversely, there seems to exist a deep connection between disturbances of embryonal life and psychotic states with various paranoid distortions of reality. Since many prenatal disturbances are caused by chemical changes in the mother's body transmitted to the child through the umbilical cord, such paranoid episodes often focus on toxic factors or invisible noxious influences of some other kind. Many psychotic patients believe that their food is being poisoned, that some venomous gases are being pumped into their house, or that a diabolical enemy is exposing them to dangerous radiation. These hostile influences often coincide with visions of various evil entities and demonic archetypal beings.

Another source of paranoid states is the beginning phase of the second perinatal matrix. This is not surprising, since the onset of delivery is a major and irreversible disturbance of the prenatal existence. Considering how unpleasant and confusing these two situations must be for the fetus, it is not difficult to imagine that emergence of the memory of the onset of birth or of a serious intrauterine perturbation into consciousness can cause feelings of all-pervading anxiety. For obvious reasons, the source of this danger cannot be identified and remains unknown. The individual then tends to project these feelings on some threatening situation in the external world—on secret underground organizations, the Nazis, Communists, Freemasons, the Ku Klux Klan, or some other potentially or actually dangerous human group, possibly even on extraterrestrial invaders. Specific content of these frightening experiences can also be drawn from corresponding areas of the collective unconscious.

BPM II in its fully developed form contributes to psychotic symptomatology the theme of profound despair and melancholia, sense of eternal damnation, and the motif of inhuman tortures and diabolic ordeals. Many psychotic patients experience never-ending suffering in hell and tortures that seem to be coming from some ingenious contraptions designed for that purpose. Psychoanalytic studies showed that the influencing machine, described by many psychotic patients as causing excruciating agony, represents the body of the "bad mother." However, these studies failed to recognize that the dangerous and torturing maternal body belongs to the delivering mother, not to the nursing mother (Tausk 1933). Other psychotic themes related to BPM II are experiences of a meaningless, bizarre, and absurd world of cardboard figures and automata and the atmosphere of grotesque circus sideshows.

BPM III adds to the clinical picture of psychotic states a rich array of experiences that represent various facets of this complex matrix. The titanic aspect manifests in the form of unbearable tensions, powerful energy flows, clashes, and discharges. The corresponding imagery and ideation is related to violent scenes of wars, revolutions, and bloody massacres. These often can reach archetypal proportions and portray scenes of enormous scope—cosmic battle between the forces of good and evil, angels battling devils, titans challenging gods, or superheroes fighting mythological monsters.

Aggressive and sadomasochistic elements of BPM III account for visions of psychotic patients involving cruelties of all kinds, as well as occasional violence, automutilations, bloody murders, and suicides. Preoccupation with aberrant sexual fantasies and visions, experiences of sexual invasion, and painful interventions on reproductive organs are also characteristic features of the third perinatal matrix. Interest in feces and other biological material and magical power attributed to excreta and excretory functions betray the involvement of the scatological facet of BPM III. The same is true for coprophilia and coprophagia, retention of urine and feces or, conversely, lack of control over the sphincters. Experiences of satanic elements, such as the Witches' Sabbath or Black Mass rituals, combine death, sex, aggression, and scatology in a way that is highly characteristic of BPM III. They are common in the experiences of psychotic patients.

The transition from BPM III to BPM IV contributes to the spectrum of psychotic experiences sequences of psychospiritual death and rebirth, apocalyptic visions of destruction and recreation of the world, and the scenes of Judgment of the Dead or Last Judgment. This can be accompanied by identification with Christ or archetypal figures representing death and resurrection and lead to ego inflation and messianic feelings. Here belong also fantasies and experiences of fathering a Divine Child or giving birth to it. Experiences of divine epiphany, visions of the Great Mother Goddess or identification with her, encounters with angelic beings and deities appearing in light, and a sense of salvation and redemption also belong to characteristic manifestations of BPM IV.

At the time when I first suggested that much of psychotic symptomatology could be understood in terms of perinatal dynamics (Grof 1975), I was not able to find any clinical studies supporting this hypothesis, or even exploring this possibility. It was astonishing how little attention researchers had given to possible relationship between psychoses and the trauma of birth. Today, a quarter of a century later, there exists ample clinical evidence that the trauma of birth plays an important role in the genesis of psychoses.

As a matter of fact, viral infections during mother's pregnancy and obstetric complications during birth, including long labors and oxygen deprivation, are among the few consistently reported risk factors for schizophrenia (Wright et al. 1997, Verdoux and Murray 1998, Kane 1999, Dalman et al. 1999, Warner 1999). Because of the strong influence of biological thinking in psychiatry, the interpretations of these data tend to favor the assumption that birth had caused some subtle brain damage undetectable by current diagnostic methods. Mainstream theoreticians and clinicians fail to acknowledge the paramount role of birth as a major psychotrauma.

While the perinatal experiences described above often represent a combination of biological memories of birth and archetypal motifs with corresponding themes, the phenomenology of psychotic states can also contain various transpersonal experiences in a pure form, without the admixture of biological perinatal elements. The most common of these are experiences of past-life memories, of contact with extraterrestrial intelligence, and of encounters with various deities and demonic beings. Occasionally, individuals diagnosed as psychotic can also have very high spiritual experiences, such as identification with God, with the Absolute, or with the Metacosmic Void.

Many of the experiences described above have been reported by mystics, saints, prophets, and spiritual teachers of all ages. It is absurd, as we have seen earlier, to attribute all these experiences to some unknown pathological process in the brain or elsewhere in the body, which is a common practice in modern psychiatry. This naturally raises the question of the relationship between psychosis and mystical experience. I have so far used the terms psychosis and psychotic, as is common in academic psychiatry. As we will see, the observations and experiences from holotropic states suggest that the concept of psychosis has to be radically redefined.

When we look at these experiences in the context of the large cartography of the psyche that is not limited to postnatal biography, but includes the perinatal and transpersonal domain, it becomes clear that the difference between mysticism and mental disorder is less in the nature and content of the experiences involved than in the attitude toward them, the individual's "experiential style," the mode of interpretation, and the ability to integrate them. Joseph Campbell often used in his lectures a quote that captures this relationship: "The psychotic drowns in the same waters in which the mystic swims with delight." My own reservations toward this otherwise very appropriate quote are related to the fact that the experiences of the mystic are often difficult and taxing and not necessarily all delightful. But the mystic is capable of seeing these challenges in the larger context of a spiritual journey that has a deeper purpose and a desirable goal.

This approach to psychoses has profound implications not only for theory, but also for therapy and, most importantly, for the course and outcome of these states. The observations from experiential therapy confirm to a great extent the revolutionary ideas of the pioneers of alternative understanding of psychosis C. G. Jung (1960c), Roberto Assagioli (1977), and Abraham Maslow (1964). We will explore this important topic in the next chapter.

CHAPTER FOUR

Spiritual Emergency: Understanding and Treatment of Crises of Transformation

One of the most important implications of the research of holotropic states is the realization that many of the conditions, which are currently diagnosed as psychotic and indiscriminately treated by suppressive medication, are actually difficult stages of a radical personality transformation and of spiritual opening. If they are correctly understood and supported, these psychospiritual crises can result in emotional and psychosomatic healing, remarkable psychological changes, and consciousness evolution (Grof and Grof 1989, 1990).

Episodes of this nature can be found in the life stories of shamans, yogis, mystics, and saints. Mystical literature of the world describes these crises as important signposts of the spiritual path and confirms their healing and transformative potential. Mainstream psychiatrists are unable to see a difference between psychospiritual crises, or even uncomplicated mystical states, and serious mental illness, because of their narrow conceptual framework. Academic psychiatry has a model of the psyche limited to postnatal biography and a strong biological bias. These are serious obstacles in understanding the nature and content of psychotic states.

The term spiritual emergency which Christina and I coined for these states alludes to their positive potential. It is a play on words suggesting a crisis, but, at the same time, an opportunity to "emerge," to rise to a higher level of psychological functioning and spiritual awareness. We often refer in this context to the Chinese character for crisis that illustrates the basic idea of spiritual emergency. This ideogram is composed of two images, one of which represents danger and the other opportunity.

Among the benefits that can result from psychospiritual crises that are allowed to run their natural course are better psychosomatic health, increased zest for life, a more rewarding life strategy, and an expanded worldview that includes the spiritual dimension of existence. Successful completion and integration of such episodes also involves a substantial reduction of aggression, increase of racial, political, and religious tolerance, ecological awareness, and deep changes in the hierarchy of values and existential priorities. It is not an exaggeration to say that successful completion and integration of psychospiritual crises can move the individual to a higher level of consciousness evolution.

In recent decades, we have seen rapidly growing interest in spiritual matters that leads to extensive experimentation with ancient, aboriginal, and modern "technologies of the sacred," mind-altering techniques that can mediate spiritual opening. Among them are various shamanic methods, Oriental meditative practices, psychedelic substances, powerful experiential psychotherapies, and laboratory methods developed by experimental psychiatry. According to public polls, the number of Americans who have had spiritual experiences has significantly increased in the second half of this century. It seems that this has been accompanied by a parallel increase of spiritual emergencies.

More and more people seem to realize that genuine spirituality based on profound personal experience is a vitally important dimension of life. In view of the escalating global crisis brought about by the materialistic orientation of Western technological civilization, it has become obvious that we are paying a great price for having denied and rejected spirituality. We have banned from our life a force that nourishes, empowers, and gives meaning to human existence.

On the individual level, the toll for the loss of spirituality is an impoverished, alienated, and unfulfilling way of life and an increase of emotional and psychosomatic disorders. On the collective level, the absence of spiritual values leads to strategies of existence that threaten the survival of life on our planet, such as plundering of nonrenewable resources, polluting the natural environment, disturbing ecological balance, and using violence as a principal means of problem-solving.

It is, therefore, in the interest of all of us to find ways of bringing spirituality back into our individual and collective life. This would have to include not only theoretical recognition of spirituality as a vital aspect of existence, but also encouragement and social sanctioning of activities that mediate experiential access to spiritual dimensions of reality. And an important part of this effort would have to be development of an appropriate support system for people undergoing crises of spiritual opening which would make it possible to utilize the positive potential of these states.

In 1980, Christina founded the Spiritual Emergency Network (SEN), an organization that connects individuals undergoing psychospiritual crises with professionals who are able and willing to provide assistance based on the new understanding of these states. Filial branches of SEN now exist in many countries of the world.

Triggers of Spiritual Emergency

In many instances, it is possible to identify the situation that precipitated the psychospiritual crisis. It can be a primarily physical factor, such as a disease, accident, or operation. At other times, extreme physical exertion or prolonged lack of sleep may appear to be the most immediate trigger. In women, it can be childbirth, miscarriage, or abortion. We have also seen situations where the onset of the process coincided with an exceptionally powerful sexual experience.

In other cases, the psychospiritual crisis begins shortly after a traumatic emotional experience. This can be loss of an important relationship, such as death of a child or another close relative, divorce, or the end of a love affair. Similarly, a series of failures or loss of a job or property can immediately precede the onset of spiritual emergency. In predisposed individuals, the "last straw" can be an experience with psychedelic substances or a session of experiential psychotherapy.

One of the most important catalysts of spiritual emergency seems to be deep involvement in various forms of meditation and spiritual practice. This should not come as a surprise, since these methods have been specifically designed to facilitate spiritual experiences. We have been repeatedly contacted by persons in whom ongoing spontaneous occurrence of holotropic states was triggered by the practice of Zen or Vipassana Buddhist meditation, Kundalini yoga, Sufi exercises, monastic contemplation, or Christian prayer.

The wide range of triggers of spiritual emergency clearly suggests that the individual's readiness for inner transformation plays a far more important role than the external stimuli. When we look for a common denominator or final common pathway of the situations described above, we find that they all involve a radical shift in the balance between the unconscious and conscious processes. Weakening of psychological defenses or, conversely, increase of the energetic charge of the unconscious dynamics, makes it possible for the unconscious (and superconscious) material to emerge into consciousness.

It is well known that psychological defenses can be weakened by a variety of biological insults, such as physical trauma, exhaustion, sleep deprivation, or intoxication. Psychological traumas can mobilize the unconscious, particularly when they involve elements that are reminiscent of earlier traumas and are part of a significant COEX system. The strong potential of delivery as a trigger of psychospiritual crisis seems to reflect the fact that childbirth combines biological weakening with specific reactivation of the perinatal memories.

Failures and disappointments in professional and personal life can undermine and thwart the outward-oriented motivations and ambitions of the individual. This makes it more difficult to use external activities as an escape from emotional problems and leads to psychological withdrawal and turning of attention to the inner world. As a result, unconscious contents can emerge into consciousness and interfere with the individual's everyday experience or even completely override it.

Diagnosis of Spiritual Emergency

When we emphasize the need to recognize the existence of spiritual emergencies, this does not mean an indiscriminate rejection of the theories and practices of mainstream psychiatry. Not all states that are currently diagnosed as psychotic are crises of psychospiritual transformation or have a healing potential. Episodes of nonordinary states of consciousness cover a very broad spectrum from purely spiritual experiences to conditions that are clearly biological in nature and require medical treatment. While mainstream psychiatrists generally tend to pathologize mystical states, there also exists the opposite error of romanticizing and glorifying psychotic states or, even worse, overlooking a serious medical problem.

Many mental health professionals who encounter the concept of spiritual emergency want to know the exact criteria by which one can make the "differential diagnosis" between spiritual emergency and psychosis. Unfortunately, it is in principle impossible to make such differentiation according to the standards used in somatic medicine. Unlike diseases treated by somatic medicine, psychotic states that are not clearly organic in nature, "functional psychoses," are not medically defined. It is actually highly questionable whether they should be called diseases at all.

Functional psychoses certainly are not diseases in the same sense as diabetes, typhoid fever, or pernicious anemia. They do not yield any specific clinical or laboratory findings that would support the diagnosis and justify the assumption that they are of biological origin. The diagnosis of these states is based entirely on the observation of unusual experiences and behaviors for which contemporary psychiatry lacks adequate explanation. The meaningless attribute "endogenous" used for these conditions is tantamount to admission of this ignorance. At present, there is no reason to refer to these conditions as "mental diseases" and assume that the experiences involved are products of a pathological process in the brain yet to be discovered by future research.

If we give it some thought, we realize it is highly unlikely that a pathological process afflicting the brain could, in and of itself, generate the incredibly rich experiential spectrum of the states currently diagnosed as psychotic. How could possibly abnormal processes in the brain generate such experiences as culturally specific sequences of psychospiritual death and rebirth, convincing identification with Christ on the cross or with the dancing Shiva, an episode involving death on the barricades in Paris during the French revolution, or complex scenes of alien abduction?

When similar experiences manifest under circumstances in which the biological changes are accurately defined, such as administration of specific dosages of chemically pure LSD-25, the nature and origin of their content remain a deep mystery. The spectrum of possible reactions to LSD is very broad and includes episodes of mystical rapture, feelings of cosmic unity, sense of oneness with God, and past-life memories, as well as paranoid states, manic episodes, apocalyptic visions, exclusively psychosomatic responses, and many others. The same dosage given to different individuals or repeatedly to the same person can induce very different experiences.

Chemical changes in the organism obviously catalyze the experience, but are not, in and of themselves, capable of creating the intricate imagery and the rich philosophical and spiritual insights, let alone mediating access to accurate new information about various aspects of the universe. The administration of LSD and other similar substances can account for the emergence of deep unconscious material into consciousness, but cannot explain its nature and contents. To understand the phenomenology of psychedelic states calls for a much more sophisticated approach than a simple reference to abnormal biochemical or biological processes in the body. This requires a comprehensive approach that has to include transpersonal psychology, mythology, philosophy, and comparative religion. The same is true in regard to psychospiritual crises.

The experiences that manifest in spiritual emergencies clearly are not artificial products of aberrant pathophysiological processes in the brain, but belong to the psyche as such. Naturally, to be able to see it this way, we have to transcend the narrow understanding of the psyche offered by mainstream psychiatry and use a vastly expanded conceptual framework. Examples of such enlarged models of the psyche are the cartography described earlier in this book, Ken Wilber's spectrum psychology (Wilber 1977), Roberto Assagioli's psychosynthesis (Assagioli 1976), and C. G. Jung's concept of the psyche as *anima mundi,* or the world soul, that includes the historical and archetypal collective unconscious (Jung 1958). Such large and comprehensive understanding of the psyche is also characteristic of the great Eastern philosophies and the mystical traditions of the world.

Since functional psychoses are not defined medically but psychologically, it is impossible to provide a rigorous differential diagnosis between spiritual emergency and psychosis in the way it is done in medical practice in relation to different forms of encephalitis, brain tumors, or dementias. Considering this fact, is it possible to make any diagnostic conclusions at all? How can we approach this problem and what can we offer in lieu of a clear and unambiguous differential diagnosis between spiritual emergency and mental disease?

A viable alternative is to define the criteria that would make it possible to determine which individual, experiencing an intense spontaneous holotropic state of consciousness, is likely to be a good candidate for a therapeutic strategy that validates and supports the process. And, conversely, we can attempt to determine under what circumstances using an alternative approach would not be appropriate and when the current practice of routine psychopharmacological suppression of symptoms would be preferable.

A necessary prerequisite for such an evaluation is a good medical examination that eliminates conditions that are organic in nature and require biological treatment. Once this is accomplished, the next important guideline is the phenomenology of the non-ordinary state of consciousness in question. Spiritual emergencies involve a combination of biographical, perinatal, and transpersonal experiences that were described earlier in the discussion of the extended cartography of the psyche. Experiences of this kind can be induced in a group of randomly selected "normal" people not only by psychedelic substances, but also by such simple means as meditation, shamanic drumming, faster breathing, evocative music, bodywork, and variety of other nondrug techniques.

Those of us who work with holotropic breathwork see such experiences daily in our workshops and seminars and have the opportunity to appreciate their healing and transformative potential. In view of this fact, it is difficult to attribute similar experiences to some exotic and yet unknown pathology when they occur spontaneously in the middle of everyday life. It makes eminent sense to approach these experiences in the same way they are approached in holotropic sessions—to encourage people to surrender to the process and to support the emergence and full expression of the unconscious material that becomes available.

Another important prognostic indicator is the person's attitude to the process and his or her experiential style. It is generally very encouraging when people who have holotropic experiences recognize that what is happening to them is an inner process, are open to experiential work, and interested to try it. Transpersonal strategies are not appropriate for individuals who lack this elementary insight, use predominantly the mechanism of projection, or suffer from persecutory delusions. The capacity to form a good working relationship with an adequate amount of trust is an absolutely essential prerequisite for psychotherapeutic work with people in crisis.

It is also very important to pay attention to the way clients talk about their experiences. The communication style, in and of itself, often distinguishes promising candidates from inappropriate or questionable ones. It is a very good prognostic indicator if the person describes the experiences in a coherent and articulate way, however extraordinary and strange their content might be. In a sense, this would be similar to hearing an account of a person who has just had a psychedelic session and intelligently describes what to an uninformed person might appear to be strange and extravagant experiences.

Varieties of Spiritual Emergency

A question that is closely related to the problem of differential diagnosis of psychospiritual crises is their classification. Is it possible to distinguish and define among them certain specific types or categories in the way it is done in the Diagnostic and Statistical Manual of Mental Disorders (DSM IV) used by traditional psychiatrists? Before we address this question, it is necessary to emphasize that the attempts to classify psychiatric disorders, with the exception of those that are clearly organic in nature, has been generally unsuccessful.

There is general disagreement about diagnostic categories among individual psychiatrists and also among psychiatric societies of different countries. Although DSM has been revised and changed a number of times, clinicians complain that they have difficulties matching the symptoms of their clients with the official diagnostic categories. Spiritual emergencies are no exception; if anything, assigning people in psychospiritual crises to well-defined diagnostic pigeon holes is particularly problematic because of the fact that their phenomenology is unusually rich and can draw on all the levels of the psyche.

The symptoms of psychospiritual crises represent a manifestation and exteriorization of the deep dynamics of the human psyche. The individual human psyche is a multidimensional and multilevel system with no internal divisions and boundaries. The elements from postnatal biography and from the Freudian individual unconscious form a continuum with the dynamics of the perinatal level and the transpersonal domain. We cannot, therefore, expect to find clearly defined and demarcated types of spiritual emergency.

And yet, our work with individuals in psychospiritual crises, exchanges with colleagues doing similar work, and study of literature have convinced us that it is possible and useful to outline certain major forms of psychospiritual crises which have sufficiently characteristic features to be differentiated from others. Naturally, their boundaries are not clear and, in practice, we will see some significant overlaps. I will first present a list of the most important varieties of psychospiritual crises we have observed and then briefly discuss each of them.

1. Shamanic crisis
2. Awakening of Kundalini
3. Episodes of unitive consciousness ("peak experiences")
4. Psychological renewal through return to the center
5. Crisis of psychic opening

6. Past-life experiences
7. Communication with spirit guides and "channeling"
8. Near-death experiences (NDEs)
9. Close encounters with UFOs and alien abduction experiences
10. Possession states
11. Alcoholism and drug addiction

Shamanic Crisis

As we discussed earlier, the career of many shamans—witch doctors or medicine men and women—in different cultures, begins with a dramatic

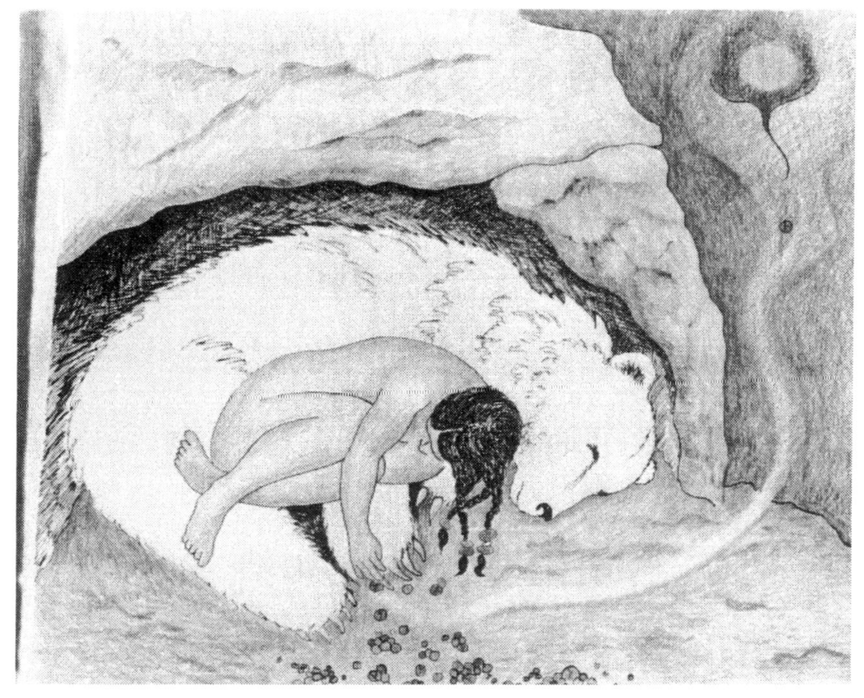

Paintings representing shamanic experiences in holotropic breathwork sessions. Above: Born of Bear on the Turquoise Moon; page 146: Guided by the Ravens to the Doorway beyond Space and Time; page 147: Initiation into Bear Tribe; page 148: Inuit Shaman Becomes Seal and Journeys to the Undersea World (Tai Ingrid Hazard).

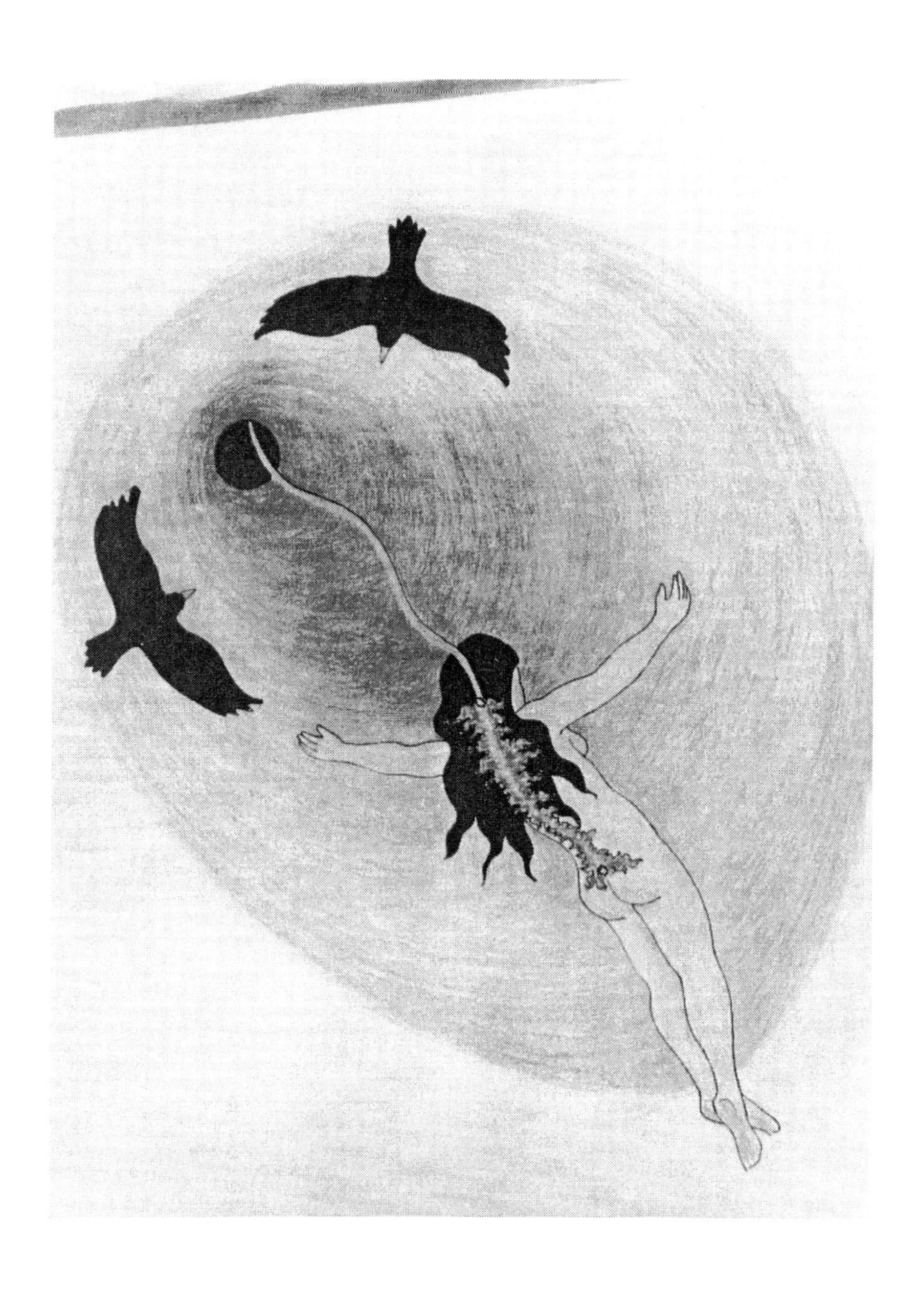

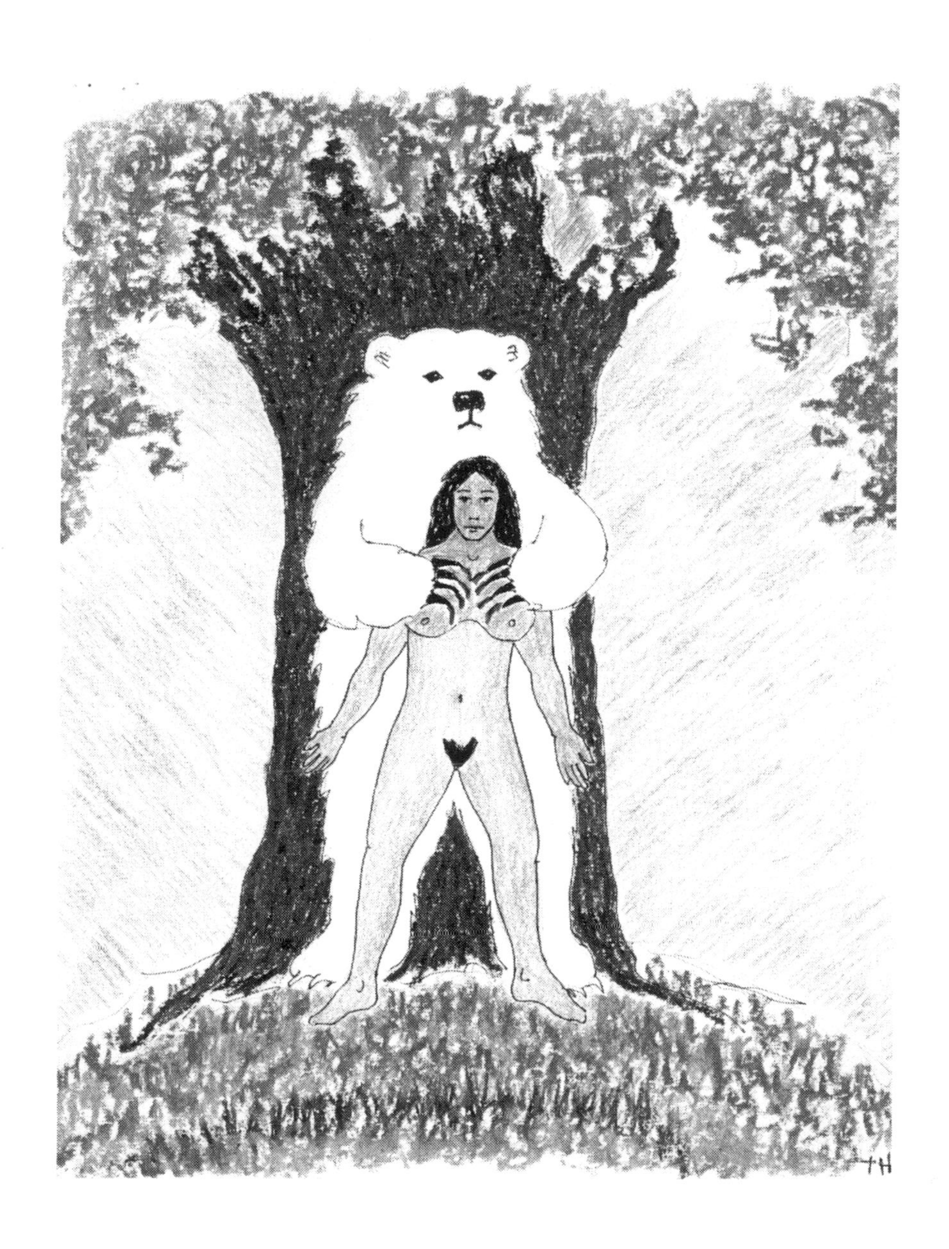

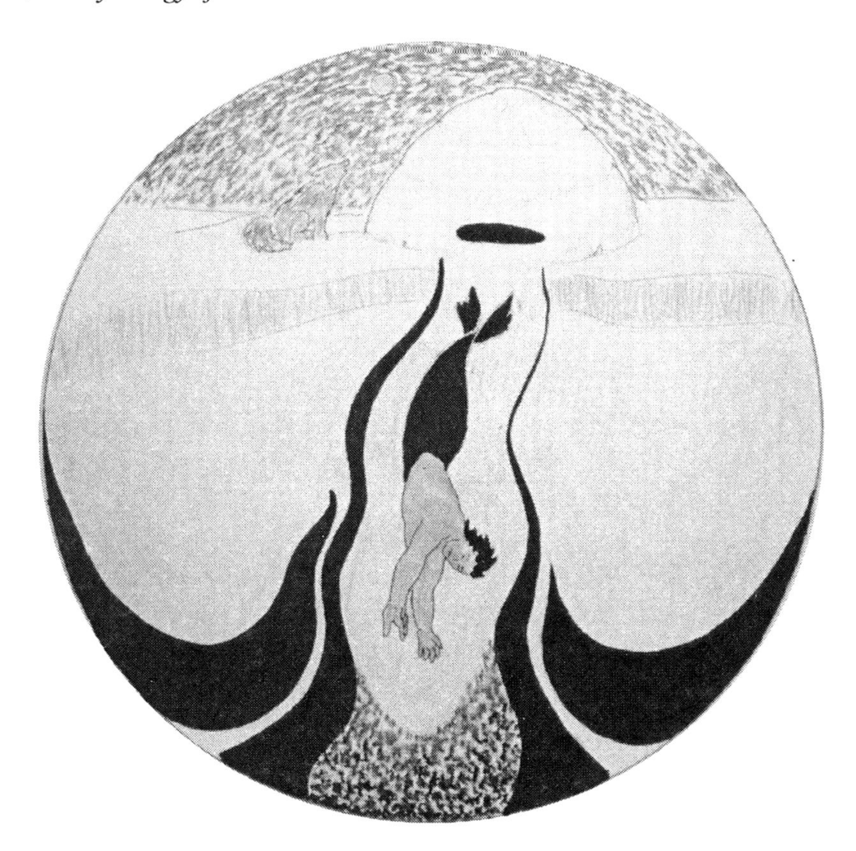

involuntary visionary state that the anthropologists call "shamanic illness." During such episodes, future shamans usually withdraw psychologically or even physically from their everyday environment and have powerful holotropic experiences. They typically undergo a journey into the underworld, the realm of the dead, where they are attacked by demons and exposed to horrendous tortures and ordeals.

This painful initiation culminates in experiences of death and dismemberment followed by rebirth and ascent to celestial regions. This might involve transformation into a bird, such as an eagle, thunderbird, or condor, and flight to the realm of the cosmic sun. The novice shaman can also have an experience of being carried by these birds into the solar region. In some cultures the motif of magic flight is replaced by that of reaching the celestial realms by climbing the world tree, a rainbow, a pole with many notches, or a ladder made of arrows.

In the course of these arduous visionary journeys, novice shamans develop deep contact with the forces of nature and with animals, both in their natural form and their archetypal versions—"animal spirits" or "power animals." When these visionary journeys are successfully completed, they can be profoundly healing. In this process, novice shamans free themselves often from emotional, psychosomatic, and even physical diseases. For this reason, shamans are frequently referred to as "wounded healers."

In many instances, the involuntary initiates attain in this experience deep insights into the energetic and transpersonal causes of diseases and learn how to heal others, as well as themselves. Following the successful completion of the initiatory crisis, the individual becomes a shaman and returns to his or her people as a fully functioning and honored member of the community. He or she assumes the combined role of a priest, visionary, and healer.

In our workshops and professional training, modern Americans, Europeans, Australians, and Asians have often experienced in their holotropic breathwork sessions episodes that bore close resemblance to shamanic crises. Besides the elements of physical and emotional torture, death, and rebirth, such states involved experiences of connection with animals, plants, and elemental forces of nature. The individuals experiencing such crises also often showed spontaneous tendencies to create rituals that were similar to those practiced by shamans of various cultures. On occasion, mental health professionals with this history have been able to use the lessons from their journeys in their work and create modern versions of shamanic procedures.

The attitude of native cultures toward shamanic crises has often been explained by the lack of elementary psychiatric knowledge and the resulting tendency to attribute every experience and behavior that these people do not understand to supernatural forces. However, nothing could be farther from truth. Shamanic cultures that recognize shamans and show them great respect, have no difficulty in differentiating them from individuals who are crazy or ill.

To be considered a shaman, the individual has to successfully complete the transformation journey and integrate the episodes of challenging holotropic states of consciousness. He or she has to be able to function at least as well as other members of the tribe. The way shamanic crises are approached and treated in these societies is an extremely useful and illustrative model of dealing with psychospiritual crises in general.

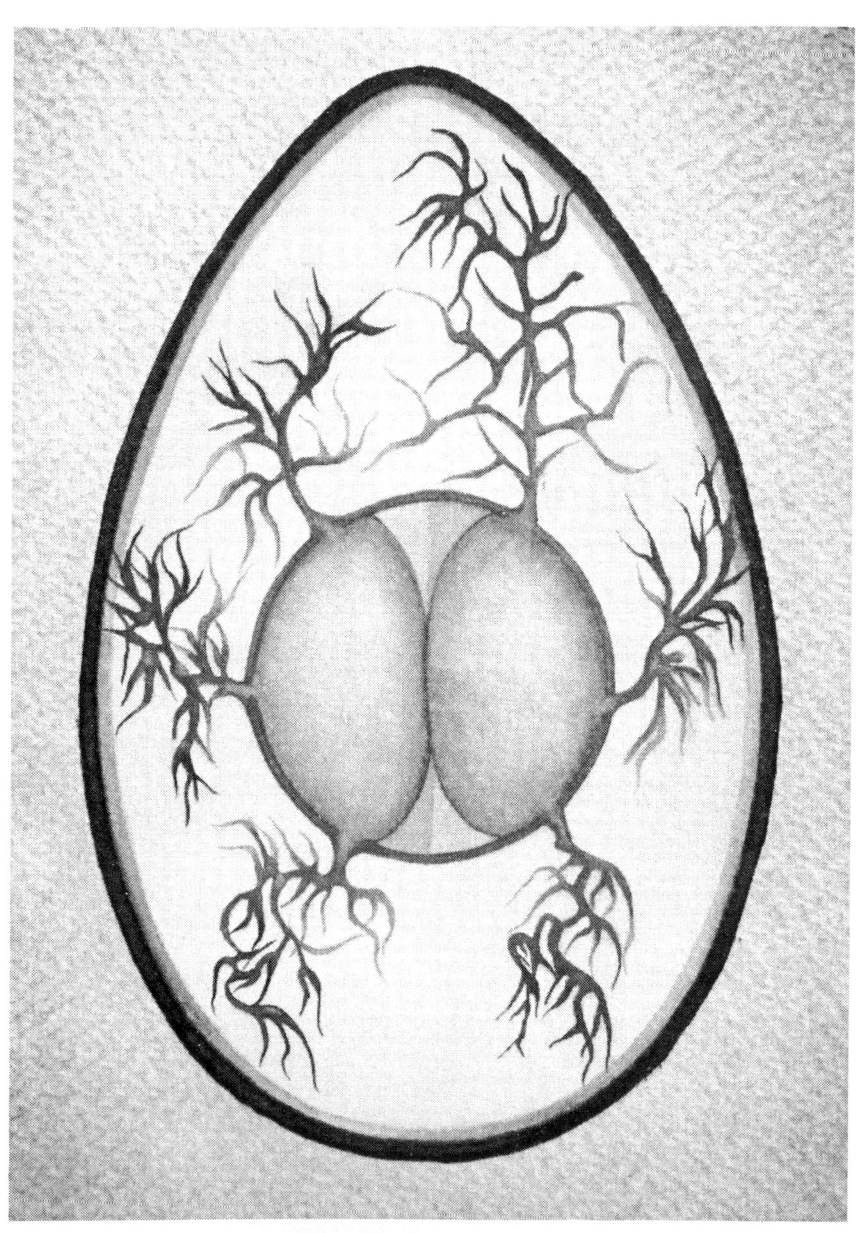

An artistic rendition of the four perinatal matrices suggesting that the four underlying patterns are manifestations of a universal archetypal sequence that does not govern only human birth, but a variety of other processes (pages 150–153).

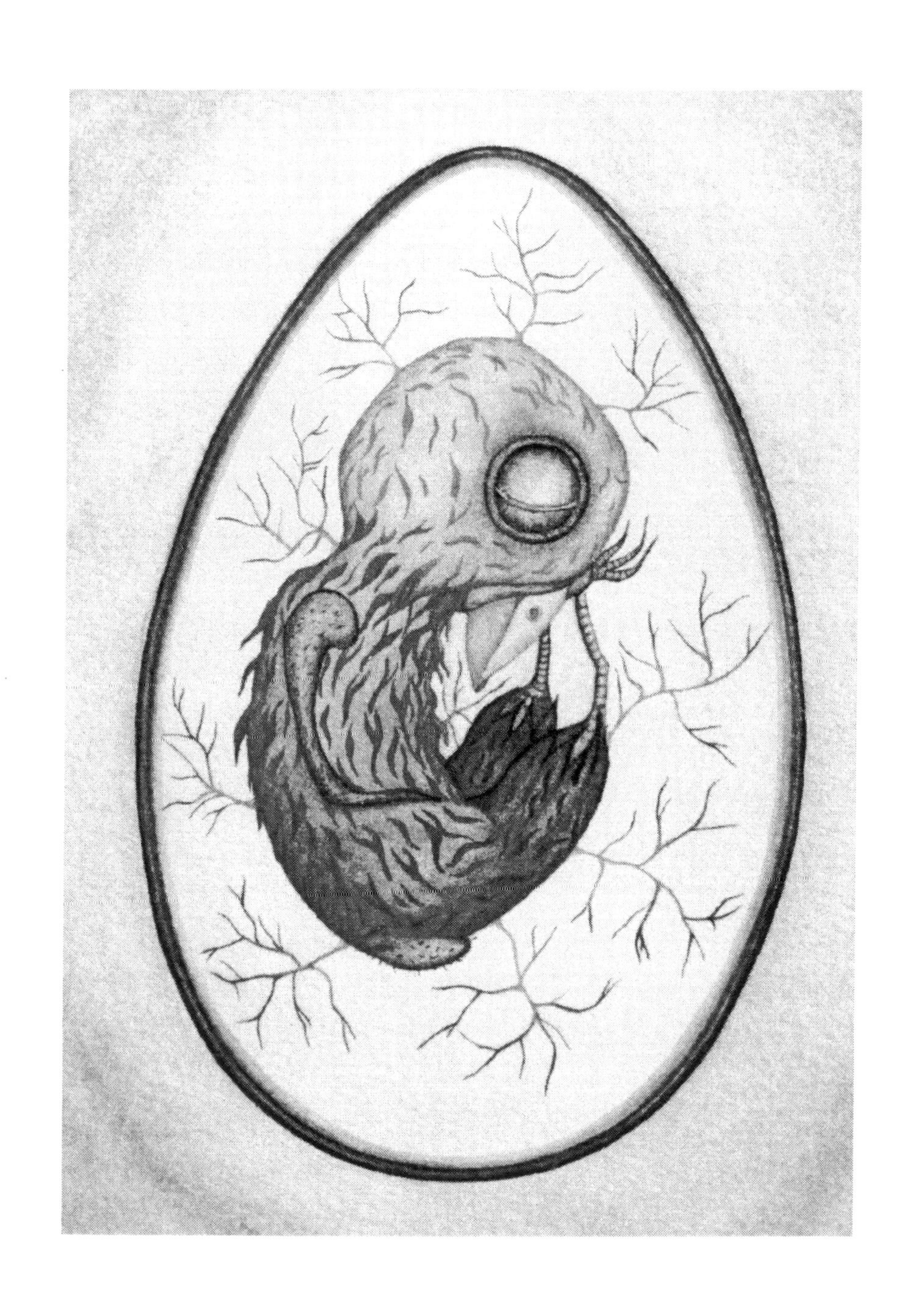

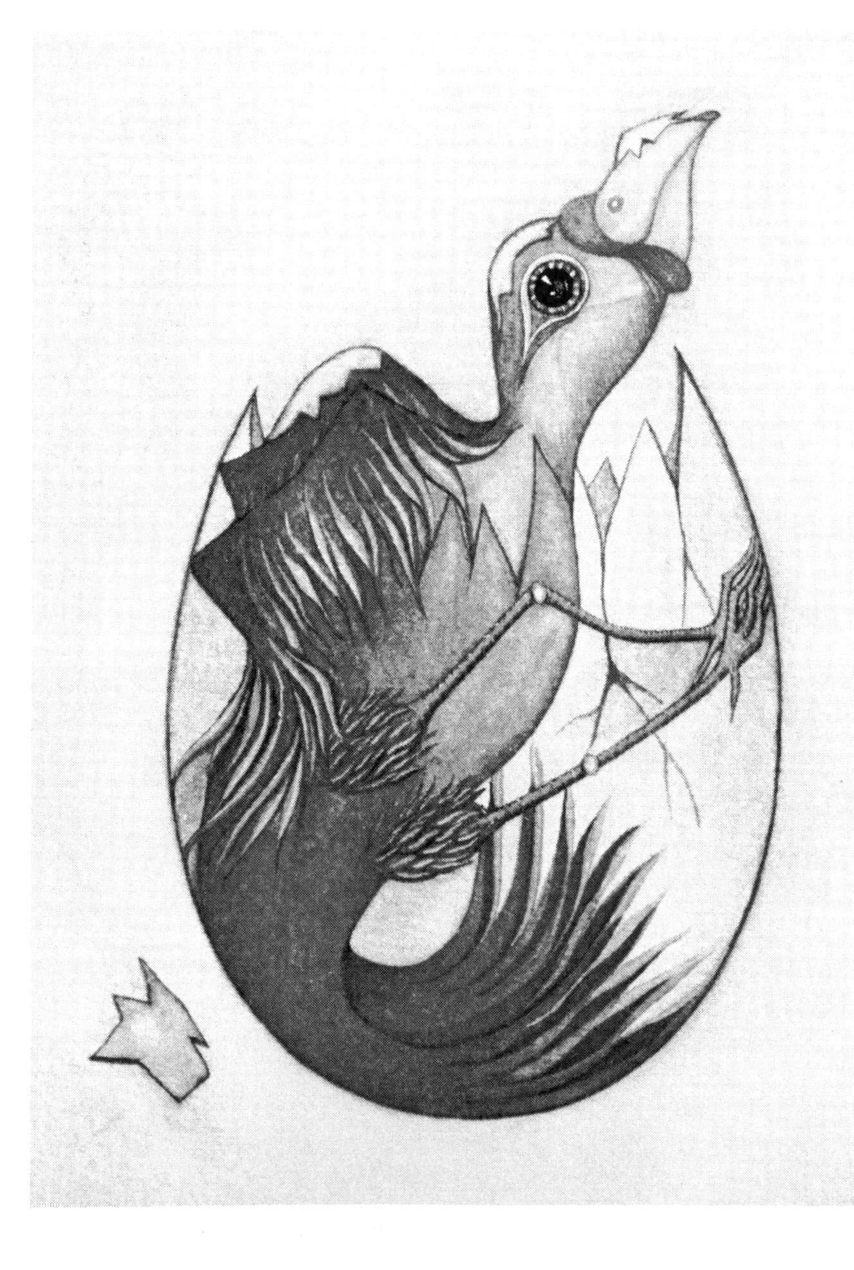

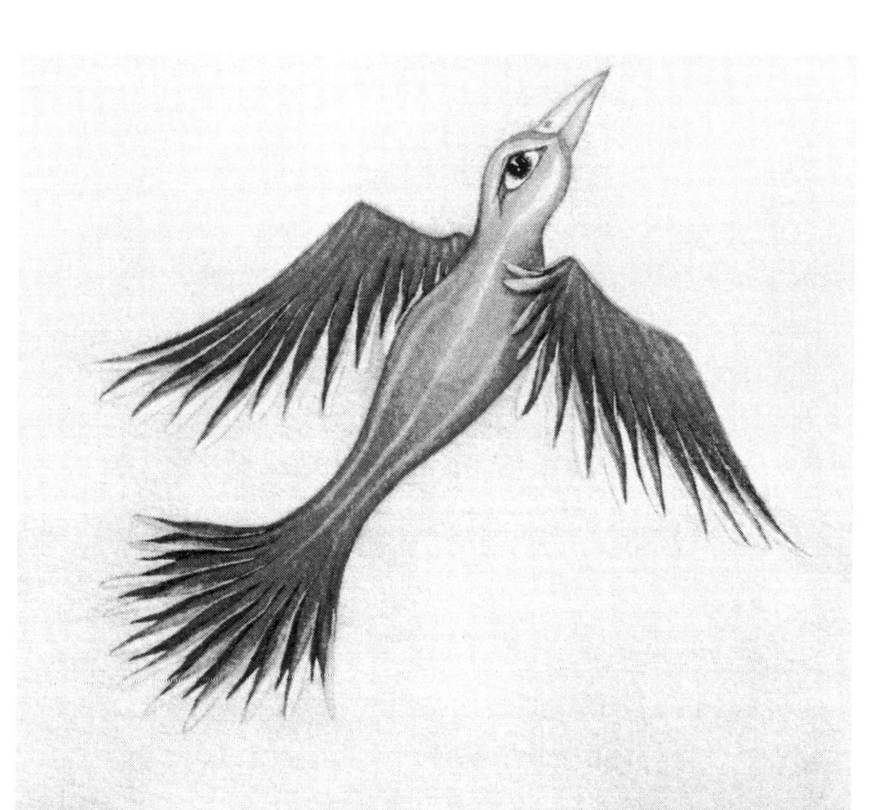

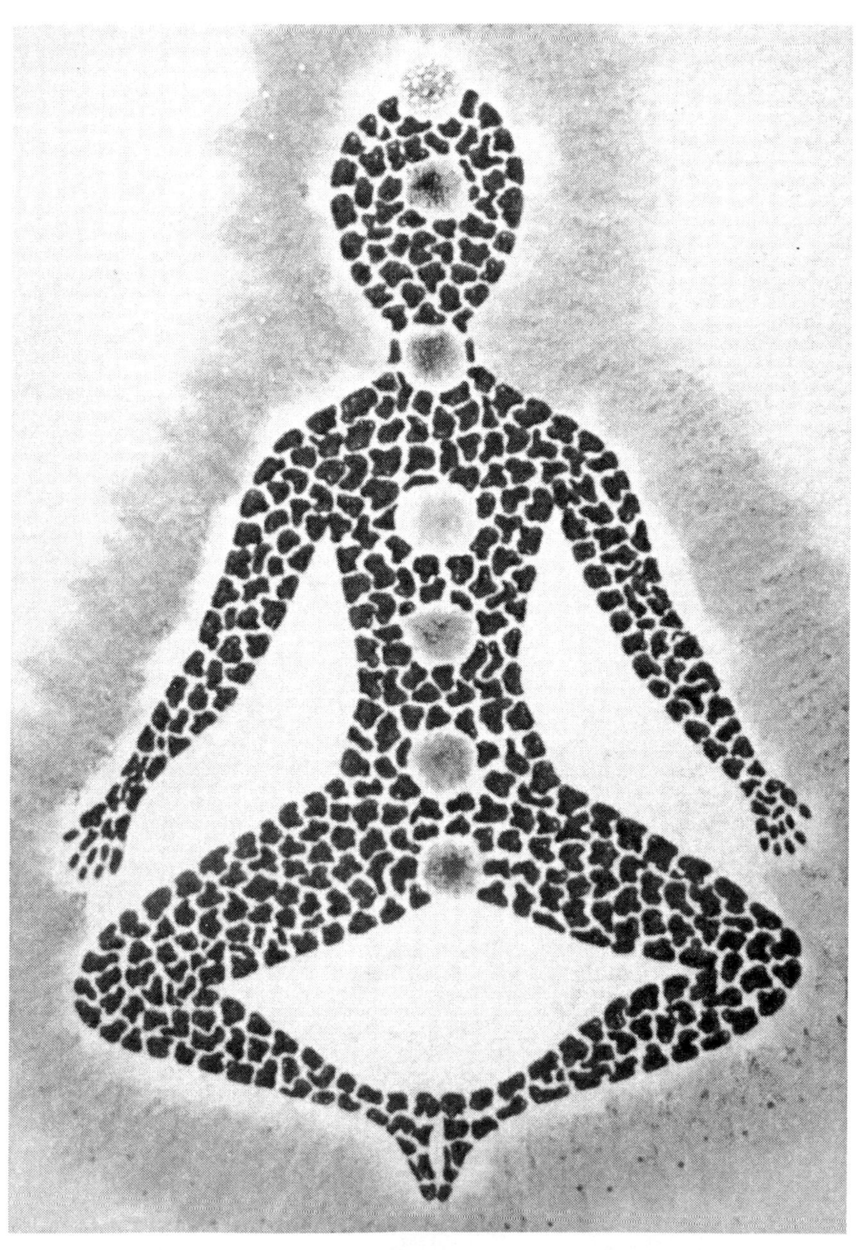

Experiences of Kundalini energy are among common manifestations in holotropic states of consciousness. Above: Experience of the chakra system and other parts of the energy body in a holotropic breathwork session.

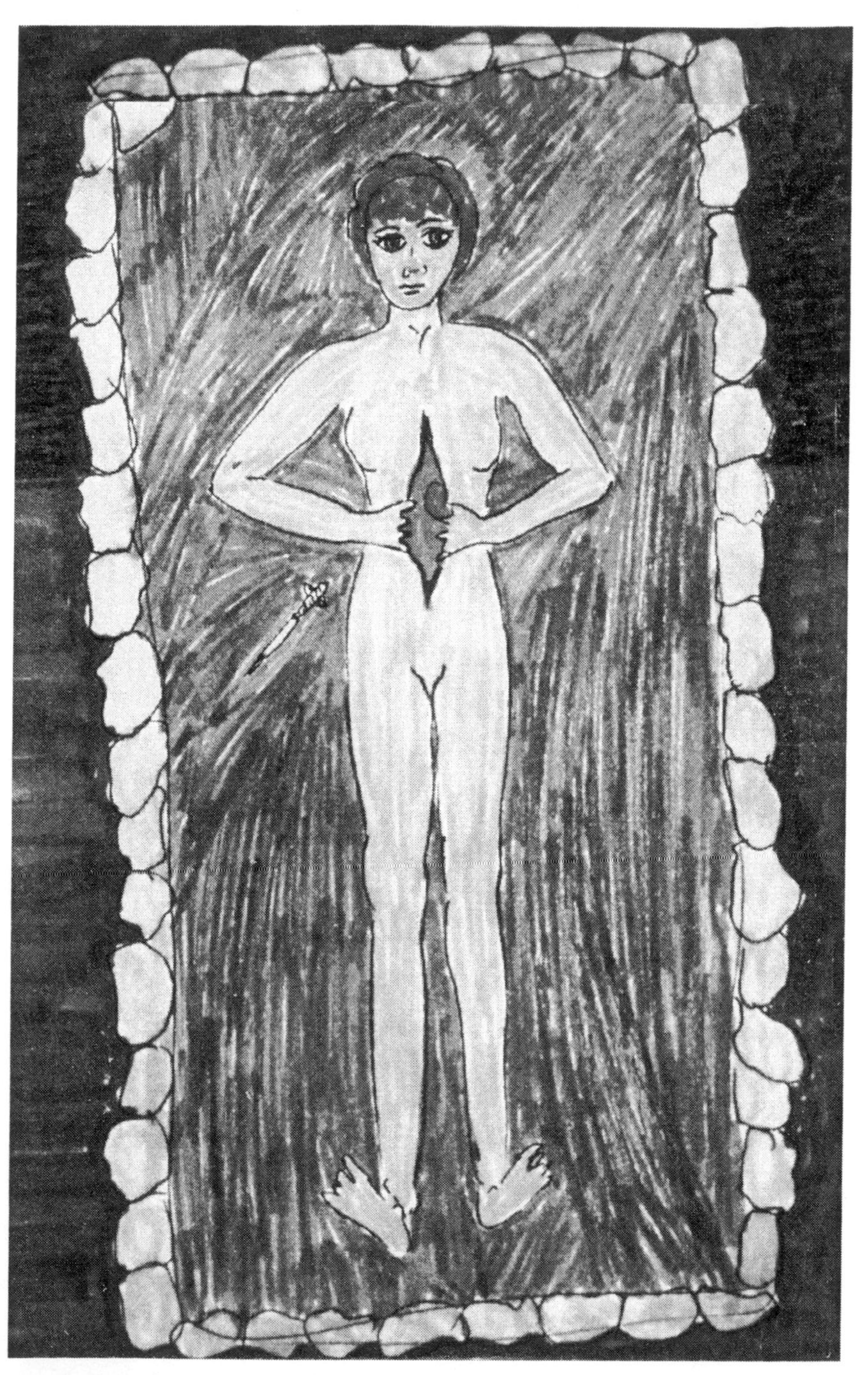

A painting depicting opening of the heart chakra in a psychedelic session.

The Awakening of Kundalini

The manifestations of this form of psychospiritual crisis resemble the descriptions of the awakening of *Kundalini,* or the Serpent Power, found in ancient Indian literature. According to the yogis, Kundalini is the generative cosmic energy, feminine in nature, that is responsible for the creation of the cosmos. In its latent form it resides at the base of the human spine in the subtle or energetic body, which is a field that pervades and permeates, as well as surrounds, the physical body. This latent energy can become activated by meditation, specific exercises, the intervention of an accomplished spiritual teacher (*guru*), a variety of emotional and physical factors, or for unknown reasons.

The activated Kundalini, called *shakti,* rises through the *nadis,* channels or conduits in the subtle body. As it ascends, it clears old traumatic imprints and opens the centers of psychic energy, called *chakras*. This process, although highly valued and considered beneficial in the yogic tradition, is not without dangers and requires expert guidance by a guru whose Kundalini is fully awakened and stabilized. The most dramatic signs of Kundalini awakening are physical and psychological manifestations called *kriyas.*

The kriyas involve intense sensations of energy and heat streaming up the spine, which can be associated with violent shaking, spasms, and twisting movements. Powerful waves of seemingly unmotivated emotions, such as anxiety, anger, sadness, or joy and ecstatic rapture, can surface and temporarily dominate the psyche. This can be accompanied by visions of brilliant light or various archetypal beings and a variety of internally perceived sounds. Many people involved in this process also have powerful experiences of what seem to be memories from past lives. Involuntary and often uncontrollable behaviors complete the picture: speaking in tongues, chanting unknown songs or sacred invocations (*mantras*), assuming yogic postures (*asanas*) and gestures (*mudras*), and making a variety of animal sounds and movements.

C. G. Jung and his co-workers dedicated to this phenomenon a series of special seminars (Jung 1996). Jung's perspective on Kundalini proved to be probably the most remarkable error of his entire career. He concluded that the awakening of Kundalini was an exclusively Eastern phenomenon and predicted that it would take at least a thousand years before this energy would be set into motion in the West as a result of depth psychology. In the last several decades, unmistakable signs of Kundalini awakening have been observed in thousands of Westerners. The credit for drawing attention to this phenomenon belongs to Californian psychiatrist and ophthalmologist Lee Sannella, who studied single-handedly nearly one thousand of such cases and summarized his findings in *The Kundalini Experience: Psychosis or Transcendence* (Sannella 1987).

Episodes of Unitive Consciousness ("Peak Experiences")

The American psychologist Abraham Maslow studied many hundreds of people who had unitive mystical experiences and coined for them the term *peak experiences* (Maslow 1964). He expressed sharp criticism of Western psychiatry's tendency to confuse such mystical states with mental disease. According to him, they should be considered supernormal, rather than abnormal, phenomena. If they are not interfered with and are allowed to run their natural course, these states typically lead to better functioning in the world and to "self-actualization" or "self-realization"—the capacity to express more fully one's creative potential and to live a more rewarding and satisfying life.

Psychiatrist and consciousness researcher Walter Pahnke developed a list of basic characteristics of a typical peak experience, based on the work of Abraham Maslow and W. T. Stace. He used the following criteria to describe this state of mind (Pahnke and Richards 1966):

Unity (inner and outer)
Strong positive emotion
Transcendence of time and space
Sense of sacredness (numinosity)
Paradoxical nature
Objectivity and reality of the insights
Ineffability
Positive aftereffects

As this list indicates, when we have a peak experience, we have a sense of overcoming the usual fragmentation of the mind and body and feel that we have reached a state of unity and wholeness. We also transcend the ordinary distinction between subject and object and experience an ecstatic union with humanity, nature, the cosmos, and God. This is associated with intense feelings of joy, bliss, serenity, and inner peace. In a mystical experience of this type, we have a sense of leaving ordinary reality, where space has three dimensions and time is linear. We enter a metaphysical, transcendent realm, where these categories no longer apply. In this state, infinity and eternity become experiential realities. The numinous quality of this state has nothing to do with previous religious beliefs; it reflects a direct apprehension of the divine nature of reality.

Descriptions of peak experiences are usually full of paradoxes. The experience can be described as "contentless, yet all-containing"; it has no specific content, but contains everything in a potential form. We can have a sense of being simultaneously everything and nothing. While our personal identity and the limited ego have disappeared, we feel that we have expanded to such an extent that our being encompasses the entire universe. Similarly, it is possible to perceive all forms as empty, or emptiness as being pregnant with forms. We can even reach a state in which we see that the world exists and does not exist at the same time.

The peak experience can convey what seems to be ultimate wisdom and knowledge in matters of cosmic relevance, which the Upanishads describe as "knowing That, the knowledge of which gives the knowledge of everything." What we have learned during this experience is ineffable; it cannot be described by words. The very nature and structure of our language seem to be inadequate for this purpose. Yet, the experience can profoundly influence our system of values and strategy of existence.

Because of the generally benign nature and positive potential of the peak experience, this is a category of spiritual emergency that should be least problematic. These experiences are by their nature transient and self-limited. There is absolutely no reason why they should have adverse consequences. And yet, due to the ignorance of our culture and misconceptions of the psychiatric profession concerning spiritual matters, many people who experience such states end up hospitalized, tranquilized, and receive pathological labels.

Psychological Renewal through Return to the Center

Another important type of transpersonal crisis was described by Californian psychiatrist and Jungian analyst John Weir Perry, who called it the "renewal process" (Perry 1974, 1976). Because of its depth and intensity, this is the type of psychospiritual crisis that is most likely diagnosed as serious mental disease. The experiences of people involved in the renewal process are so strange, extravagant, and far from everyday reality that it seems obvious that some serious pathological process must be affecting the functioning of their brains.

The individuals involved in this kind of crisis experience their psyche as a colossal battlefield where a cosmic combat is being played out between the forces of Good and Evil, or Light and Darkness. They are preoccupied with the theme of death—ritual killing, sacrifice, martyrdom, and afterlife. The problem of opposites fascinates them, particularly issues related to the differences between sexes. They experience themselves as the center of fantastic events that have cosmic relevance and are important for the future of the world. Their visionary states tend to take them farther and farther back—through their own history and the history of humanity, all the way to the creation of the world and the original ideal state of paradise. In this process, they seem to strive for perfection, trying to correct things that went wrong in the past.

After a period of turmoil and confusion, the experiences become more and more pleasant and start moving toward a resolution. The process often culminates in the experience of *hieros gamos*, or "sacred marriage," in which the individual is elevated to an illustrious or even divine status and experiences union with an equally distinguished partner. This indicates that the masculine and the feminine aspects of the personality are reaching a new balance. The sacred union can be experienced either with an imaginal archetypal figure, or is projected onto an idealized person from one's life, who then appears to be a karmic partner or a soul mate.

At this time, one can also have experiences involving what Jungian psychology interprets as symbols representing the Self, the transpersonal center that reflects our deepest and true nature and is related to, but not totally identical with, the Hindu concept of Atman-Brahman, the Divine Within. In visionary states, it can appear in the form of a source of light of supernatural beauty, precious stones, pearls, radiant jewels, and other similar symbolic representations. Examples of this development from painful and challenging experiences to the discovery of one's divinity can be found in John Perry's books (Perry 1953, 1974, 1976) and in *The Stormy Search for the Self,* our book on spiritual emergencies (Grof and Grof 1990).

At this stage of the process, these glorious experiences are interpreted as a personal apotheosis, a ritual celebration that raises one's experience of oneself to a highly exalted human status or to a state above the human condition altogether—a great leader, a world savior, or even the Lord of the Universe. This is often associated with a profound sense of spiritual rebirth that replaces the earlier preoccupation with death. At the time of completion and integration, one usually envisions an ideal future—a new world governed by love and justice, where all ills and evils have been overcome.

As the intensity of the process subsides, the person realizes that the entire drama was a psychological transformation that was limited to the inner world and did not necessarily involve external reality.

According to John Perry, the renewal process moves the individual in the direction of what Jung called "individuation"—a full realization and expression of one's deep potential. One aspect of Perry's research deserves special notice, since it produced what is probably the most convincing evidence against simplistic biological understanding of psychoses. He was able to show that the experiences involved in the renewal process exactly match the main themes of royal dramas that were enacted in many ancient cultures on New Year's Day.

In all these cultures, such ritual dramas celebrating the advent of the new year were performed during what Perry calls "the archaic era of incarnated myth." This was the period in the history of these cultures when the rulers were considered to be incarnated gods. Examples of such God/kings were the Egyptian pharaohs, the Peruvian Incas, the Hebrew and Hittite kings, or the Chinese and Japanese emperors (Perry 1966). The positive potential of the renewal process and its deep connection with archetypal symbolism and with specific periods of human history represents a very compelling argument against the theory that these experiences are chaotic pathological products of diseased brains.

The Crisis of Psychic Opening

An increase in intuitive abilities and the occurrence of psychic or paranormal phenomena are very common during spiritual emergencies of all kinds. However, in some instances, the influx of information from nonordinary sources, such as precognition, telepathy, or clairvoyance, becomes so overwhelming and confusing that it dominates the picture and constitutes a major problem, in and of itself.

Among the most dramatic manifestations of psychic opening are out-of-body experiences. In the middle of everyday life, and often without any noticeable trigger, one's consciousness can seem to detach from the body and witness what is happening in the surroundings of the body or in various remote locations. The information attained during these episodes by extrasensory perception often proves to correspond to consensus reality. Out-of-body experiences occur with extraordinary frequency in near-death situations, where the accuracy of this "remote viewing" has been established by systematic studies (Ring 1982, 1985, Ring and Valarino 1998).

People experiencing intense psychic opening might be so much in touch with the inner processes of others that they exhibit remarkable telepathic abilities. They might indiscriminately verbalize accurate incisive insights into other people's minds concerning various issues that these individuals are trying to hide. This can frighten, irritate, and alienate others so severely that it often becomes a significant factor contributing to unnecessary hospitalization. Similarly, accurate precognition of future situations and clairvoyant perception, particularly occurring repeatedly in impressive clusters, can seriously disturb the persons in crisis, as well as those around them, since it undermines their notion of reality.

In experiences that can be called "mediumistic," one has a sense of losing one's own identity and taking on the identity of another person. This can involve assuming the other person's body image, posture, gestures, facial expression, feelings, and even thought processes. Accomplished shamans, psychics, and spiritual healers can use such experiences in a controlled and productive way. Unlike the persons in spiritual emergency, they are capable of taking on the identity of others at will and also resuming their own separate identity after they accomplish the task of the session. During the crises of psychic opening, the sudden, unpredictable, and uncontrollable loss of one's ordinary identity can be very frightening.

People in spiritual crisis often experience uncanny coincidences that link the world of inner realities, such as dreams and visionary states, to happenings in everyday life. This phenomenon was first recognized and described by C. G. Jung, who gave it the name *synchronicity* and explored it in a special essay (Jung 1960a). The study of synchronistic events helped Jung realize that archetypes were not principles limited to the intrapsychic domain. It became clear to him that they have what he called "psychoid" quality, which means they govern not only the psyche, but also happenings in the world of consensus reality. I have explored this fascinating topic in my other writings (Grof 1988, 1992).

Jungian synchronicities represent authentic phenomena and cannot be ignored and discounted as accidental coincidences. They also should not be indiscriminately dismissed as pathological distortions of reality—perception of meaningful relations where, in actuality, there are none. This is a common practice in contemporary psychiatry where any allusion to meaningful coincidences is automatically diagnosed as "delusion of reference." In the case of true synchronicities, any open-minded witnesses, who have access to all the relevant information, recognize that the coincidences involved are beyond any reasonable statistical probability. Extraordinary synchronicities accompany many forms of spiritual emergency, and in crises of psychic opening they are particularly common.

Past-Life Experiences

Among the most dramatic and colorful transpersonal experiences occurring in holotropic states are what appear to be memories from previous incarnations. These are sequences that take place in other historical periods and other countries and are usually associated with powerful emotions and physical sensations. They often portray in great detail the persons, circumstances, and historical settings involved. Their most remarkable aspect is a convincing sense of remembering and reliving something that one has already seen (*déjà vu*) or experienced (*déjà vecu*) at some time in the past. This is clearly the same type of experience that in India and many other countries of the world inspired the belief in reincarnation and the law of karma.

The rich and accurate information that these "past-life memories" provide, as well as their healing potential, impels us to take them seriously. When the content of a karmic experience fully emerges into consciousness, it can suddenly provide an explanation for many otherwise incomprehensible aspects of one's daily life. Strange difficulties in relationships with certain people, unsubstantiated fears, and peculiar idiosyncrasies and attractions, as well as otherwise incomprehensible emotional and psychosomatic symptoms now seem to make sense as karmic carry-overs from a previous lifetime. These problems typically disappear when the karmic pattern in question is fully and consciously experienced. We will return to the intriguing subject of past-life experiences later in this book.

Past-life experiences can complicate life in several different ways. Before their content emerges fully into consciousness and reveals itself, one can be haunted in everyday life by strange emotions, physical feelings, and visions without knowing where these are coming from or what they mean. Experienced out of context, these experiences naturally appear incomprehensible and irrational. Another kind of complication occurs when a particularly strong karmic experience starts emerging into consciousness in the middle of everyday activities and interferes with normal functioning.

One might also feel compelled to act out some of the elements of the karmic pattern before it is fully experienced and understood or completed. For instance, it might suddenly seem that a certain person in one's present life played an important role in a previous incarnation, the memory of which is emerging into consciousness. When this happens, one may seek emotional contact with a person who now appears to be a "soul-mate" from one's karmic past or, conversely, confrontation and show-down with an adversary from another lifetime. This kind of activity can lead to unpleasant complications, since the alleged karmic partners usually have no basis in their own experiences for understanding this behavior.

Even if one manages to avoid the danger of embarrassing acting-out, the problems are not necessarily over. After a past-life memory has fully emerged into consciousness and its content and implications have been revealed to the experiencer, there remains one more challenge. One has to reconcile this experience with the traditional beliefs and values of the Western civilization. Denial of the possibility of reincarnation represents a rare instance of complete agreement between the Christian church and materialistic science. Therefore, in Western culture, acceptance and intellectual integration of a past-life memory is a difficult task for either an atheist or a traditionally religious person.

Assimilation of past-life experiences into one's belief system can be a relatively easy task for someone who does not have a strong commitment to Christianity or the materialistic worldview. The experiences are usually so convincing that one simply accepts their message and might even feel excited about this new discovery. However, fundamentalist Christians and those who have a strong investment in rationality and the traditional scientific perspective can be catapulted into period of confusion when they are confronted with convincing personal experiences that seem to challenge their belief system.

Communication with Spirit Guides and "Channeling"

Occasionally, one can encounter in a holotropic experience a being who seems to show interest in a personal relationship and assumes the position of a teacher, guide, protector, or simply a convenient source of information. Such beings are usually perceived as discarnate humans, suprahuman entities, or deities existing on higher planes of consciousness and endowed with extraordinary wisdom. Sometimes they take on the form of a person; at other times they appear as radiant sources of light, or simply let their presence be sensed. Their messages are usually received in the form of direct thought transfer or through other extrasensory means. In some instances, communication can take the form of verbal messages.

A particularly interesting phenomenon in this category is *channeling,* which has in recent years received much attention from the public and mass media. A "channeling" person transmits to others messages received from a source that appears to be external to his or her individual consciousness. It occurs through speaking in a trance, using automatic writing, or recording telepathically received thoughts. Channeling has played an important role in the history of humanity. Among the channeled spiritual teachings are many scriptures of enormous cultural influence, such as the ancient Indian Vedas, the Qur'an, and the Book of Mormon. A remarkable modern example of a channeled text is *A Course in Miracles,* recorded by psychologist Helen Schucman (Anonymous 1975).

Experiences of channeling can precipitate a serious psychological and spiritual crisis. One possibility is that the individual involved can interpret the experience as an indication of beginning insanity. This is particularly likely if the channeling involves hearing voices, a well-known symptom of paranoid schizophrenia. The quality of the channeled material varies from trivial and questionable chatter to extraordinary information. On occasion, channeling can provide consistently accurate data about subjects to which the recipient was never exposed. This fact can then appear to be a particularly convincing proof of the involvement of supernatural realities and can lead to serious philosophical confusion for an atheistic layperson or a scientist with a materialistic worldview.

Spirit guides are usually perceived as advanced spiritual beings on a high level of consciousness evolution, who are endowed with superior intelligence and extraordinary moral integrity. This can lead to highly problematic ego inflation in the channeler, who might feel chosen for a special mission and see it as a proof of his or her own superiority.

Near-Death Experiences (NDEs)

World mythology, folklore, and spiritual literature abound in vivid accounts of the experiences associated with death and dying. Special sacred texts have been dedicated exclusively to descriptions and discussions of the posthumous journey of the soul, such as the *Tibetan Book of the Dead* (*Bardo Thödol*), the *Egyptian Book of the Dead* (*Pert em hru*), and their European counterpart, *Ars Moriendi* (*The Art of Dying*) (Grof 1994).

In the past, this funeral mythology was discounted by Western scholars as a product of fantasy and wishful thinking of primitive people who were unable to face the fact of impermanence and their own mortality.

This situation changed dramatically after the publication of Raymond Moody's international best-seller *Life After Life,* which brought scientific confirmation of these accounts and showed that an encounter with death can be a fantastic adventure in consciousness. Moody's book was based on reports of 150 people who had experienced a close confrontation with death, or were actually pronounced clinically dead, but regained consciousness and lived to tell their stories (Moody 1975).

Moody reported that people who had near-death experiences (NDEs) frequently witnessed a review of their entire lives in the form of a colorful, incredibly condensed replay occurring within only seconds of clock time. Consciousness often detached from the body and floated freely above the scene, observing it with curiosity and detached amusement, or traveled to distant locations. Many people described passing through a dark tunnel or funnel toward a divine light of supernatural brilliance and beauty.

This light was not physical in nature, but had distinctly personal characteristics. It was a Being of Light, radiating infinite, all-embracing love, forgiveness, and acceptance. In a personal exchange, often perceived as an audience with God, these individuals received lessons regarding existence and universal laws and had the opportunity to evaluate their past by these new standards. Then they chose to return to ordinary reality and live their lives in a new way congruent with the principles they had learned. Since their publication, Moody's findings have been repeatedly confirmed by other researchers.

Most survivors emerge from their near-death experiences profoundly changed. They have a universal and all-encompassing spiritual vision of reality, a new system of values, and a radically different general strategy of life. They have deep appreciation for being alive and feel kinship with all living beings and concern for the future of humanity and the planet. However, the fact that the encounter with death has a great positive potential does not mean that this transformation is easy.

Near-death experiences very frequently lead to spiritual emergencies. A powerful NDE can radically undermine the worldview of the people involved, because it catapults them abruptly and without warning into a reality that is diametrically different. A car accident in the middle of rush-hour traffic or a heart attack during jogging can launch someone within a matter of seconds into a fantastic visionary adventure that tears his or her ordinary reality asunder. Following an NDE, people might need special counseling and support to be able to integrate these extraordinary experiences into their everyday life.

Close Encounters with UFOs and Alien Abduction Experiences

The experiences of encounters with extraterrestrial spacecrafts and of abduction by alien beings can often precipitate serious emotional and intellectual crises that have much in common with spiritual emergencies. This fact requires an explanation, since most people consider UFOs simply in terms of four alternatives: actual visitation of the earth by alien spacecraft, hoax, misperception of natural events and devices of terrestrial origin, and psychotic hallucinations. Alvin Lawson also has made an attempt to interpret UFO abduction experiences as misinterpretations of the trauma of birth, using my own clinical material (Lawson 1984).

Descriptions of UFO sightings typically refer to lights that have an uncanny, supernatural quality. These lights resemble those mentioned in many reports of visionary states. C. G. Jung, who dedicated a special study to the problem of "flying saucers," suggested that these phenomena might be archetypal visions originating in the collective unconscious of humanity, rather than psychotic hallucinations or visits by extraterrestrials from distant civilizations (Jung 1964). He supported his thesis by careful analysis of legends about flying discs that have been told throughout history and reports about actual apparitions that have occasionally caused crises and mass panic.

It has also been pointed out that the extraterrestrial beings involved in these encounters have important parallels in world mythology and religion, systems having their roots in the collective unconscious. The alien spacecrafts and cosmic flights depicted by those who were allegedly abducted or invited for a ride also have their parallels in spiritual literature, such as the chariot of the Vedic god Indra or Ezekiel's flaming machine described in the Bible. The fabulous landscapes and cities visited during these journeys resemble the visionary experiences of paradise, celestial realms, and cities of light.

The abductees often report that the aliens took them into a special laboratory and subjected them to various experiments and painful examinations using various exotic instruments. This can involve probing the cavities of the body with special emphasis on the sexual organs. There are frequent references to genetic experiments with the goal of producing hybrid offspring. These interventions are very painful and occasionally border on torture. This brings the experiences of the abductees close to the initiatory crises of the shamans and to the ordeals of the neophytes in the aboriginal rites of passage.

There is an additional reason why a UFO experience can precipitate a spiritual crisis. It is similar to the problem we have discussed earlier in relation to spirit guides and channeling. The alien visitors are usually seen as representatives of civilizations that are incomparably more advanced than ours, not only technologically but intellectually, morally, and spiritually. Such contact often has very powerful mystical undertones and is associated with insights of cosmic relevance. It is thus easy for the recipients of such special attention to interpret it as an indication of their own uniqueness.

Abductees might feel that they have attracted the interest of superior beings from an advanced civilization because they themselves are in some way exceptional and particularly suited for a special purpose. In Jungian psychology, a situation in which the individual claims the luster of the archetypal world for his or her own person is referred to as "ego inflation." For all these reasons, experiences of "close encounters" can lead to serious transpersonal crises.

People who have experienced the strange world of UFO experiences and alien abduction need professional help from someone who has general knowledge of archetypal psychology and who is also familiar with the specific characteristics of the UFO phenomenon. Experienced researchers, such as Harvard psychiatrist John Mack, have brought ample evidence that the alien abduction experiences represent a serious conceptual challenge for Western psychiatry and materialistic science in general and that it is naive and undefendable to see them as manifestations of mental disease or discard them altogether (Mack 1994, 1999).

Over the years, I have worked with many individuals who had powerful experiences of alien abduction in psychedelic sessions, holotropic breathwork, and spiritual emergencies. Almost without exception, these episodes were extremely powerful and experientially convincing; on occasion, they also had definite psychoid features. In view of my observations, I am convinced that these experiences represent phenomena *sui generis* and deserve to be seriously studied. The position of mainstream psychiatrists who see them as products of an unknown pathological process in the brain is clearly oversimplistic and highly implausible.

The alternative involving actual visits of aliens from other worlds is equally implausible. An extraterrestrial civilization capable of sending spaceships to our planet would have to have technical means that we cannot even imagine. We have enough information about the planets of the solar system to know that they are unlikely sources of such an expedition. The distance from the nearest celestial bodies outside the solar system amounts to many light years. Negotiating such distances would require velocities approaching the speed of light or interdimensional travel through hyperspace. A civilization capable of such achievments would very likely have technology that would make it impossible for us to differentiate between hallucinations and reality. Until more reliable information is available, it seems most plausible to see the UFO experiences as manifestations of archetypal elements from the collective unconscious.

Possession States

People in this type of transpersonal crisis have a distinct feeling that their psyche and body have been invaded and that they are being controlled by an evil entity or energy with personal characteristics. They perceive it as coming from outside their own personality and as being hostile and disturbing. It can appear to be a confused discarnate entity, a demonic being, or the consciousness of a wicked person invading them by means of black magic and hexing procedures.

There are many different types and degrees of such conditions. In some instances, the true nature of this disorder remains hidden. The problem manifests as serious psychopathology, such as antisocial or even criminal behavior, suicidal depression, murderous aggression or self-destructive behavior, promiscuous and deviant sexual impulses and acting-out, or excessive use of alcohol and drugs. It is often not until such a person starts experiential psychotherapy that "possession" is identified as a condition underlying these problems.

In the middle of an experiential session, the face of a possessed person can become cramped and take the form of a "mask of evil," and the eyes can assume a wild expression. The hands and body might develop strange contortions, and the voice may become altered and take on an otherworldly quality. When this situation is allowed to develop, the session can bear a striking resemblance to exorcisms in the Catholic Church, or exorcist rituals in various aboriginal cultures. The resolution often comes after dramatic episodes of choking, projectile vomiting, and frantic physical activity, or even temporary loss of control. Sequences of this kind can be unusually healing and transformative and often result in a deep spiritual conversion of the person involved. A detailed description of the most dramatic episode of this kind I have observed during my entire professional career can be found in my previous publication (the case of Flora) (Grof 1980).

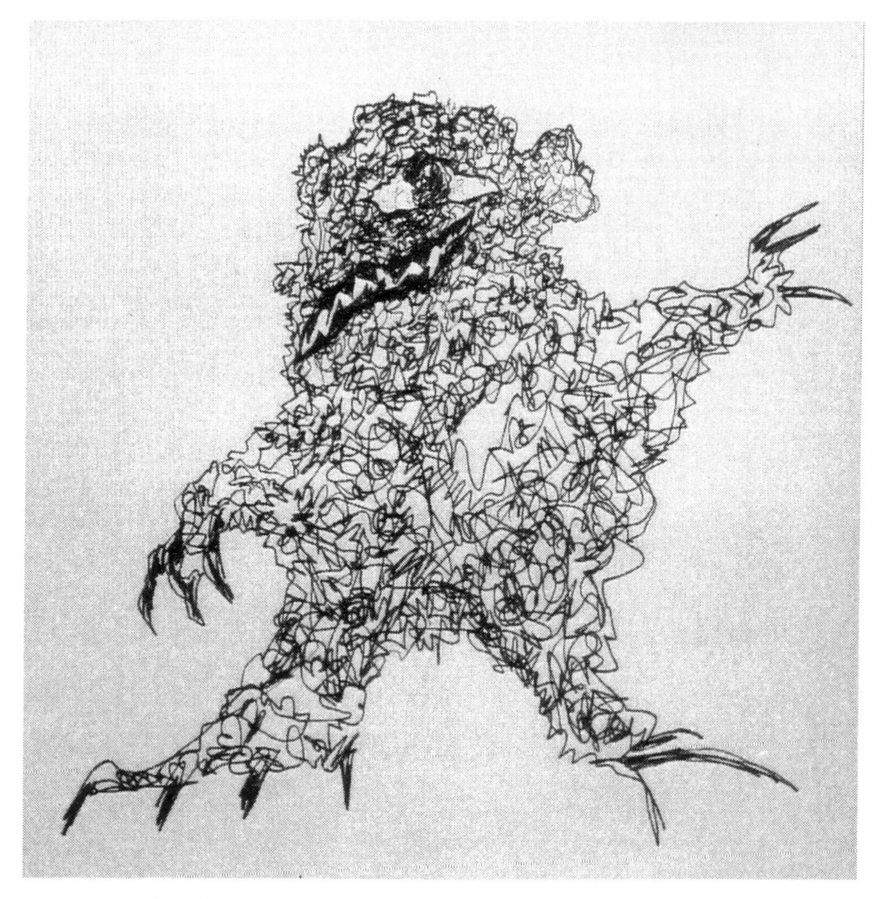

Drawing of a demonic figure encountered in a holotropic breathwork session. It was related to the power of the mind to separate us from our true nature.

Other times, the possessed person is aware of the presence of the "evil entity" and spends much effort trying to fight it and control its influence. In the extreme version of the possession state, the problematic energy can spontaneously manifest and take over in the middle of everyday life. This situation resembles the one described earlier for experiential sessions, but the individual here lacks the support and protection provided by the therapeutic context. Under such circumstances, he or she can feel extremely frightened and desperately alone. Relatives, friends, and often even therapists tend to withdraw from the "possessed" individual and respond with a strange mixture of metaphysical fear and moral rejection. They often label the person as evil and refuse further contact.

This condition clearly belongs in the category of "spiritual emergency," in spite of the fact that it involves negative energies and is associated with many objectionable forms of behavior. The demonic archetype is by its very nature transpersonal, since it represents the negative mirror image of the divine. It also often appears to be a "gateway phenomenon," comparable to the terrifying guardians flanking the doors of Oriental temples. It hides access to a profound spiritual experience, which often follows after a possession state has been successfully resolved. With the help of somebody who is not afraid of its uncanny nature and is able to encourage its full conscious manifestation, this energy can be dissipated, and remarkable healing occurs.

Alcoholism and Drug Addiction as Spiritual Emergency

It makes good sense to describe addiction as a form of spiritual emergency, in spite of the fact that it differs in its external manifestations from more obvious types of psychospiritual crises. In addiction, like in the possession states, the spiritual dimension is obscured by the destructive and self-destructive nature of the disorder. While in other forms of spiritual emergency people encounter problems because of their difficulty to cope with mystical experiences, in addiction the source of the problem is strong spiritual longing and the fact that the contact with the mystical dimension has not been made.

There exists ample evidence that behind the craving for drugs or alcohol is unrecognized craving for transcendence or wholeness. Many recovering people talk about their restless search for some unknown missing element or dimension in their lives and describe their unfulfilling and frustrating pursuit of substances, foods, relationships, possessions, or power that reflects an unrelenting effort to satiate this craving (Grof 1993).

We discussed earlier a certain superficial similarity that exists between mystical states and intoxication by alcohol or hard drugs. Both of these conditions share the sense of dissolution of individual boundaries, disappearance of disturbing emotions, and transcendence of mundane problems. Although the intoxication with alcohol or drugs lacks many important characteristics of the mystical state, such as serenity, numinosity, and richness of philosophical insights, the experiential overlap is sufficient to seduce alcoholics and addicts into abuse.

William James was aware of this connection and wrote about it in *Varieties of Religious Experience:* "The sway of alcohol over mankind is unquestionably due to its power to stimulate the mystical faculties of human nature, usually crushed to earth by the cold facts and criticisms of the sober hour. Sobriety diminishes, discriminates, and says no; drunkenness expands, unites and says yes" (James 1961). He also saw the implications of this fact for therapy, which he expressed very succinctly in his famous statement: "The best treatment for dipsomania (an archaic term for alcoholism) is religiomania."

C. G. Jung's independent insight in this regard was instrumental in the development of the worldwide network of Twelve Step Programs. It is not generally known that Jung played a very important role in the history of Alcoholics Anonymous (AA). The information about this little-known aspect of Jung's work can be found in a letter that Bill Wilson, the cofounder of AA, wrote to Jung in 1961 (Wilson and Jung 1963).

Jung had a patient, Roland H., who came to him after having exhausted other means of recovery from alcoholism. Following a temporary improvement after a year's treatment with Jung, he suffered a relapse. Jung told him that his case was hopeless and suggested that his only chance was to join a religious community and hope for a profound spiritual experience. Roland H. joined the Oxford Group, an evangelical movement emphasizing self-survey, confession, and service. There he experienced a religious conversion that freed him from alcoholism. He then returned to New York City and became very active in the Oxford Group there. He was able to help Bill Wilson's friend, Edwin T., who in turn helped Bill Wilson in his personal crisis. In his powerful spiritual experience, Bill Wilson had a vision of a worldwide chain-style fellowship of alcoholics helping each other.

Years later, Wilson wrote Jung a letter, in which he brought to his attention the important role that Jung played in the history of AA. In his answer, Jung wrote in reference to his patient: "His craving for alcohol was the equivalent, on a low level, of the spiritual thirst of our being for wholeness, expressed in medieval language: the union with God." Jung pointed out that in Latin, the term *spiritus* covers both meanings—alcohol and spirit. He then expressed succinctly in the sentence "spiritus contra spiritum" his belief that only a deep spiritual experience can save people from the ravages of alcohol. James's and Jung's insight have since been confirmed by clinical research (Grof 1980).

Treatment of Spiritual Emergencies

Psychotherapeutic strategy for individuals undergoing spiritual crises reflects the principles that we discussed earlier in this book. It is based on the realization that these states are not manifestations of an unknown pathological process, but results of a spontaneous movement in the psyche that has healing and transformative potential. Understanding and appropriate treatment of spiritual emergencies requires a vastly extended model of the psyche that includes the perinatal and transpersonal dimensions.

The nature and degree of the therapeutic assistance that is necessary depends on the intensity of the psychospiritual process involved. In mild forms of spiritual emergency the person in crisis is usually able to cope with the holotropic experiences in the course of everyday life. All that he or she needs is an opportunity to discuss the process with a transpersonally oriented therapist, who provides constructive feedback and helps the client to integrate the experiences into everyday life.

If the process is more active, it might require regular sessions of experiential therapy to facilitate emergence of the unconscious material and full expression of emotions and blocked physical energies. The general strategy of this approach is identical with that used in holotropic breathwork sessions. When the experiences are very intense, all we have to do is to encourage the client to surrender to the process. If we encounter strong psychological resistance, we might occasionally use releasing bodywork like in the termination periods of breathwork sessions. Holotropic breathwork as such is indicated only if the natural unfolding of the process reaches an impasse.

These intense experiential sessions can be complemented with Gestalt practice, Dora Kalff's Jungian sandplay, or bodywork with a psychologically experienced practitioner. A variety of auxiliary techniques can also prove extremely useful under these circumstances. Among them are writing of a log, painting of mandalas, expressive dancing, and jogging, swimming, or other sport activities. If the client is able to concentrate on reading, transpersonally oriented books, particularly those specifically focusing on the problem of psychospiritual crises or some specific aspect of his or her inner experiences, can be extremely helpful.

People whose experiences are so intense and dramatic that they cannot be handled on an out-patient basis, represent a special problem. There exist practically no facilities offering twenty-four-hour supervision without the use of routine, suppressive psychopharmacological intervention.

Several experimental facilities of this kind that existed in the past in California, such as John Perry's Diabasis in San Francisco and Chrysalis in San Diego or Barbara Findeisen's Pocket Ranch in Geyserville were short-lived. Creation of such alternative centers is a necessary prerequisite for effective therapy of spiritual emergencies in the future.

In some places, helpers have tried to overcome this deficiency by creating teams of trained assistants who take shifts in the client's home for the time of the duration of the episode. Management of intense acute forms of spiritual emergency requires some extraordinary measures, whether it occurs in a special facility or in a private home. Extended episodes of this kind can last days or weeks and can be associated with a lot of physical activity, intense emotions, loss of appetite, and insomnia. This brings a danger of dehydration, vitamin and mineral deficiency, and exhaustion. Insufficient supply of food can induce hypoglycemia that is known to weaken psychological defenses and bring additional material from the unconscious. This can lead to a vicious circle that perpetuates the acute condition. Tea with honey, bananas, or another form of food containing glucose can be of great help in grounding the process.

A person in intense psychospiritual crisis is usually so deeply involved in his or her experience that they forget about food, drink, and elementary hygiene. It is thus up to the helpers to take care of the client's basic needs. Since the care for people undergoing the most acute forms of spiritual emergency is unusually demanding, the helpers have to take shifts of reasonable duration to protect their own mental and physical health. To guarantee comprehensive and integrated care under these circumstances, it is necessary to keep a log and carefully record the intake of food, liquids, and vitamins.

Sleep deprivation, like fasting, tends to weaken the defenses and facilitate the influx of unconscious material into consciousness. This can also lead to a vicious circle that needs to be interrupted. It might, therefore, be necessary to give the client occasionally a minor tranquilizer or a hypnotic to secure sleep. In this context, medication is seen as a purely palliative measure and is not considered therapy, which is the way tranquilizing medication is often presented in mainstream psychiatry. The administration of minor tranquilizers or hypnotics interrupts the vicious circle and gives the client the necessary rest and the energy to continue the following day with the uncovering process.

In later stages of spiritual emergency, when the intensity of the process subsides, the person no longer requires constant supervision. He or she gradually returns to everyday activities and resumes the responsibility concerning basic care. The overall duration of the stay in a protected environment depends on the rate of stabilization and integration of the process. If necessary, we might schedule occasional experiential sessions and recommend the use of selected complementary and auxiliary techniques described earlier. Regular discussions about the experiences and insights from the time of the episode can be of great help in integrating the material.

The treatment of alcoholism and drug addiction presents some specific problems and has to be discussed separately from that of other spiritual emergencies. It is particularly the element of physiological addiction and the progressive nature of the disorder that requires special measures. Before dealing with the psychological problems underlying addiction, it is imperative to break the chemical cycle that perpetuates the use of substances. The individual has to go through a period of withdrawal and detoxification in a special residential facility.

Once this is accomplished, the focus can turn to the psychospiritual roots of the problem. As we have seen, alcoholism and drug addiction represent a misguided search for transcendence. For this reason, to be successful, the therapeutic program has to include as an integral part a strong emphasis on the spiritual dimension of the problem. Historically, most successful in combating addiction have been the programs of Alcoholics Anonymous (AA) and Narcotics Anonymous (NA), fellowships offering a comprehensive approach based on the Twelve Step philosophy outlined by Bill Wilson.

Following the program step by step, the alcoholic or addict recognizes and admits that they have lost control over their lives and have become powerless. They are encouraged to surrender and let a higher power of their own definition take over. A painful review of their personal history produces an inventory of their wrongdoings. This provides the basis for making amends to all the people whom they have hurt by their addiction. Those who have reached sobriety and are in recovery are then urged to carry the message to other addicts and to help them to overcome their habit.

The Twelve Step Programs are invaluable in providing support and guidance for alcoholics and addicts from the beginning of treatment throughout the years of sobriety and recovery. Since the focus of this book is the healing potential of holotropic states, we will now explore whether and in what way these states can be useful in the treatment of addiction. This question is closely related to the Eleventh Step that emphasizes the need "to improve through prayer and meditation our conscious contact with God as we understand God." Since holotropic states can facilitate mystical experiences, they clearly fit into this category.

Over the years, I have had extensive experience with the use of holotropic states in the treatment of alcoholics and addicts and also in the work with recovering people who used them to improve the quality of their sobriety. I participated in a team at the Maryland Psychiatric Research Center in Baltimore that conducted large, controlled studies of psychedelic therapy in alcoholics and hard drug addicts (Grof 1980). I have also had the opportunity to witness the effect of serial holotropic breathwork sessions on many recovering people in the context of our training. I will first share my own observations and experiences from this work and then discuss the problems involved in the larger context of the Twelve Step movement.

In my experience, it is highly unlikely that either holotropic breathwork or psychedelic therapy can help alcoholics and addicts at the time when they are actively using. Even deep and meaningful experiences do not seem to have the power to break the chemical cycle involved. Therapeutic work with holotropic states should be introduced only after alcoholics and addicts have undergone detoxification, overcome the withdrawal symptoms, and reached sobriety. Only then can they benefit from holotropic experiences and do some deep work on the psychological problems underlying their addiction. At this point, holotropic states can be extremely useful in helping them to confront traumatic memories, process difficult emotions associated with them, and obtain valuable insights into the psychological roots of their abuse.

Holotropic experiences can also mediate the process of psychospiritual death and rebirth that is known as "hitting bottom" and is a critical turning point in the life of many alcoholics and addicts. The experience of ego death happens here in a protected situation where it does not have the dangerous physical, interpersonal, and social consequences it would have if it happened spontaneously in the client's natural surroundings. And finally, holotropic states can mediate experiential access to profound spiritual experiences, the true object of the alcoholic's or addict's craving, and make it thus less likely that they will seek unfortunate surrogates in alcohol or narcotics.

The programs of psychedelic therapy for alcoholics and addicts conducted at the Maryland Psychiatric Research Center were very successful, in spite of the fact that the protocol limited the number of psychedelic sessions to a maximum of three. At a six-month follow-up, over 50 percent of chronic alcoholics and one-third of narcotic drug addicts participating in these programs were still sober and were considered "essentially rehabilitated" by an independent evaluation team (Pahnke et al. 1970, Savage and McCabe 1971, Grof 1980). Recovering people in our training and workshops, almost without exception, see holotropic breathwork as a way of improving the quality of their sobriety and facilitating their psychospiritual growth.

In spite of the evidence of its beneficial effects, the use of holotropic states in recovering people found strong opposition among some conservative members of the Twelve Step movement. These people assert that alcoholics and addicts seeking any form of a "high" are experiencing a "relapse." They pass this judgment not only when the holotropic state involves the use of psychedelic substances, but extend it also to experiential forms of psychotherapy and even to meditation, an approach explicitly mentioned in the description of the Eleventh Step.

It is likely that this extremist attitude has its roots in the history of AA. Bill Wilson, the co-founder of AA, participated after twenty years of sobriety in a psychedelic program and had several LSD sessions. He considered these experiences very useful and made an effort to introduce supervised psychedelic sessions into Alcoholics Anonymous. This caused a major turmoil in the movement and was eventually rejected.

We are confronted with two conflicting perspectives on the relationship between holotropic states and addiction. One of them sees any effort to depart from the ordinary state of consciousness to be unacceptable for an addicted person and qualifying as relapse. The contrary view is based on the idea that seeking a spiritual state is a legitimate and natural tendency of human nature and that striving for transcendence is the most powerful motivating force in the psyche (Weil 1972). Addiction then is a misguided and distorted form of this effort and the most effective remedy for it is facilitating access to a genuine experience of the divine.

The future will decide which of these two approaches will be adopted by professionals and by the recovering community. In my opinion, the most promising development would be a marriage of the Twelve Step Programs, the most effective method for treating alcoholism and drug addiction, with transpersonal psychology that can provide a solid theoretical background for spiritually grounded therapy. Responsible use of holotropic therapy would be a very logical integral part of such a comprehensive treatment.

My wife and I organized in the 1980s two meetings of the International Transpersonal Association (ITA) in Eugene, Oregon, and Atlanta, Georgia, that demonstrated the feasibility and usefulness of bringing together the Twelve Step Programs and transpersonal psychology. The empirical and theoretical justification for such merging was discussed in several publications (Grof 1987, Grof 1993, Sparks 1993).

The concept of "spiritual emergency" is new and will undoubtedly be complemented and refined in the future. However, we have repeatedly seen that even in its present form, as defined by Christina and myself, it has been of great help to many individuals in crises of transformation. We have observed that when these conditions are treated with respect and receive appropriate support, they can result in remarkable healing, deep positive transformation, and a higher level of functioning in everyday life. This has often happened in spite of the fact that, in the present situation, the conditions for treating people in psychospiritual crises are far from ideal.

In the future, the success of this endeavor could increase considerably, if people capable of assisting individuals in spiritual emergencies could have at their disposal a network of twenty-four-hour centers for those whose experiences are so intense that they cannot be treated on an out-patient basis. At present, the absence of such facilities and lack of support from the insurance companies for unconventional approaches represent the most serious obstacles in effective application of the new therapeutic strategies.

CHAPTER FIVE

New Perspectives in Psychotherapy and Self-Exploration

As we have seen, the research of holotropic states has revolutionized the understanding of emotional and psychosomatic disorders. It has shown that psychopathological symptoms and syndromes of psychogenic origin cannot be adequately explained by traumatic events in postnatal biography. Observations from deep experiential psychotherapy have revealed that these conditions have a multilevel dynamic structure which regularly includes significant elements from the perinatal and transpersonal domains of the psyche.

This discovery, in and of itself, paints a very pessimistic picture of psychotherapy as we usually understand it. It explains why verbal, biographically oriented approaches have been generally very disappointing as tools for dealing with serious clinical problems. Because of their conceptual and technical limitations, these methods are unable to reach the deeper roots of the conditions they are attempting to heal. Fortunately, the work with holotropic states does more than just reveal that emotional and psychosomatic disorders have significant perinatal and transpersonal dimensions. It also provides access to new effective therapeutic mechanisms operating on these deep levels of the psyche.

The approach to therapy and self-exploration based on the insights from the study of holotropic states and utilizing their healing potential can be referred to as *holotropic strategy of psychotherapy*. This strategy represents an important alternative to the techniques of various schools of depth psychology which emphasize verbal exchange between the therapist and the client. It also differs significantly from the experiential therapies developed by humanistic psychologists, which encourage direct emotional expression and engage the body, but are conducted in the ordinary state of consciousness.

What all the traditional schools of psychotherapy have in common is the effort to understand how the psyche functions, why the symptoms develop, and what they mean. This theoretical knowledge is then used in developing a technique that the therapist employs in his or her interaction with the client to correct the deviant psychodynamic processes. Although the client's cooperation is an essential part of the therapeutic process, it is the therapist who is seen as the active agent and the source of knowledge necessary for successful outcome.

This approach, although seldom seriously questioned by theoreticians and practitioners, is fraught with some major problems. The world of psychotherapy is fragmented into many schools that show a remarkable lack of agreement concerning the most fundamental theoretical issues, as well as the appropriate therapeutic measures. This is true not only for treatment modalities that are based on a priori incompatible philosophical and scientific assumptions, such as behaviorist deconditioning and psychoanalysis, but also for most schools of depth psychology that were inspired by Freud's original work. They disagree considerably in regard to the motivating forces of the psyche and to the factors that are responsible for the development of psychopathology. Consequently, they differ in their views concerning the strategy of psychotherapy and the nature of therapeutic interventions.

Under these circumstances, the therapist's activities and interventions are inevitably more or less arbitrary, since they are influenced by his or her basic training, as well as personal philosophy. The basic tenet of holotropic therapy is that symptoms of emotional and psychosomatic disorders represent an attempt of the organism to free itself from old traumatic imprints, heal itself, and simplify its functioning. They are not only a nuisance and complication of life, but also a major opportunity. Effective therapy then consists in temporary activation, intensification, and subsequent resolution of the symptoms. The facilitator then simply supports the process that has been spontaneously set in motion.

This is a principle that holotropic therapy shares with *homeopathy*. A homeopathic therapist has the task to identify and apply the remedy that in healthy individuals during the so-called *proofing* produces the symptoms that the client manifests (Vithoulkas 1980). The holotropic state of consciousness tends to function as a universal homeopathic remedy in that it activates any existing symptoms and exteriorizes the symptoms that are latent.

I have described earlier the "radar function" that operates in holotropic states and that automatically brings to the surface those unconscious contents that have a strong emotional charge and are most readily available for processing. This is an extremely useful and important mechanism that saves the therapist from the impossible task of determining what are the truly relevant aspects of the material the client is presenting,

At this point, it seems appropriate to say a few words about the attitude and approach to symptoms that exists in mainstream psychiatry. Under the influence of the medical model that dominates psychiatric thinking, psychiatrists generally tend to see the intensity of symptoms as an indicator of the seriousness of emotional and psychosomatic disorders. Intensification of symptoms is thus seen as "worsening" of the clinical condition and amelioration of symptoms as "improvement."

This is a common practice in everyday clinical work, in spite of the fact that it is in conflict with the experience from dynamic psychiatry. In the course of systematic psychotherapy, intensification of symptoms suggests emergence of important unconscious material and often heralds major progress in therapy. It is also well known that acute and dramatic emotional states rich in symptoms usually have a much better clinical prognosis than slowly and insidiously developing conditions with less conspicuous symptoms. The confusion of seriousness of the condition with the intensity of symptoms, together with some other factors, such as the work load of most psychiatrists, economic concerns, and the convenience of pharmacological interventions, is responsible for the fact that much of psychiatric therapy focuses almost exclusively on the suppression of symptoms.

Although this practice reflects the influence of the medical model on psychiatry, in somatic medicine such exclusive focus on suppression of symptoms would actually be considered very bad medical practice. In the treatment of physical diseases, symptomatic therapy is applied only if we simultaneously administer causal measures. For example, applying ice and feeding aspirin to a patient with high fever without establishing the etiology of the febrile condition obviously would not be acceptable medical practice. The only exception to this rule is therapy of incurable diseases, which is limited to symptomatic treatment, because causal treatment is not known.

In one of his lectures in the 1970s, Fritjof Capra used an interesting parable to illustrate the fallacy of focusing on the symptoms rather than the underlying problem. Imagine that you are driving a car and suddenly a red light appears on the dash board. It happens to be the light indicating that your oil is dangerously low. You do not understand the functioning of the car, but you know that a red light on the dash board means trouble. You take your car to the garage and present the problem to the mechanic. The mechanic takes a look and says: "Red light? Piece of cake!" He reaches for the wire and pulls it out. The red light disappears and he sends you back on the road.

We would not have a very high opinion of a mechanic who would offer this type of "solution." We expected an intervention that would fix the problem and leave the signaling system intact, not elimination of the mechanism that would warn us if there were a problem. Similarly, the goal of real therapy of emotional disorders is to attain a situation in which symptoms do not manifest, because there is no reason for them to manifest, not one in which they cannot appear because the signaling system is out of commission.

This is a solution that the holotropic strategy of therapy aims for. When we encourage, facilitate, and support full emergence of the material underlying the symptoms, the process accomplishes what the organism was attempting to achieve—liberation from traumatic imprints and release of pent-up emotional and physical energies associated with them. As we saw in the chapter on spiritual emergency, this understanding of the therapeutic process does not apply only to neuroses and psychosomatic disorders, but also to many conditions that mainstream psychiatrists would diagnose as psychotic and see as manifestations of serious mental disease.

The inability to recognize the healing potential of such extreme states reflects the narrow conceptual framework of Western psychiatry that is limited to postnatal biography and the individual unconscious. Experiences for which this narrow framework does not have a logical explanation are then attributed to a pathological process of unknown origin. The extended cartography of the psyche that includes the perinatal and transpersonal domains provides a natural explanation for the intensity and content of such extreme states.

Another important assumption of holotropic therapy is that an average person of our culture operates in a way that is far below his or her real potential and capacity. This impoverishment is due to the fact that he or she identifies with only a small fraction of their being—the physical body and the ego. This false identification leads to an inauthentic, unhealthy, and unfulfilling way of life and contributes to the development of emotional and psychosomatic disorders of psychological origin. The appearance of distressing symptoms that do not have any organic basis can be seen as an indication that the individual operating on false premises has reached a point where it became obvious that the old way of being in the world does not work any more and has become untenable.

When it becomes clear that the orientation toward the external world has failed, the individual psychologically withdraws into his or her inner world and strongly emotionally charged contents of the unconscious start emerging into consciousness. This invasion of disturbing material tends to interfere with the individual's ability to function in everyday life. Such a breakdown can occur in a certain limited area of life—such as marriage and sexual life, professional activity, or pursuit of various personal ambitions—or afflict simultaneously all segments and aspects of the individual's life.

The extent and depth of this breakdown depend on the timing of important traumas that the individual suffered in infancy and childhood; they determine whether the process reaches neurotic or psychotic proportions. Traumatization in later stages of postnatal life cause disposition to a neurotic breakdown that afflicts only certain segments of the individual's interpersonal and social functioning. Process that reaches psychotic proportions involves all areas of life; it usually indicates serious disturbances in the early stages of infancy.

The resulting situation represents a crisis or even emergency, but also a great opportunity. The main objective of holotropic therapy is to support the unconscious activity or even further mobilize it and bring into full consciousness the memories of repressed and forgotten traumas. In this process, the energy bound in emotional and psychosomatic symptoms is liberated and discharged and symptoms are converted into a stream of experiences. The content of these experiences can be drawn from any level of the psyche—biographical, perinatal, or transpersonal.

The task of the facilitator or therapist in holotropic therapy is to support the experiential process with full trust in its healing nature, without trying to direct it or change it in any way. The process is guided by the client's own inner healing intelligence. The term *therapist* is used here in the sense of the Greek *therapeutes,* which means the person assisting in the healing process, not an active agent whose task is to "fix the client." It is important for the therapist to support the experiential unfolding, even if he or she does not rationally understand it.

Some powerful healing and transforming experiences might not have any specific content at all; they consist of sequences of intense build-up of emotions or physical tensions and subsequent deep release and relaxation. Frequently the insights and specific contents emerge later in the process, or even in the following sessions. In some instances the resolution occurs on the biographical level, in others in connection with perinatal material or with various transpersonal themes. Dramatic healing and personality transformation with lasting effects often result from experiences that altogether elude rational understanding.

The most powerful technique of inducing holotropic states for therapeutic purposes is, without any doubt, the use of psychedelic plants or substances. At this time, there are only a few official research projects involving these substances and psychedelic therapy is not generally available anywhere in the world. I will, therefore, focus our discussion on an approach that can induce holotropic states by nonpharmacological means and is not associated with complicated political, administrative, and legal problems.

Theory and Practice of Holotropic Breathwork

In the last twenty-five years, my wife Christina and I have developed an approach to therapy and self-exploration that we call "holotropic breathwork." It induces very powerful holotropic states by a combination of very simple means— accelerated breathing, evocative music, and a technique of bodywork that helps to release residual bioenergetic and emotional blocks. In its theory and practice, this method brings together and integrates various elements from ancient and aboriginal traditions, Eastern spiritual philosophies, and Western depth psychology.

The Healing Power of Breath

The use of various breathing techniques for religious and healing purposes can be traced back to the dawn of human history. In ancient and preindustrial cultures, breath and breathing have played a very important role in cosmology, mythology, and philosophy, as well as an important tool in ritual and spiritual practice. Since earliest history, virtually every major psychospiritual system seeking to comprehend human nature has viewed breath as a crucial link between the body, mind, and spirit. This is clearly reflected in the words many languages use for breath.

In the ancient Indian literature, the term *prana* meant not only physical breath and air, but also the sacred essence of life. Similarly, in traditional Chinese medicine, the word *chi* refers to the cosmic essence and the energy of life, as well as the natural air we breathe by our lungs. In Japan, the corresponding word is *ki*. Ki plays an extremely important role in Japanese spiritual practices and martial arts. In ancient Greece, the word *pneuma* meant both air or breath and spirit or the essence of life. The Greeks also saw breath as being closely related to the psyche. The term *phren* was used both for the diaphragm, the largest muscle involved in breathing, and mind (as we see in the term *schizophrenia* = split mind). In the old Hebrew tradition, the same word, *ruach,* denoted both breath and creative spirit, which were seen as identical. In Latin the same name was used for breath and spirit—*spiritus*. Similarly, in Slavic languages, spirit and breath have the same linguistic root.

It has been known for centuries that it is possible to influence consciousness by techniques that involve breathing. The procedures that have been used for this purpose by various ancient and non-Western cultures cover a very wide range from drastic interferences with breathing to subtle and sophisticated exercises of various spiritual traditions. Thus the original form of baptism practiced by the Essenes involved forced submersion of the initiate under water for an extended period of time. This resulted in a powerful experience of death and rebirth. In some other groups, the neophytes were half-choked by smoke, by strangulation, or compression of the carotid arteries.

Profound changes in consciousness can be induced by both extremes in the breathing rate, hyperventilation and prolonged withholding of breath, as well as by using them in an alternating fashion. Very sophisticated and advanced methods of this kind can be found in the ancient Indian science of breath, or *pranayama*. Specific techniques involving intense breathing or withholding of breath are also part of various exercises in Kundalini Yoga, Siddha Yoga, the Tibetan Vajrayana, Sufi practice, Burmese Buddhist and Taoist meditation, and many others.

More subtle techniques which emphasize special awareness in relation to breathing rather than changes of the respiratory dynamics have a prominent place in Soto Zen Buddhism (*shikan taza*) and certain Taoist and Christian practices. Indirectly, the depth and rhythm of breathing gets profoundly influenced by such ritual artistic performances, as the Balinese monkey chant or Ketjak, the Inuit Eskimo throat music, and singing of kirtans, bhajans, or Sufi chants.

In materialistic science, breathing lost its sacred meaning and was stripped of its connection to the psyche and spirit. Western medicine reduced it to an important physiological function. The physical and psychological manifestations that accompany various respiratory maneuvers, have all been pathologized. The psychosomatic response to faster breathing, the so-called *hyperventilation syndrome,* is considered a pathological condition, rather than what it really is, a process that has an enormous healing potential. When hyperventilation occurs spontaneously, it is routinely suppressed by administration of tranquilizers, injections of intravenous calcium, and application of a paperbag over the face to increase the concentration of carbon dioxide and combat the alkalosis caused by faster breathing.

In the last few decades, Western therapists rediscovered the healing potential of breath and developed techniques that utilize it. We have ourselves experimented in the context of our month-long seminars at the Esalen Institute in Big Sur, California, with various approaches involving breathing. These included both breathing exercises from ancient spiritual traditions under the guidance of Indian and Tibetan teachers and techniques developed by Western therapists. Each of these approaches has a specific emphasis and uses breath in a different way. In our own search for an effective method of using the healing potential of breath, we tried to simplify this process as much as possible.

We came to the conclusion that it is sufficient to breathe faster and more effectively than usual and with full concentration on the inner process. Instead of emphasizing a specific technique of breathing, we follow even in this area the general strategy of holotropic work, to trust the intrinsic wisdom of the body and follow the inner clues. In holotropic breathwork, we encourage people to begin the session with faster and somewhat deeper breathing, tying inhalation and exhalation into a continuous circle of breath. Once in the process, they find their own rhythm and way of breathing.

We have been able to confirm repeatedly Wilhelm Reich's observation that psychological resistances and defenses are associated with restricted breathing (Reich 1961). Respiration is an autonomous function, but it can also be influenced by volition. Deliberate increase of the pace of breathing typically loosens psychological defenses and leads to a release and emergence of unconscious (and superconscious) material. Unless one has witnessed or experienced this process personally, it is difficult to believe on theoretical grounds alone the power and efficacy of this technique.

The Healing Potential of Music

In holotropic breathwork, the consciousness-altering effect of breath is combined with evocative music. Like breathing, music and other forms of sound technology have been used for millenia as powerful tools in ritual and spiritual practice. Since time immemorial, monotonous drumming, chanting, and other forms of sound-producing techniques have been the principle tools of shamans in many different parts of the world. Many preindustrial cultures have developed quite independently drumming rhythms that in laboratory experiments have remarkable effect on the electric activity of the brain (Jilek 1974; Neher 1961 and 1962). The archives of cultural anthropologists contain countless examples of trance-inducing methods of extraordinary power combining instrumental music, chanting, and dancing.

In many cultures, sound technology has been used specifically for healing purposes in the context of intricate ceremonies. The Navajo healing rituals conducted by trained singers have astounding complexity that has been compared to that of the scripts of Wagnerian operas. The trance dance of the !Kung Bushmen of the African Kalahari Desert has enormous healing power, as has been documented in many anthropological studies and movies (Lee and DeVore 1976; Katz 1976). The healing potential of the syncretistic religious rituals of the Caribbean and South America, such as the Cuban *santeria* or Brazilian *umbanda* is recognized by many professionals in these countries who have traditional Western education. Remarkable instances of emotional and psychosomatic healing occur in the meetings of Christian groups using music, singing, and dance, such as the Snake Handlers, or the Holy Ghost People, and the revivalists or members of the Pentecostal Church.

Some great spiritual traditions have developed sound technologies that do not induce just a general trance state, but have a more specific effect on consciousness. Here belong above all the Tibetan multivocal chanting, the sacred chants of various Sufi orders, the Hindu bhajans and kirtans, and particularly the ancient art of *nada yoga* or the way to union by sound. The Indian teachings postulate a specific connection between sounds of specific frequencies and the individual chakras. With the systematic use of this knowledge, it is possible to influence the state of consciousness in a predictable and desirable way. These are just a few examples of the extensive use of music for ritual, healing, and spiritual purposes.

We used music systematically in the program of psychedelic therapy at the Maryland Psychiatric Research Center in Baltimore and have learned much about its extraordinary potential for psychotherapy. Carefully selected music seems to be of particular value in holotropic states of consciousness, where it has several important functions. It mobilizes emotions associated with repressed memories, brings them to the surface, and facilitates their expression. It helps to open the door into the unconscious, intensifies and deepens the therapeutic process, and provides a meaningful context for the experience. The continuous flow of music creates a carrier wave that helps the subject move through difficult experiences and impasses, overcome psychological defenses, surrender, and let go. In holotropic breathwork sessions, which are usually conducted in groups, music has an additional function: it masks the noises made by the participants and weaves them into a dynamic esthetic Gestalt.

To use music as a catalyst for deep self-exploration and experiential work, it is necessary to learn a new way of listening to music and relating to it that is alien to our culture. In the West, we employ music frequently as an acoustic background that has little emotional relevance. Typical examples would be use of popular music in cocktail parties or piped music (muzak) in shopping areas and work spaces. An approach quite characteristic for more sophisticated audiences is the disciplined and intellectualized listening to music in theaters and concert halls. The dynamic and elemental way of using music characteristic of rock concerts comes closer to the use of music in holotropic therapy. However, the attention of participants in such events is usually extroverted and the experience lacks an element that is essential in holotropic therapy or self-exploration—sustained focused introspection.

In holotropic therapy, it is essential to surrender completely to the flow of music, let it resonate in one's entire body, and respond to it in a spontaneous and elemental fashion. This includes manifestations that would be unthinkable in a concert hall, where even crying or coughing might be a source of embarrassment. Here one has to give full expression to whatever the music is bringing out, whether it is loud screaming or laughing, babytalk, animal noises, shamanic chanting, or talking in tongues. It is also important not to control any physical impulses, such as bizarre grimacing, sensual movements of the pelvis, violent shaking, or intense contortions of the entire body. Naturally, there are exceptions to this rule; destructive behavior directed toward oneself, others, and the physical environment is not permissible.

We also encourage participants to suspend any intellectual activity, such as trying to guess the composer of the music or the culture from which the music comes. Other ways of avoiding the emotional impact of the music involve engaging one's professional expertise—judging the performance of the orchestra, guessing which instruments are playing, and criticizing the technical quality of the recording or the music equipment in the room. When we can avoid these pitfalls, music can become a very powerful tool for inducing and supporting holotropic states of consciousness. For this purpose, the music has to be of superior technical quality and sufficient volume to drive the experience. The combination of music with faster breathing has a remarkable mind-altering power.

As far as the specific choice of music is concerned, I will outline here only the general principles and give a few suggestions based on our experience. After a certain time, each therapist or therapeutic team develops a list of their favorite pieces for various stages of the sessions. The basic rule is to respond sensitively to the phase, intensity, and content of the participants' experience, rather than trying to program it. This is in congruence with the general philosophy of holotropic therapy, particularly the deep respect for the wisdom of the inner healer, for the collective unconscious, and for the autonomy and spontaneity of the healing process.

In general, it is important to use music that is powerful, evocative, and conducive to a positive experience. We try to avoid selections that are jarring, dissonant, and anxiety-provoking. Preference should be given to music of high artistic quality that is not well known and has little concrete content. One should avoid playing songs and other vocal pieces in languages known to the participants, which would through their verbal content convey a specific message or suggest a specific theme. When vocal compositions are used, they should be in foreign languages so that the human voice is perceived just as another musical instrument. For the same reason, it is preferable to avoid pieces which evoke specific intellectual associations and tend to program the content of the session, such as Wagner's or Mendelssohn's wedding marches and overture to Bizet's Carmen.

The session typically begins with activating music that is dynamic, flowing, and emotionally uplifting and reassuring. As the session continues, the music gradually increases in intensity and moves to powerful trance-inducing pieces, preferably drawn from ritual and spiritual traditions of various native cultures. Although many of these performances can be esthetically pleasing, the main purpose of the human groups that developed them is not entertainment, but induction of holotropic experiences.

About an hour and a half into the session of holotropic breathwork, when the experience typically culminates, we introduce what we call "breakthrough music." The selections used at this time range from sacred music—masses, oratoria, requiems, and other powerful orchestral pieces—to excerpts from dramatic movie soundtracks. In the second half of the session, the intensity of the music gradually decreases and we bring in loving and emotionally moving pieces ("heart music"). Finally, in the termination period of the session, the music has a soothing, flowing, timeless, and meditative quality.

Most practitioners of holotropic breathwork collect musical recordings and tend to create their own favorite sequences for the five consecutive phases of the session: (1) opening music (2) trance-inducing music (3) breakthrough music (4) heart music, and (5) meditative music. Some of them use music programs prerecorded for the entire session; this allows the facilitators to be more available for the group, but makes it impossible to flexibly adjust the selection of the music to the energy of the group. Table 5.1 lists the pieces of music that are most frequently used in holotropic breathwork and most popular among breathworkers. It is based on the results of a poll that psychologist Steven Dinan, a certified facilitator of holotropic breathwork, conducted with the community of other practitioners.

TABLE 5.1 **Favorite Pieces of Music for Holotropic Breathing (Based on a poll conducted by Steven Dinan among HB facilitators)**

Album	Artist
Nomad	Nomad
Dorje Ling	David Parsons
1492	Vangelis (soundtrack)
Globalarium	James Asher
Passion	Peter Gabriel
Dance the Devil Away	Outback
Feet in the Soil	James Asher
Mission	Ennio Morricone (soundtrack)
Power of One	Hans Zimmer (soundtrack)
Last of the Mohicans	Trevor Jones (soundtrack)
Egypt	Mickey Hart
Passage in Time	Dead Can Dance
Antarctica	Vangelis (soundtrack)
Deep Forest	Deep Forest
Jiva Mukti	Nada Shakti & Bruce Becvar
Legends of the Fall	James Homer (soundtrack)
Mustt-Mustt	Nusrat Fateh Ali Khan

TABLE 5.1 Favorite Pieces of Music for Holotropic Breathing (*continued*)

Album	Artist
Planet Drum	Mickey Hart
Shaman's Breath	Professor Trance & the Energizers
Themes	Vangelis
Trancendance	Tulku
X	Klaus Schultze
All One Tribe	Scott Fitzgerald
Baraka	Michael Stearns (soundtrack)
Bones	Gabrielle Roth
Braveheart	James Horner (soundtrack)
Direct	Vangelis
Dynamic/Kundalini	Osho
Earth Tribe Rhythms	Brent Lewis
Music to Disappear In	Raphael
Schindler's List	John Williams (soundtrack)
Tana Mana	Ravi Shankar
Thunderdrums	Scott Fitzgerald
All Hearts Beating	Barbara Borden
Closer to Far Away	Douglas Spotted Eagle
Distant Drums Approach	Michael Uyttebroek
Drums of Passion	Babatunde Olatunji
Gula Gula	Mari Boine Persen
Heaven and Earth	Kitaro/soundtrack
Journey of the Drums	Prem Das,Muruga, & Shakti
Kali's Dream	Alex Jones
Lama's Chant	Lama Gyurme & Rykiel
Mishima	Philip Glass (soundtrack)
Powaqqatsi	Philip Glass (soundtrack)
Rendezvous	Jean-Michel Jarre
Skeleton Woman	Flesh & Bone
Songs of Sanctuary	Adiemus
Transfer Station Blue	Michael Shrieve
Voices	Vangelis
Waves	Gabrielle Roth
Anima	010
At the Edge	Mickey Hart
Divine Songs	Alice Coltrane
Drummers of Burundi	The Drummers of Burundi
Drums of Passion: The Beat	Babatunde Olatunji
Exotic Dance	Anugamo & Sabastian
Force Majeure	Tangerine Dream
From Spain to Spain	Vox
Gnawa Music of Marrakesh	Night Spirit Masters
House of India	d.j. Cheb I Sabbah

TABLE 5.1 **Favorite Pieces of Music for Holotropic Breathing (*continued*)**

Album	Artist
Little Buddha	Ryuichi Sakamoto (soundtrack)
Mask	Vangelis
Meeting Pool	Baka Beyond
Miracle Mile	Tangerine Dream
Out of Africa	Dan Wallin et al.(soundtrack)
Oxygene	Jean Michel Jarre
Pangea	Dan Lacksman
Piano	Michael Nyman (soundtrack)
Planets	Gustav Holst
Private Music of. .	Tangerine Dream
Rai Rebels	various
Rhythm Hunter	Brent Lewis
Sacred Site	Michael Stearns
Serpent's Egg	Dead Can Dance
Stellamara	Sonya Drakulich & Jeff Stott
Tibetan Tantric Choir	The Gyuto Monks
Tongues	Gabrielle Roth
Totem	Gabrielle Roth
Whirling	Omar Faruk Tekbilek
Winds of Warning	Adam Plack & Johnny White Ant

The Use of Bodywork

The physical response to holotropic breathwork varies considerably from one person to another. In most instances, faster breathing brings, at first, more or less dramatic psychosomatic manifestations. The textbooks of respiratory physiology refer to this response as the "hyperventilation syndrome." They describe it as a stereotypical pattern of physiological responses that consists primarily of tensions in the hands and feet ("carpopedal spasms"). We have now conducted the breathing sessions with over thirty thousand persons and have found the traditional understanding of the effects of faster breathing to be incorrect.

There exist many individuals in whom fast breathing carried over a period of three to four hours does not lead to a classical hyperventilation syndrome, but to progressive relaxation, intense sexual feelings, or even mystical experiences. Others develop tensions in various parts of the body, but do not show signs of the carpopedal spasms. Moreover, in those who develop tensions, continued faster breathing does not lead to progressive increase of the tensions, but tends to be self-limited. It typically reaches a climactic culmination followed by profound relaxation. The pattern of this sequence has a certain resemblance to a sexual orgasm.

In repeated holotropic sessions, this process of intensification of tensions and subsequent resolution tends to move from one part of the body to another in a way that varies from person to person. The overall amount of muscular tensions and of intense emotions tends to decrease with the number of sessions. What happens in this process is that faster breathing extended for a long period of time changes the chemistry of the organism in such a way that blocked physical and emotional energies associated with various traumatic memories are released and become available for peripheral discharge and processing. This makes it possible for the previously repressed content of these memories to emerge into consciousness and be integrated. It is thus a healing process that should be encouraged and supported and not a pathological process that needs to be suppressed, as it is commonly practiced in mainstream medicine.

Physical manifestations that develop during the breathing in various areas of the body are not simple physiological reactions to hyperventilation. They have a complex psychosomatic structure and usually have specific psychological meaning for the individuals involved. Sometimes they represent an intensified version of tensions and pains, which the person knows from everyday life, either as a chronic problem or as symptoms that appear at times of emotional or physical stress, fatigue, lack of sleep, weakening by an illness, or the use of alcohol or marijuana. Other times, they can be recognized as reactivation of old symptoms that the individual suffered from in infancy, childhood, puberty, or some other time of his or her life.

The tensions that we carry in our body can be released in two different ways. The first of them involves *catharsis* and *abreaction*—discharge of pent-up physical energies through tremors, twitches, dramatic body movements, coughing, gagging, and vomiting. Both catharsis and abreaction also typically include release of blocked emotions through crying, screaming, or other types of vocal expression. These are mechanisms that are well known in traditional psychiatry since the time when Sigmund Freud and Joseph Breuer published their studies in hysteria (Freud and Breuer 1936). Various abreactive techniques have been used in traditional psychiatry in the treatment of traumatic emotional neuroses, and abreaction also represents an integral part of the new experiential psychotherapies, such as the neo-Reichian work, Gestalt practice, and primal therapy.

The second mechanism that can mediate release of physical and emotional tensions plays an important role in holotropic breathwork, rebirthing, and other forms of therapy using breathing techniques. It represents a new development in psychiatry and psychotherapy and seems to be in many ways more effective and interesting. Here the deep tensions surface in the form of *transient muscular contractions of various duration.* By sustaining these muscular tensions for extended periods of time, the organism consumes enormous amounts of previously pent-up energy and simplifies its functioning by disposing of them. The deep relaxation that typically follows the temporary intensification of old tensions or appearance of previously latent ones bears witness to the healing nature of this process.

These two mechanisms have their parallels in sport physiology, where it is well known that it is possible to do work and train the muscles in two different ways, by *isotonic* and *isometric* exercises. As the name suggest, during isotonic exercises the tension of the muscles remains constant while their length oscillates. During isometric exercises, the tension of the muscles changes, but their length remains the same all the time. A good example of isotonic activity is boxing, while weight-lifting is distinctly isometric. Both of these mechanisms are extremely effective in releasing and resolving muscular tension. In spite of their superficial differences, they have thus much in common and in holotropic breathwork they complement each other very effectively.

In many instances, the difficult emotions and physical manifestations that emerge from the unconscious during holotropic sessions get automatically resolved and the breathers end up in a deeply relaxed meditative state. In that case, no external interventions are necessary and they remain in this state until they return to an ordinary state of consciousness. After a brief check with the facilitators, they move to the art room room to draw a mandala.

If the breathing, in and of itself, does not lead to a good completion and there are residual tensions or unresolved emotions, facilitators offer participants a specific form of bodywork which helps them to reach a better closure for the session. The general strategy of this work is to ask the breather to focus his or her attention on the area where there is a problem and do whatever is necessary to intensify the existing physical sensations. The facilitator then helps to intensify these feelings even further by appropriate external intervention.

While the attention of the breather is focused on the energetically charged problem area, he or she is encouraged to find a spontaneous response to this situation. This response should not reflect a conscious choice of the breather, but be fully determined by the unconscious process. It often takes an entirely unexpected and surprising form—voice of a specific animal, talking in tongues or an unknown foreign language, shamanic chant from a particular culture, gibberish, or baby talk. Equally frequent are completely unexpected physical reactions, such as violent tremors, jolts, coughing, and vomiting, as well as typically animal movements. It is essential that the facilitators simply support this process, rather than apply some technique offered by a particular school of therapy. This work continues until the facilitator and the breather reach an agreement that the session has been adequately closed.

Nourishing Physical Contact

In holotropic breathwork, we also use a different form of physical intervention, one that is designed to provide support on a deep preverbal level. This is based on the observation that there exist two fundamentally different forms of trauma and that they require diametrically different approaches. The first of these can be referred to as *trauma by commission.* It is the result of external intrusions that had damaging impact on the future development of the individual. Here belong such insults as physical or sexual abuse, frightening situations, destructive criticism, or ridicule. These traumas represent foreign elements in the unconscious that can be brought into consciousness, energetically discharged, and resolved.

Although this distinction is not recognized in conventional psychotherapy, the second form of trauma, *trauma by omission,* is radically different. It actually involves the opposite mechanism—lack of positive experiences that are essential for a healthy emotional development. The infant, as well as an older child, has strong primitive needs for instinctual satisfaction and security that pediatricians and child psychiatrists call *anaclitic* (from the Greek *anaklinein* meaning to lean upon). These involve the need to be held, caressed, comforted, be played with, and be the center of human attention. When these needs are not met, it has serious consequences for the future of the individual.

Many people have a history of emotional deprivation, abandonment, and neglect that resulted in serious frustration of the anaclitic needs. The only way to heal this type of trauma is to offer a corrective experience in the form of supportive physical contact in a holotropic state of consciousness.

For this approach to be effective, the individual has to be deeply regressed to the infantile stage of development, otherwise the corrective measure would not reach the developmental level on which the trauma occurred. Depending on circumstances and on previous agreement, this physical support can range from simple holding of the hand or touching the forehead to full body contact.

Use of nourishing physical contact is a very effective way of healing early emotional trauma. However, it requires following strict ethical rules. We have to explain to the breathers before the session the rationale of this technique and get their approval to use it. Under no circumstances can this approach be practiced without previous consent and no pressures can be used to obtain this permission. For many people with a history of sexual abuse, physical contact is a very sensitive and charged issue. Very often those who need it most have the strongest resistance to it. It can sometimes take a long time before a person develops enough trust toward the facilitators and the group to be able to accept this technique and benefit from it.

Supportive physical contact has to be used exclusively to satisfy the needs of the breathers and not those of the sitters or facilitators. By this I do not mean only sexual needs or needs for intimacy which, of course, are the most obvious issues. Equally problematic can be a strong need to be needed, loved, or appreciated, unfulfilled maternal need, and other less extreme forms of emotional wants and desires. I remember an incident from one of our workshops at the Esalen Institute in Big Sur, California, which can serve as a good example.

At the beginning of our five-day seminar, one of the participants, a postmenopausal woman, shared with the group how much she had always wanted to have children and how much she suffered because this had not happened. In the middle of the holotropic session, in which she was a sitter for a young man, she suddenly pulled the upper part of her partner's body into her lap and started to rock and comfort him. Her timing could not have been worse; as we found out later during the sharing, he was at the time in the middle of a past-life experience that featured him as a powerful Viking warrior on a military expedition.

It is usually quite easy to recognize when a breather is regressed to early infancy. In a really deep age regression, all the wrinkles in the face tend to disappear and the individual might actually look and behave like an infant. This can involve various infantile postures and gestures, as well as hypersalivation and sucking. Other times, the appropriateness of offering physical contact is obvious from the context, for example, when the breather just finished reliving biological birth and looks lost and forlorn. The maternal needs of the woman in the Esalen workshop were so strong that they took over and she was unable to objectively assess the situation and act appropriately.

Before closing this section on bodywork, I would like to address one question that often comes up in the context of holotropic workshops or lectures on experiential work: "Since reliving of traumatic memories is typically very painful, why should it be therapeutic rather than represent a retraumatization?" I believe that the best answer can be found in the article "Unexperienced Experience" by the Irish psychiatrist Ivor Browne and his team (McGee et al. 1984). They suggested that we are not dealing here with an exact replay or repetition of the original traumatic situation, but with the first full experience of the appropriate emotional and physical reaction to it. This means that, at the time when they happen, the traumatic events are recorded in the organism, but not fully consciously experienced, processed, and integrated.

In addition, the person who is confronted with the previously repressed traumatic memory is not any more the helpless and vitally dependent child or infant he or she was in the original situation, but a grown-up adult. The holotropic state induced in powerful experiential forms of psychotherapy thus allows the individual to be present and operate simultaneously in two different sets of spacetime coordinates. Full age regression makes it possible to experience all the emotions and physical sensations of the original traumatic situation from the perspective of the child, but at the same time analyze and evaluate the memory in the therapeutic situation from a mature adult perspective.

The Course of Holotropic Sessions

The nature and course of holotropic sessions varies considerably from person to person and in the same person also from session to session. Some individuals remain entirely quiet and almost motionless. They might have very profound experiences, yet give the impression to an external observer that nothing is happening or that they are sleeping. Others are agitated and show rich motor activity. They experience violent shaking and complex twisting movements, roll and flail around, assume fetal positions, behave like infants struggling in the birth canal, or look and act like newborns. Also crawling, swimming, digging, or climbing movements are quite common.

Occasionally, the movements and gestures can be extremely refined, complex, quite specific, and differentiated. They can take the form of strange animal movements emulating snakes, birds, or feline predators and be associated with corresponding sounds. Sometimes breathers assume spontaneously various yogic postures and gestures (*asanas* and *mudras*) that they are not intellectually familiar with. Occasionally, the automatic movements and/or sounds resemble ritual or theatrical performances from different cultures—shamanic practices, Javanese dances, the Balinese monkey chant, Japanese Kabuki, or talking in tongues reminiscent of the Pentecostal meetings.

The emotional qualities observed in holotropic sessions cover a very wide range. On one side of the spectrum, one can encounter feelings of extraordinary well-being, profound peace, tranquillity, serenity, bliss, cosmic unity, or ecstatic rapture. On the other side of the same spectrum are episodes of indescribable terror, consuming guilt, or murderous aggression, and a sense of eternal doom. The intensity of these extraordinary emotions can transcend anything that can be experienced or even imagined in the everyday state of consciousness. These extreme emotional states are usually associated with experiences that are perinatal or transpersonal in nature.

In the middle band of the experiential spectrum observed in holotropic breathwork sessions are less extreme emotional qualities that are closer to what we know from our daily existence—episodes of anger, anxiety, sadness, hopelessness, and feelings of failure, inferiority, shame, guilt or disgust. These are typically linked to biographical memories; their sources are traumatic experiences from infancy, childhood, and later periods of life. Their positive counterparts are feelings of happiness, emotional fulfillment, joy, sexual satisfaction, and general increase in zest.

As I mentioned earlier, in some instances, faster breathing does not induce any physical tensions or difficult emotions, but leads directly to increasing relaxation, sense of expansion and well-being, and visions of light. The breather can feel flooded with feelings of love and experiences of mystical connection to other people, nature, the entire cosmos, and God. More frequently, these positive emotional states arise at the end of the holotropic sessions, after the challenging and turbulent parts of the experience have subsided.

It is surprising how many people in our culture, because of strong Protestant ethics or for some other reasons, have great difficulties accepting ecstatic experiences, unless they follow suffering and hard work, or even then. They often respond to them with a strong sense of guilt or with a feeling that they do not deserve them. It is also common, particularly in mental health professionals, to react to positive experiences with mistrust and suspicion that they hide and mask some particularly painful and unpleasant material. It is very important under these circumstances to reassure the breathers that positive experiences are extremely healing and encourage them to accept them without reservation as unexpected grace.

A typical result of a holotropic breathwork session is profound emotional release and physical relaxation. After a successful and well-integrated session, many people report that they feel more relaxed than they have ever felt in their life. Continued accelerated breathing thus represents an extremely powerful and effective method of stress reduction and it is conducive to emotional and psychosomatic healing. Another frequent result of this work is connection with the numinous dimensions of one's own psyche and of existence in general. This is also the understanding that one finds in the spiritual literature of many cultures and ages.

The healing potential of breath is particularly strongly emphasized in Kundalini yoga. There episodes of faster breathing are used in the course of meditative practice (*bastrika*) or occur spontaneously as part of the emotional and physical manifestations known as *kriyas*. This is consistent with my own view that similar spontaneous episodes occurring in psychiatric patients and referred to as the *hyperventilation syndrome,* are attempts at self-healing. They should be encouraged and supported rather than routinely suppressed, which is the common medical practice.

Holotropic breathwork sessions vary in their duration from individual to individual and, in the same individual, also from session to session. It is essential for the best possible integration of the experience that the facilitators and sitters stay with the breather as long as he or she is in process and has unusual experiences. In the terminal stage of the session, good bodywork can significantly facilitate emotional and physical resolution. Intimate contact with nature can also have a very calming and grounding effect and help the integration of the session. Particularly effective in this regard is exposure to water, such as a stay in a hot tub or swim in a pool, a lake, or in the ocean.

Mandala Drawing and the Sharing Groups

When the session is completed and the breather returns to the ordinary state of consciousness, the sitter accompanies him or her to the mandala room. This room is equipped with a variety of art supplies, such as pastels, magic markers, and water colors, as well as large drawing pads. On the sheets of these pads are pencil drawings of circles about the size of dinner plates. The breathers are asked to sit down, meditate on their experience, and then find a way of expressing what happened to them during the session.

There are no specific guidelines for the mandala drawing. Some people simply produce color combinations, others construct geometrical mandalas or figurative drawings or paintings. The latter might represent a vision that occurred during the session or a pictorial travelogue with several distinct sequences. On occasion, the breather decides to document a single session with several mandalas reflecting different aspects or stages of the session. In rare instances, the breather has no idea what he or she is going to draw and produces an automatic drawing.

We have seen instances when the mandala did not illustrate the immediately preceding session, but actually anticipated the session that followed. This is in congruence with C. G. Jung's idea that the products of the psyche cannot be fully explained from preceding historical events. In many instances, they have not just a retrospective, but also a prospective aspect. Some mandalas thus reflect a movement in the psyche that Jung called *the individuation process* and reveal its forthcoming stage. A possible alternative to mandala drawing is sculpting with clay. We introduced this method when we had in our group participants who were blind and could not draw a mandala. It was interesting to see that some of the other participants preferred to use this medium, when it was available, or opted for a combination mandala/three-dimensional figure.

Later during the day, breathers bring their mandalas to a sharing session, in the course of which they talk about their experiences. The strategy of the facilitators who lead the group is to encourage maximum openness and honesty in sharing the experience. Willingness of participants to reveal the content of their sessions, including various intimate details, is conducive to bonding and development of trust in the group. It deepens, intensifies, and expedites the therapeutic process.

In contrast with the practice of most therapeutic schools, facilitators abstain from interpreting the experiences of participants. The reason for it is the lack of agreement concerning the functioning of the psyche among the existing schools. We discussed earlier that under these circumstance any interpretations are questionable and arbitrary. Another reason for staying away from interpretations is the fact that psychological contents are overdetermined and meaningfully related to several levels of the psyche. Giving a supposedly definitive explanation or interpretation carries the danger of freezing the process and interfering with therapeutic progress.

A more productive alternative is to ask questions that help to elicit additional information from the perspective of the client who, being the experiencer, is the ultimate expert as far as his or her experience is concerned. When we are patient and resist the temptation to share our own impressions, participants very often find their own explanations that best reflect their experiences. On occasion, it can be very helpful to share our observations from the past concerning similar experiences or point out connections with experiences of other members of the group. When the experiences contain archetypal material, using C. G. Jung's method of *amplification*—pointing out parallels between a particular experience and similar mythological motifs from various cultures—or consulting a good dictionary of symbols might be very helpful.

On the days following intense sessions that involved a major emotional breakthrough or opening, a wide variety of complementary approaches can facilitate integration. Among them are discussions about the session with an experienced facilitator, writing down the content of the experience, or drawing more mandalas. Good bodywork with a practitioner who allows emotional expression, jogging, swimming, and other forms of physical exercise, or expressive dancing can be very useful, if the holotropic experience freed excess of previously pent-up physical energy. A session of Gestalt therapy or Dora Kalff's Jungian sandplay can be of great help in refining insights into the holotropic experience and understanding its content.

Therapeutic Potential of Holotropic Breathwork

Christina and I have developed and practiced holotropic breathwork outside of the professional setting—in our monthlong seminars and shorter workshops at the Esalen Institute, in various breathwork workshops in many other parts of the world, and in our training program for facilitators. I have not had the opportunity to test the therapeutic efficacy of this method in the same way I had been able to do in the past when I conducted psychedelic therapy. The psychedelic research at the Maryland Psychiatric Research Center involved controlled clinical studies with psychological testing and a systematic, professionally conducted follow-up.

However, the therapeutic results of holotropic breathwork have often been so dramatic and meaningfully connected with specific experiences in the sessions that I have no doubt holotropic breathwork is a viable form of therapy and self-exploration. We have seen over the years numerous instances when participants in the workshops and the training were able to break out of depression that had lasted several years, overcome various phobias, free themselves from consuming irrational feelings, and radically improve their self-confidence and self-esteem. We have also witnessed on many occasions disappearance of severe psychosomatic pains, including migraine headaches, and radical and lasting improvements or even complete clearing of psychogenic asthma. On many occasions, participants in the training or workshops favorably compare their progress in several holotropic sessions to years of verbal therapy.

When we talk about evaluating the efficacy of powerful forms of experiential psychotherapy, such as work with psychedelics or holotropic breathwork, it is important to emphasize certain fundamental differences between these approaches and verbal forms of therapy. Verbal psychotherapy often extends over a period of years and major exciting breakthroughs are rare exceptions rather than commonplace events. When changes of symptoms occur, it happens on a broad time scale and it is difficult to prove their causal connection with specific events in therapy or the therapeutic process in general. By comparison, in a psychedelic or holotropic session, powerful changes can occur in the course of a few hours and they can be convincingly linked to a specific experience.

The changes observed in holotropic therapy are not limited to conditions traditionally considered emotional or psychosomatic. In many cases, holotropic breathwork sessions lead to dramatic improvement of physical conditions that in medical handbooks are described as organic diseases. Among them was clearing of chronic infections (sinusitis, pharyngitis, bronchitis, and cystitis) after bioenergetic unblocking opened blood circulation in the corresponding areas. Unexplained to this day remains solidification of bones in a woman with osteoporosis that occurred in the course of holotropic training.

We have also seen restitution of full peripheral circulation in several people suffering from Raynaud's disease, a disorder that involves coldness of hands and feet accompanied by dystrophic changes of the skin. In several instances, holotropic breathwork led to striking improvement of arthritis. In all these cases, the critical factor conducive to healing seemed to be release of excessive bioenergetic blockage in the afflicted parts of the body followed by vasodilation. The most astonishing observation in this category was a dramatic remission of advanced symptoms of Takayasu arteritis, a disease of unknown etiology, characterized by progressive occlusion of arteries in the upper part of the body. It is a condition that is usually considered progressive, incurable, and potentially lethal.

In a few instances, the therapeutic potential of holotropic breathwork was confirmed in clinical studies conducted by practitioners who had been trained by us and independently use this method in their work. We have also had on many occasions the opportunity to receive informal feedback from people years after their emotional, psychosomatic, and physical symptoms improved or disappeared after holotropic sessions in our training or in our workshops. This has shown us that the improvements achieved in holotropic sessions are often lasting. It is anticipated that the efficacy of this interesting method of self-exploration and therapy will be in the future confirmed by well designed clinical research.

Physiological Mechanisms Involved in Holotropic Breathwork

In view of the powerful effect holotropic breathwork has on consciousness, it is interesting to consider the physiological and biochemical mechanisms that might be involved. Many people believe that when we breathe faster, we simply bring more oxygen into the body and the brain. But the situation is actually much more complicated. It is true that faster breathing brings more air and thus oxygen into the lungs, but it also eliminates carbon dioxide (CO_2) and causes vasoconstriction in certain parts of the body.

Since CO_2 is acidic, reducing its content in blood increases the alkalinity of the blood (so called pH) and in an alkaline setting relatively less oxygen is transferred to the tissues. This triggers a homeostatic mechanism that works in the opposite direction: the kidneys excrete urine that is more alkaline to compensate for this change. The brain is one of the areas in the body that tends to respond to faster breathing by vasoconstriction. Since the degree of gas exchange does not depend only on the rate of breathing, but also on its depth, the situation is quite complex and it is not easy to assess the overall situation in an individual case without a battery of specific laboratory examinations.

However, if we take all the above physiological mechanisms into consideration, the situation of people during holotropic breathwork very likely resembles that in high mountains, where there is less oxygen and the

CO_2 level is decreased by compensatory faster breathing. The cerebral cortex, being the youngest part of the brain from an evolutionary point of view, is generally more sensitive to a variety of influences (such as alcohol and anoxia) than the older parts of the brain. This situation would thus cause inhibition of the cortical functions and intensified activity in the archaic parts of the brain, making the unconscious processes more available.

It is interesting that many individuals, and entire cultures, who lived in extreme altitudes, were known for their advanced spirituality. We can think in this context of the yogis in the Himalayas, the Tibetan Buddhists, and the Peruvian Incas. It is tempting to attribute it to the fact that, in an atmosphere with a lower content of oxygen, they had easy access to transpersonal experiences. However, an extended stay in high elevations leads to physiological adaptations, for example, hyperproduction of red blood cells. The acute situation during holotropic breathwork might, therefore, not be directly comparable to an extended stay in high mountains.

In any case, there is a long way from the description of the physiological changes in the brain to the extremely rich array of phenomena that holotropic breathwork induces, such as authentic experiential identification with animals, archetypal visions, or past-life memories. This situation is similar to the problem of the psychological effects of LSD. The fact that both of these methods can induce transpersonal experiences in which there is access to accurate new information about the universe through extrasensory channels, shows that these contents are not stored in the brain.

Aldous Huxley, after having experienced psychedelic states, came to the conclusion that our brain cannot possibly be the source of these experiences. He suggested that it functions more like a reducing valve that shields us from an infinitely larger cosmic input. The concepts, such as "memory without a material substrate" (von Foerster 1965), Sheldrake's "morphogenetic fields" (Sheldrake 1981), and Laszlo's "psi field" (Laszlo 1993) bring important support for Huxley's idea and make it increasingly plausible.

Holotropic Therapy and Other Treatment Modalities

After several decades of work with holotropic states, I have no doubt that the new insights concerning the nature of consciousness, dimensions of the human psyche, and the architecture of emotional and psychosomatic disorders that we have explored in the preceding chapters have general validity and are of lasting value. In my opinion, they should be incorporated into the theory of psychiatry and psychology and become part of the conceptual framework of all therapists, without regard to the level or type of therapy that they practice.

As Frances Vaughan so eloquently articulated in her discussion of transpersonal psychotherapy, the content and focus of therapeutic work at any particular time is determined by what the client brings into the session. The specific contribution of the therapist is that he or she has a conceptual framework large enough to provide a meaningful context for anything that emerges in the process. A transpersonal therapist can thus follow the clients to any domain or level of the psyche where their process takes them (Vaughan 1979).

If the theoretical framework of the therapist is limited, he or she will not be able to understand phenomena that lie outside of it and will tend to interpret them as derivatives of something that is part of their own narrow worldview. This will lead to serious distortions and will seriously affect the quality and efficacy of the therapeutic process, whether it is experiential or involves verbal means. Since I mentioned these two basic forms of psychotherapy, it might be useful to look at their indications and potential, as well as limitations.

Certain important aspects of emotional and psychosomatic disorders, particularly those associated with blockages of emotional and physical energy, require experiential approach and attempts to influence them by verbal therapy represent waste of time. It is also generally impossible to reach the perinatal and transpersonal roots of emotional problems by therapy limited to verbal means alone. However, talking therapy is certainly an important complement to deep experiential sessions. It helps to integrate the material that emerged in holotropic states into the clients' everyday life, whether it is a biographical trauma, perinatal sequence, or deep spiritual experience. The same is true for experiences emerging spontaneously in episodes of spiritual emergency.

Verbal psychotherapy can be extremely important in its own right for clearing communication problems and interpersonal dynamics of a couple or an entire family. Conducted on a one-to-one basis, it can provide a corrective experience and help develop trust in human relations in people who experienced rejection or abuse in their early history. It can also interrupt and heal vicious circles in interpersonal interaction, based on generalization, anticipation of disappointment, and resulting self-fulfilling prophecy.

Systematic work with holotropic states is compatible and can be combined with a broad spectrum of other uncovering therapies, such as Gestalt practice, various forms of bodywork, expressive painting and dancing, Jacob Moreno's psychodrama, Dora Kalff's sandplay, Francine Shapiro's eye movement desensitization and reprocessing (EMDR), and many others. In combination with physical exercise, meditation and movement meditation, such as jogging, swimming, Hatha Yoga, Vipassana, tai-chi, or chi-gong, this can be a very effective therapeutic package that over time can result not only in emotional and psychosomatic healing, but also permanent positive changes of personality.

CHAPTER SIX

Spirituality and Religion

The area in which the research of holotropic states brought probably the most radical new perspectives is spirituality and its relation to religion. The understanding of human nature and of the cosmos developed by Western materialistic science is substantially different from that found in ancient and preindustrial societies. Over the centuries, scientists have systematically explored various aspects of the material world and accumulated an impressive amount of information that had not been available in the past. They have replaced, corrected, and complemented earlier concepts about nature and the universe.

However, the most striking difference between the two worldviews is not in the amount and accuracy of data about material reality; that is a natural and expected result of scientific progress. The most profound disagreement revolves around the question whether existence has a sacred or spiritual dimension. This is clearly an issue of great significance that has far-reaching implications for human existence. The way we answer this question will profoundly influence our hierarchy of values, our strategy of existence, and our day-to-day behavior toward other people and nature. And the answers these two human groups give in this regard are diametrically opposite.

All the human groups of the preindustrial era were in agreement that the material world, which we perceive and in which we operate in our everyday life, is not the only reality. Their worldview included the existence of hidden dimensions of reality inhabited by various deities, demons, discarnate entities, ancestral spirits, and power animals. Preindustrial cultures had a rich ritual and spiritual life that revolved around the possibility of achieving direct experiential contact with these ordinarily hidden domains and beings and to receive from them important information or assistance. They believed that it was an important and useful way to influence the course of material events.

In these societies, the activities of everyday life were based not only on the information received through the senses, but also on the input from these invisible dimensions. Anthropologists doing field research in native cultures have been baffled by what they called the "double logic" of the human groups they studied. The natives clearly exhibited extraordinary skills and possessed ingenious implements that were perfectly adequate as means for sustenance and survival. Yet, they combined their practical activities, such as hunting, fishing, and farming with rituals addressing various realms and entities that for the anthropologists were imaginary and nonexistent.

For materialistically oriented anthropologists, who had no experience with holotropic states of consciousness, such behavior was irrational and utterly incomprehensible. Unlike their conservative colleagues, whose methodology was limited to external observation of the cultures they studied, open-minded and adventurous anthropologists ("visionary anthropologists") realized that to understand these cultures, it was essential to participate in their rituals involving holotropic states.

These researchers, such as Michael Harner, Richard Katz, Barbara Meyerhoff, or Carlos Castaneda, had no problems understanding the double logic of the natives. Their experiences showed them that tool making and practical skills are related to material reality that we perceive in our ordinary state of consciousness. Ritual activity addresses the hidden realities, the existence of which is revealed in holotropic states. The worldview of academic anthropology (the "etic approach") is limited to external observations of material reality, the perspective of the natives ("emic approach") includes information from holotropic experience of inner realities. The two perspectives are not mutually exclusive, but complementary.

The descriptions of the sacred dimensions of reality and the emphasis on spiritual life are in sharp conflict with the belief system that dominates the industrial world. According to Western mainstream academic science, only matter really exists. The history of the universe is the history of developing matter. Life, consciousness, and intelligence are more or less accidental and insignificant epiphenomena of this development. They

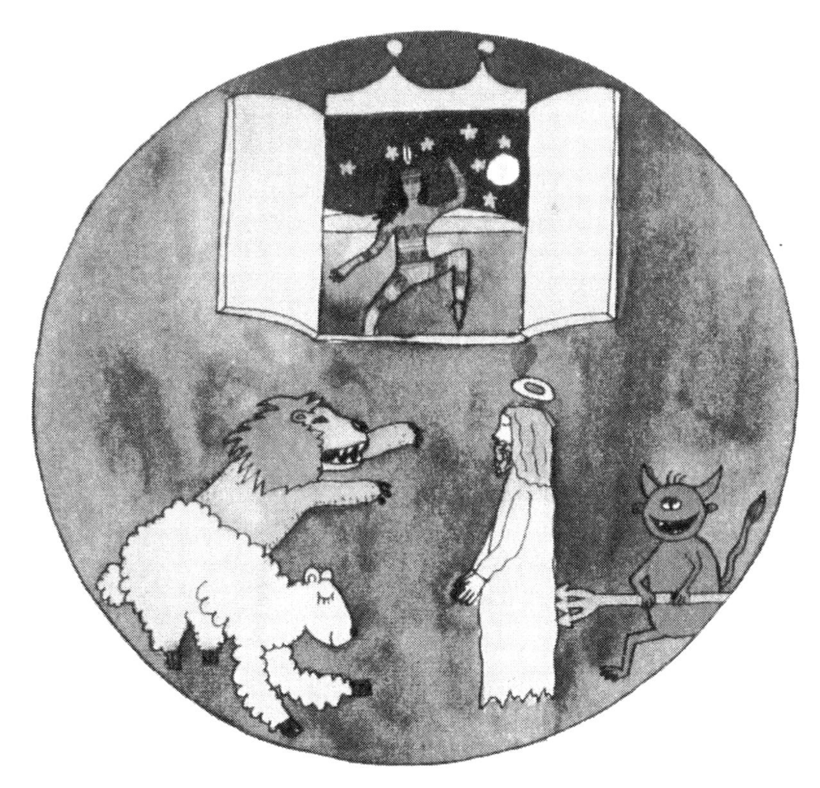

Above and right: Drawings illustrating experiences in a session with psychedelic mushrooms. These experiences exposed and mocked morbid and righteous religiosity, fake spirituality that is intolerant of other creeds and hostile toward the human body and nature. They portrayed and celebrated universal, all-embracing, and nature-oriented spirituality. The power and vitality of this approach to life is symbolized by the lion emerging out of a lamb and a Native American dancer.

appeared on the scene after billions of years of evolution of passive and inert matter in a trivially small part of an immense universe. It is obvious that in a universe of this kind there is no place for spirituality.

According to Western neuroscience, consciousness is a product of the physiological processes in the brain, and thus critically dependent on the body. Very few people, including most scientists, realize that we have absolutely no proof that consciousness is actually produced by the brain and that we do not have even a remote notion how something like that

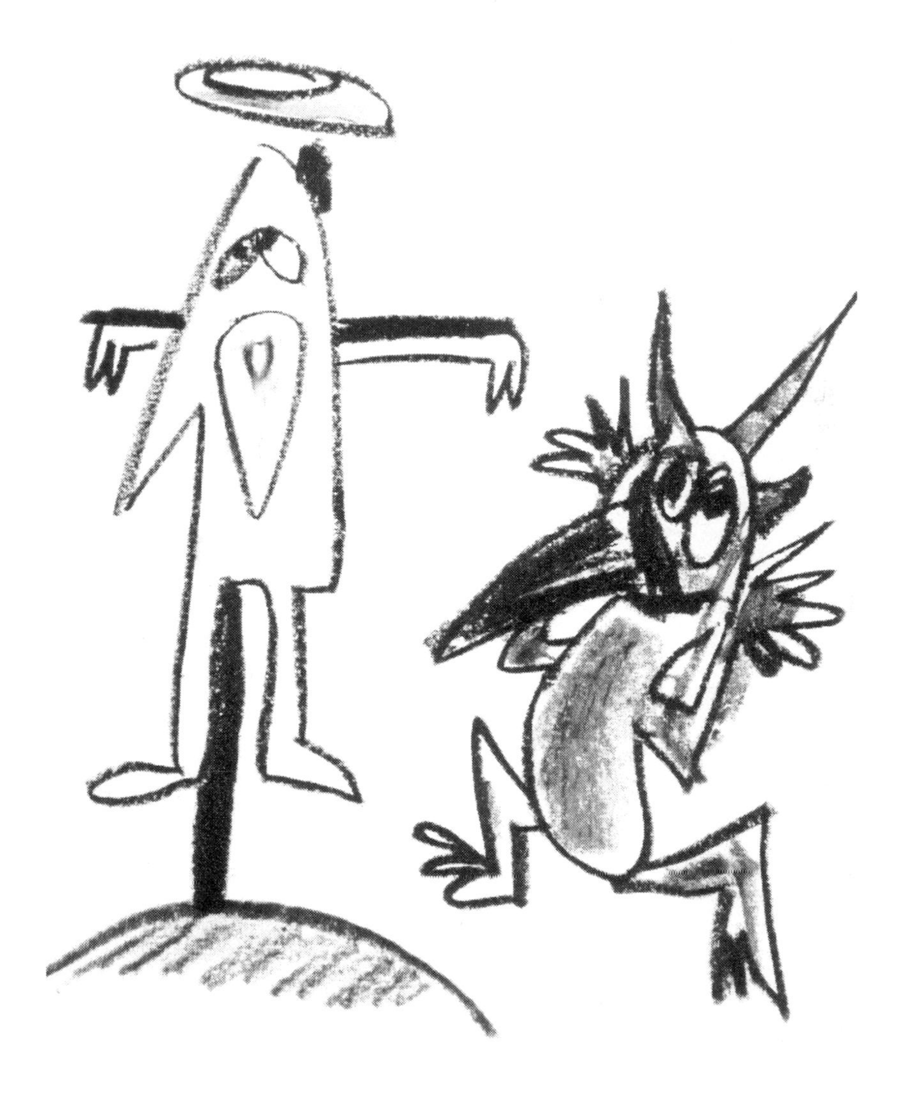

could possibly happen. In spite of it, this basic metaphysical assumption remains one of the leading myths of Western materialistic science and has profound influence on our entire society.

In light of the observations from the study of holotropic states, the current contemptuous dismissal and pathologization of spirituality characteristic of monistic materialism appears untenable. In holotropic states, the spiritual dimensions of reality can be directly experienced in a way that is as convincing as our daily experience of the material world. It is also possible to describe step by step procedures that facilitate access to these experiences. Careful study of transpersonal experiences shows that they are ontologically real and inform us about important aspects of existence that are ordinarily hidden.

In general, the study of holotropic states confirms C. G. Jung's insight that the experiences originating on deeper levels of the psyche (in my own terminology, "perinatal" and "transpersonal" experiences) have a certain quality that he called (after Rudolph Otto) *numinosity.* The term *numinous* is relatively neutral and thus preferable to other similar names, such as religious, mystical, magical, holy, or sacred, which have often been used in problematic contexts and are easily misleading. The sense of numinosity is based on direct apprehension of the fact that we are encountering a domain that belongs to a superior order of reality, one which is sacred and radically different from the material world.

To prevent misunderstanding and confusion that in the past compromised many similar discussions, it is critical to make a clear distinction between spirituality and religion. Spirituality is based on direct experiences of nonordinary aspects and dimensions of reality. It does not require a special place or an officially appointed person mediating contact with the divine. The mystics do not need churches or temples. The context in which they experience the sacred dimensions of reality, including their own divinity, are their bodies and nature. And instead of officiating priests, they need a supportive group of fellow seekers or the guidance of a teacher who is more advanced on the inner journey than they are themselves.

Direct spiritual experiences appear in two different forms. The first of these, the experience of *the immanent divine,* involves subtly, but profoundly transformed perception of the everyday reality. A person having this form of spiritual experience sees people, animals, and inanimate objects in the environment as radiant manifestations of a unified field of cosmic creative energy and realizes that the boundaries between them are illusory and unreal. This is a direct experience of nature as god, Spinoza's *deus sive natura.* Using the analogy with television, this experience could be likened to a situation where a black and white picture would suddenly change into one in vivid, "living color." In both cases, much of the old perception of the world remains in place, but is radically redefined by the addition of a new dimension.

The second form of spiritual experience, that of *the transcendent divine,* involves manifestation of archetypal beings and realms of reality that are ordinarily transphenomenal, unavailable to perception in the everyday state of consciousness. In this type of spiritual experience, entirely new elements seem to "unfold" or "explicate," to borrow terms from David Bohm, from another level or order of reality. When we return to the analogy with television, this would be like discovering that there exist channels other than the one we have been previously watching.

For many people, the first encounter with the sacred dimensions of existence occurs in the context of the death-rebirth process, when the experiences of different stages of birth are accompanied by visions and scenes from the archetypal domain of the collective unconscious. However, the full connection with the spiritual realm is made when the process moves to the transpersonal level of the psyche. When that happens, various spiritual experiences appear in their pure form, independently of the fetal elements. In some instances, the holotropic process bypasses the biographical and perinatal levels altogether and provides direct access to the transpersonal realm.

Spirituality involves a special kind of relationship between the individual and the cosmos and is, in its essence, a personal and private affair. By comparison, organized religion is institutionalized group activity that takes place in a designated location, a temple or a church, and involves a system of appointed officials who might or might not have had personal experiences of spiritual realities. Once a religion becomes organized, it often completely loses the connection with its spiritual source and becomes a secular institution that exploits human spiritual needs without satisfying them.

Organized religions tend to create hierarchical systems focusing on the pursuit of power, control, politics, money, possessions, and other secular concerns. Under these circumstances, religious hierarchy as a rule dislikes and discourages direct spiritual experiences in its members, because they foster independence and cannot be effectively controlled. When this is the case, genuine spiritual life continues only in the mystical branches, monastic orders, and ecstatic sects of the religions involved.

Brother David Steindl-Rast, a Benedictine monk and Christian philosopher, uses a beautiful metaphor to illustrate this situation. He compares the original mystical experience to the glowing magma of an exploding volcano, which is exciting, dynamic, and alive. After we have this experience, we feel the need to put it into a conceptual framework and formulate a *doctrine*. The mystical state represents a precious memory and we might create a *ritual* that will remind us of this momentous event. The experience connects us with the cosmic order and this has profound direct impact on our *ethics*—system of values, moral standards, and behavior.

For a variety of reasons, in the course of its existence, organized religion tends to lose connection with its original spiritual source. When it gets disconnected from its experiential matrix, its doctrines degenerate into *dogmas,* rituals into empty *ritualism,* and cosmic ethics into *moralism.* In Brother David's simile, the remains of what once was a vital spiritual system now resemble much more the encrusted lava than the electrifying magma of the mystical experience that created it.

People who have experiences of the immanent or transcendent divine open up to spirituality found in the mystical branches of the great religions of the world or in their monastic orders, not necessarily in their mainstream organizations. If these experiences take a Christian form, the individual would feel resonance with St. Teresa of Avila, St. John of the Cross, Meister Eckhart, or St. Hildegarde von Bingen. Such experiences would not result in appreciation for the Vatican hierarchy and the edicts of the popes, nor would they convey understanding of the position of the Catholic Church on contraception or of its ban on women in the clergy.

A spiritual experience of the Islamic variety would bring the person close to the teachings of various Sufi orders and instigate interest in their practice. It would not generate sympathy for the religiously motivated politics of some Moslem groups and passion for *jihad,* the Holy War against infidels. Similarly, a Judaic form of this experience would connect the individual to the Jewish mystical tradition, as expressed in the Cabala or the Hassidic movement, and not to fundamentalist Judaism or Sionism. A deep mystical experience tends to dissolve the boundaries between religions, while dogmatism of organized religions tends to emphasize differences and engender antagonism and hostility.

True spirituality is universal and all-embracing and is based on personal mystical experience rather than on dogma or religious scriptures. Mainstream religions might unite people within their own radius, but tend to be divisive on a larger scale, because they set their group against all the others and attempt either to convert them or eradicate them. The epithets "pagans," "goyim," and "infidels" and the conflicts between the Christians and Jews, Moslems and Jews, Christians and Moslems, or Hindus and Sikhs, are just a few salient examples. In today's troubled world, religions in their present form are part of the problem rather than part of the solution. Ironically, even differences between various factions of the same religion can become a sufficient reason for serious conflict and bloodshed, as exemplified by the history of the Christian church and the ongoing violence in Ireland.

There is no doubt that the dogmas of organized religions are generally in fundamental conflict with science, whether this science uses the mechanistic-materialistic model or is anchored in the emerging paradigm. However, the situation is very different in regard to authentic mysticism based on spiritual experiences. The great mystical traditions have amassed extensive knowledge about human consciousness and about the spiritual realms in a way that is similar to the method that scientists use in acquiring knowledge about the material world. It involves methodology for inducing transpersonal experiences, systematic collection of data, and intersubjective validation.

Spiritual experiences, like any other aspect of reality, can be subjected to careful open-minded research and studied scientifically. There is nothing unscientific about unbiased and rigorous study of transpersonal phenomena and of the challenges they present for materialistic understanding of the world. Only such an approach can answer the critical question about the ontological status of mystical experiences: Do they reveal deep truth about some basic aspects of existence, as maintained by perennial philosophy, or are they products of superstition, fantasy, or mental disease, as Western materialistic science sees them?

The main obstacle in the study of spiritual experiences is the fact that traditional psychology and psychiatry are dominated by materialistic philosophy and lack genuine understanding of religion and spirituality. Western psychiatry makes no distinction between a mystical experience and a psychotic experience and sees both as manifestations of mental disease. In its rejection of religion, it does not differentiate between primitive folk beliefs or the fundamentalist literal interpretations of religious scriptures and sophisticated mystical traditions or Eastern spiritual philosophies based on centuries of systematic introspective exploration of the psyche.

An extreme example of this lack of discrimination is Western science's rejection of Tantra, a system that offers deep understanding of the human psyche and an extraordinary spiritual vision of existence in the context of a comprehensive and sophisticated scientific worldview. Tantric scholars developed a profound understanding of the universe that has been in many ways validated by modern science. It included sophisticated models of space and time, the concept of the Big Bang, and such elements as a heliocentric system, interplanetary attraction, spherical shape of the earth and planets, and entropy. This knowledge preceded by centuries corresponding discoveries in the West.

Additional achievments of Tantra included advanced mathematics and the invention of the decimal count with a zero. Tantra also had a profound psychological theory and experiential method, based on maps of the subtle or energy body involving psychic centers (*chakras*) and conduits (*nadis*). It has developed highly refined abstract and figurative spiritual art and a complex ritual (Mookerjee and Khanna 1977).

The seeming incompatibility of science and spirituality is quite remarkable. Throughout history, spirituality and religion had played a critical and vital role in human life, until their influence was undermined by the scientific and industrial revolution. Science and religion represent extremely important parts of human life, each in its own way. Science is the most powerful tool for obtaining information about the world we live in and spirituality is indispensable as a source of meaning in our life. And the religious impulse certainly has been one of the most compelling forces driving human history and culture.

It is hard to imagine that this would have been possible if ritual and spiritual life were based on psychotic hallucinations, delusions, and on entirely unfounded superstitions and fantasies. To exert such a powerful influence on the course of human affairs, religion clearly has to reflect an authentic and very profound aspect of human nature, however problematic and distorted expressions this genuine core might have found in the course of human history. Let us now look at this dilemma in the light of the observations from consciousness research. All great religions of the world were inspired by powerful holotropic experiences of the visionaries, who initiated and sustained these creeds, and by divine epiphanies of the prophets, mystics, and saints. These experiences, revealing the existence of sacred dimensions of reality, served as a vital source of all religious movements.

Gautama Buddha, meditating in Bodh Gaya under the Bo tree, had a dramatic visionary experience of Kama Mara, the master of the world illusion, who tried to detract him from his spiritual quest. He first used his three seductive daughters in an effort to divert Buddha's interest from spirituality to sex. When this attempt had failed, he brought in his menacing army to instigate in Buddha the fear of death, intimidate him, and prevent him from reaching enlightenment. Buddha successfully overcame these obstacles and experienced illumination and spiritual awakening. On other occasions, he also envisioned a long chain of his previous incarnations and experienced a profound liberation from karmic bonds.

The Islamic text *Miraj Nameh*, gives a description of the "miraculous journey of Mohammed," a powerful visionary state during which archangel

Gabriel escorted Mohammed through the seven Moslem heavens, Paradise, and Hell (Gehenna). During this visionary journey, Mohammed experienced in the seventh heaven an "audience" with Allah. In a state, described as "ecstasy approaching annihilation," he received from Allah a direct communication. This experience and additional mystical states that Mohammed had over a period of twenty-five years became the basis for the *suras* of the Qur'an and for the Moslem faith.

In the Judeo-Christian tradition, the Old Testament offers a colorful account of Moses' experience of Yahwe in the burning bush, description of Abraham's interaction with the angel, and other visionary experiences. The New Testament describes Jesus' experience of the temptation by the devil during his stay in the desert. Similarly, Saul's blinding vision of Christ on the way to Damascus, St. John's apocalyptic revelation in his cave on the island Patmos, Ezechiel's observation of the flaming chariot, and many other episodes clearly are transpersonal experiences in holotropic states of consciousness. The Bible provides many other examples of direct communication with God and with the angels. In addition, the descriptions of the temptations of St. Anthony and of the visionary experiences of other saints and Desert Fathers are well-documented parts of Christian history.

Modern mainstream psychiatrists interpret such visionary experiences as manifestations of serious mental diseases, although they lack adequate medical explanation and the laboratory data supporting this position. Psychiatric literature contains numerous articles and books that discuss what would be the most appropriate clinical diagnoses for many of the great figures of spiritual history. St. John of the Cross has been called "hereditary degenerate," St. Teresa of Avila dismissed as a severe hysterical psychotic, and Mohammed's mystical experiences have been attributed to epilepsy.

Many other religious and spiritual personages, such as the Buddha, Jesus, Ramakrishna, and Shri Ramana Maharshi have been seen as suffering from psychoses, because of their visionary experiences and "delusions." Similarly, some traditionally trained anthropologists have argued whether shamans should be diagnosed as schizophrenics, ambulant psychotics, epileptics, or hysterics. The famous psychoanalyst Franz Alexander, known as one of the founders of psychosomatic medicine, wrote a paper in which even Buddhist meditation is described in psychopathological terms and referred to as "artificial catatonia" (Alexander 1931).

In the industrial civilization, people who have direct experiences of spiritual realities are thus seen as mentally ill. Mainstream psychiatrists make no distinction between mystical experiences and psychotic experiences and see both categories as manifestations of psychosis. The kindest judgment about mysticism that has so far come from official academic circles was the statement of the Committee on Psychiatry and Religion of the Group for the Advancement of Psychiatry entitled *Mysticism: Spiritual Quest or Psychic Disorder?* This document published in 1976 conceded that mysticism might be a phenomenon that lies somewhere between normalcy and psychosis.

Religion and spirituality have been extremely important forces in the history of humanity and civilization. Had the visionary experiences of the founders of religions been nothing more than products of brain pathology, it would be difficult to explain the profound impact they have had on millions of people over the centuries and the glorious architecture, paintings, sculptures, music, and literature they have inspired. There does not exist a single ancient or preindustrial culture in which ritual and spiritual life did not play a pivotal role. The current approach of Western psychiatry and psychology thus pathologizes not only spiritual but also cultural life of all human groups throughout centuries except the educated elite of the Western industrial civilization that shares the materialistic and atheistic worldview.

The official position of psychiatry in regard to spiritual experiences also creates a remarkable split in our own society. In the United States, religion is officially tolerated, legally protected, and even righteously promoted by certain circles. There is a Bible in every motel room, politicians pay lip-service to God in their speeches, and collective prayer is a standard part of the presidential inauguration ceremony. However, in the light of materialistic science, people who take seriously spiritual beliefs of any kind appear to be uneducated, suffering from shared delusions, or emotionally immature.

And if somebody in our culture would have during divine service in the church a spiritual experience of the kind that inspired every major religion of the world, an average minister would very likely send him or her to a psychiatrist. We go to church and listen to stories about mystical experiences had by people two thousand and more years ago. At the same time, similar experiences that occur to contemporary people are seen as signs of mental disease. It has happened on many occasions that people who had been brought to psychiatric facilities as a result of having had intense spiritual experiences were hospitalized, subjected to tranquilizing medication or even shock treatments, and received psychopathological diagnostic labels that stigmatized them for the rest of their lives.

In the present climate, even the suggestion that spiritual experiences deserve systematic study and should be critically examined appears absurd to conventionally trained scientists. Showing serious interest in this area, in and of itself, can be considered a sign of poor judgment and blemishes the researcher's professional reputation. In actuality, there exists no scientific "proof" that the spiritual dimension does *not* exist. The refutation of its existence is essentially a metaphysical assumption of Western science, based on an incorrect application of an outdated paradigm. As a matter of fact, the study of holotropic states, in general, and transpersonal experiences, in particular, provides more than enough data suggesting that postulating such a dimension makes good sense (Grof 1985, 1988).

By pathologizing holotropic states of consciousness, Western science has pathologized the entire spiritual history of humanity. It assumed a disrespectful and arrogant attitude toward spiritual, ritual, and cultural life of pre-industrial societies throughout centuries, as well as spiritual practice of people in our own society. In this view, of all the human groups in history only the intellectual elite of Western civilization that subscribes to monistic materialism of Western science has an accurate and reliable understanding of existence. All those who do not share this view are seen as primitive, ignorant, or deluded.

Systematic study of various forms of holotropic states conducted in the last few decades by clinicians using psychedelic therapy and powerful experiential psychotherapies, thanatologists, anthropologists, Jungian analysts, researchers of meditation and biofeedback, and others has shown that Western psychology and psychiatry have made a serious error in dismissing mystical experiences as manifestations of brain pathology of unknown etiology. The new findings have inspired the development of transpersonal psychology, a discipline that has undertaken unbiased scientific research of spirituality on its own terms, rather than seeing it through the prism of the materialistic paradigm.

Transpersonal psychology seriously studies and respects the entire spectrum of human experience, including holotropic states, and all the domains of the psyche—biographical, perinatal and transpersonal. As a result, it is more culturally sensitive and offers a way of understanding the psyche that is universal and applicable to any human group and any historical period. It also honors the spiritual dimensions of existence and acknowledges the deep human need for transcendental experiences. In this context, spiritual search appears to be an understandable and legitimate human activity.

The differences between the understanding of the universe, nature, human beings, and consciousness developed by Western science and that found in the ancient and preindustrial societies are usually explained in terms of superiority of materialistic science over superstition and primitive magical thinking of native cultures. In this context, atheism is seen as a sophisticated and enlightened view of reality that the native cultures have yet to achieve when they receive the benefit of Western education. Careful analysis of this situation reveals that the reason for this difference is not the superiority of Western science, but ignorance and naivité of the industrial societies in regard to holotropic states of consciousness.

All preindustrial cultures held these states in high esteem and spent much time and energy trying to develop effective and safe ways of inducing them. They possessed deep knowledge of these states, systematically cultivated them, and used them as the major vehicle of their ritual and spiritual life. The worldviews of these cultures reflected not only the experiences and observations made in the everyday state of consciousness, but also those from deep visionary states. Modern consciousness research and transpersonal psychology have shown that many of these experiences are authentic disclosures of ordinarily hidden dimensions of reality and cannot be dismissed as pathological distortions.

In visionary states, the experiences of other realities or of new perspectives on our everyday reality are so convincing and compelling that the individuals who have had them have no other choice than to incorporate them into their worldview. It is thus systematic experiential exposure to holotropic states of consciousness, on the one side, and the absence thereof, on the other, that sets the native cultures and technological societies ideologically so far apart. I have not yet met a single European, American, or member of one of the other technologized societies, who has had a deep experience of the transcendental realms and continues to subscribe to the worldview of Western materialistic science. This development is quite independent of the level of intelligence, type and degree of education, or professional credentials of the individuals involved.

CHAPTER SEVEN

The Experience of Death and Dying: Psychological, Philosophical, and Spiritual Perspectives

Research of holotropic states brought much clarity into another area that has in the past been subject to much denial, discord, and confusion—the problems related to death and dying. The beginnings of this controversy can be found in the conceptual development of Sigmund Freud. In his early writings, Freud considered the issue of death to be irrelevant for psychology. The reason for this attitude was his belief that the id operated in a realm that lay beyond time and space and, therefore, did not know and acknowledge death. In this context, problems that appeared to be death related, such as fear of death, actually masked some other issues—death wishes toward somebody else, fear of castration, concerns about loss of control, or fright of an overwhelming sexual orgasm (Fenichel 1945).

During these early years Freud also believed that the primary motivating force in the psyche was what he called the "pleasure principle," a tendency to avoid discomfort and seek satisfaction. Later, when he discovered the existence of phenomena to which this principle did not apply, such as masochism, self-mutilation, and need for punishment, this understanding of the psyche became untenable. Struggle with the conceptual challenges involved made him realize that the phenomena that are "beyond the pleasure principle" could not be understood without bringing in the problem of death.

He eventually formulated an entirely new psychology, in which the psyche was not any more a battlefield between the libidinal forces and the self-preservation drive, but between libido and what he called the "death instinct" (Libido and Destrudo or Eros and Thanatos). Although Freud himself saw these two principles as biological instincts, they had actually definite mythological features, not unlike the Jungian archetypes (Freud 1955 and 1964). This revision, considered by Freud to be the most definitive formulation of his ideas, did not evoke much enthusiasm in his followers. A "statistical survey" conducted by Brun showed that about 94 per cent of Freud's followers had rejected the death instinct theory (Brun 1953).

The work with holotropic states confirmed Freud's general intuition about the psychological importance of death, but it substantially revised, modified, and expanded his views. It did not confirm the existence of an independent death instinct, but showed that life-threatening events, such as injuries, operations, near drowning, or prenatal and perinatal crises, play an important role in the development of personality and as sources of serious psychopathology. This work also revealed that death has important representation on the transpersonal level of the psyche in the form of past-life memories, eschatological deities and domains, and complex archetypal motifs, such as that of the Apocalypse or the Nordic Ragnarok.

Conversely, it became clear that experiential confrontation with death in the course of therapy has important healing, transformative, and evolutionary potential. This research also revealed that the attitude toward death and coming to terms with it has important implications for the quality of one's life, hierarchy of values, and strategy of existence. Experiential encounter with death, whether it is symbolic (in meditation, psychedelic sessions, spiritual emergency, or holotropic breathwork) or real (in an accident, in war, in a concentration camp, or during a heart attack) can lead to a powerful spiritual opening.

The research of holotropic states has brought many fascinating insights into various problems related to death and dying, such as phenomenology of near-death experiences, fear of death and its role in human life, survival of consciousness after death, and reincarnation. These insights are of great importance not only for scientific disciplines such as psychiatry, psychology, anthropology, and thanatology, but for all of us as individuals. It would be difficult to find a subject that is more universal and more personally relevant for every single individual than death and dying.

In the course of our life, we all will lose acquaintances, friends, and relatives and eventually face our own biological demise. In view of this fact, it is quite astonishing that, until the late 1960s, the Western industrial civilization showed an almost complete lack of interest in the subject of death and dying. This was true not only for the general population, but also for scientists and professionals involved in disciplines that should be interested in this subject, such as medicine, psychiatry, psychology, anthropology, philosophy, and theology. The only plausible explanation for this situation is that, for some reason, technological societies developed a massive psychological denial of death.

This disinterest is even more striking, when we compare the situation in our society with that in the ancient and preindustrial cultures and realize that their attitude to death and dying was diametrically different. Death played an extremely critical and central role in their cosmologies, philosophies, spiritual and ritual life, and mythologies, as well as everyday life. The practical importance of this difference becomes obvious when we compare the situation of a person facing death in these two historical and cultural environments.

A person brought up in one of the Western industrial societies typically has a pragmatic and materialistic worldview, or is at least very profoundly influenced by the exposure to that worldview. According to Western neuroscience, consciousness is an epiphenomenon of matter, a product of the physiological processes in the brain, and thus critically dependent on the body. From this perspective, there cannot be any doubt that death of the body, particularly of the brain, is the absolute end of any form of conscious activity. When we accept the basic premise about the primacy of matter, this conclusion is logical, obvious, and unquestionable. Belief in any form of consciousness after death, posthumous journey of the soul, or reincarnation seems naive and ridiculous. It is dismissed as a product of wishful thinking of people who are unable to accept the obvious biological imperative of death.

The undermining effect of materialistic science is not the only factor that has weakened the influence of religion in our culture. As we have seen earlier, Western religion has also largely lost its experiential component and with it the connection to its deep spiritual sources. As a result, it has become empty, meaningless, and increasingly irrelevant in our life. In this form, it cannot compete with the persuasiveness of materialistic science backed up by its technological triumphs. Religion ceases to be a vital force during our life, as well as at the time of dying and death. Its references to afterlife and the abodes of the beyond, such as heaven and hell, have been relegated to the realm of fairy tales and handbooks of psychiatry.

This attitude effectively inhibited scientific interest in the experiences of dying patients and of individuals in near-death situations until the 1970s. The rare reports on this subject received very little attention, whether they came in the form of books for general public, such as Jess E. Weisse's *The Vestibule* (Weisse 1972) and Jean-Baptiste Delacour's *Glimpses of the Beyond* (Delacour 1974), or scientific research, such as the study of death-bed observations of physicians and nurses conducted by Karlis Osis (Osis et al. 1961). Since the publication of Raymond Moody's international bestseller *Life after Life* in 1975, Ken Ring, Michael Sabom, and other pioneers of thanatology have amassed impressive evidence about the striking characteristics of near-death experiences from accurate extrasensory perception during out-of-body experiences to profound personality changes following them (Sabom 1982, Greyson and Flynn 1984, Ring and Valarino 1998).

The material from these studies has been widely publicized in numerous television talk shows featuring thanatologists and near-death experiencers, in best-selling books, and even in many Hollywood movies. Yet, these remarkable and potentially paradigm-shattering observations, which could revolutionize our understanding of the nature of consciousness and its relationship to the brain, are still being dismissed by most professionals as irrelevant hallucinations caused by biological crises of the organism.

It is also well known that near-death experiences have a profound impact on the survivors' psychological and physical well-being, as well as their worldview and behavior. And yet, these events are not routinely discussed with the patients and information about them is not considered an important part of the patients' history and included in the medical records. In most medical facilities, no specific psychological support is being offered that would help to integrate these challenging experiences.

People undergoing the process of dying in Western societies also often lack effective human support that would ease their transition. We try to protect ourselves from the emotional discomfort that death induces. The industrial world tends to remove sick and dying people into hospitals and nursing homes. The emphasis is on life-support systems and mechanical prolongation of life, often beyond any reasonable limits, rather than the human environment and the quality of the experience during the remaining days. The family system has disintegrated and children often live far from parents and grandparents. At the time of medical crisis, the contact is often formal and minimal.

With a few exceptions, mental health professionals, who have developed specific forms of psychological support and counseling for a large variety of emotional crises, have given little attention to the dying. Those facing the most profound of all imaginable crises, one that affects simultaneously the biological, emotional, interpersonal, social, philosophical, and spiritual aspects of the individual, remain the only ones for whom meaningful help is not available. A promising development in this regard is the growing network of hospices, inspired by the pioneering work of Cicely Saunders (Saunders 1967), that provide warm human environment for the dying.

All this occurs in the much larger context of collective denial of impermanence and mortality that characterizes Western industrial civilization. Much of our encounter with death is sanitized by teams of professionals who mitigate its immediate impact. In its extreme expression, it includes postmortem barbers and hairdressers, tailors, make-up experts, and plastic surgeons who make a wide variety of cosmetic adjustments on the corpse before it is shown to relatives and friends.

The media help create more distance from death by diluting it into empty statistics, reporting in a matter-of-fact way about the thousands of victims who die in wars, revolutions, and natural catastrophes. Movies and TV shows further trivialize death by capitalizing on violence. They anesthetize modern audiences against its emotional relevance by exposing them to countless scenes of dying, killing, and murder in the context of entertainment.

In general, the conditions of life existing in modern technological countries do not offer much ideological or psychological support for people who are facing death. This contrasts very sharply with the situation encountered by those dying in one of the ancient and preindustrial societies. Their cosmologies, philosophies, mythologies, as well as spiritual and ritual life, contain a clear message that death is not the absolute and irrevocable end of everything. They provide assurance for the dying that life or existence continues in some form beyond the biological demise.

Eschatological mythologies are in general agreement that the soul of the deceased undergoes a complex series of adventures in consciousness. The posthumous journey of the soul is sometimes described as a travel through fantastic landscapes that bear some similarity to those on earth, other times as encounters with various archetypal beings, or as moving through a sequence of holotropic states of consciousness. In some cultures the soul reaches a temporary realm in the Beyond, such as the Christian purgatory or the *lokas* of Tibetan Buddhism, in others an eternal abode—heaven, hell, paradise, or the sun realm. Many cultures have independently developed a belief system in metempsychosis or reincarnation that includes return of the unit of consciousness to another physical lifetime on earth.

Preindustrial societies all seemed to agree that death was not the ultimate defeat and end of everything, but an important transition. The experiences associated with death were seen as visits to important dimensions of reality that deserved to be experienced, studied, and carefully mapped. The dying were familiar with the eschatological cartographies of their cultures, whether these were shamanic maps of the funeral landscapes or sophisticated descriptions of the Eastern spiritual systems, such as those found in the *Tibetan Book of the Dead* (*Bardo Thödol*).

This important text of Tibetan Buddhism represents an interesting counterpoint to the exclusive pragmatic emphasis on productive life and denial of death characterizing the Western civilization. It describes the time of death as a unique opportunity for spiritual liberation from the cycles of death and rebirth or, in the event that we do not achieve liberation, a period that determines the nature of our next incarnation. In this context, it is possible to see the intermediate states between lives (*bardos*) as being in a way more important than incarnate existence. It is then essential to prepare for this time by systematic spiritual practice during our lifetime.

Another characteristic aspect of ancient and preindustrial cultures that colors the experience of dying is their acceptance of death as an integral part of life. Throughout their lives, people living in these cultures get used to spending time around dying people, handling corpses, observing cremation, and living with the remnants of the dead. For a Westerner, a visit to a place like Benares where this attitude is expressed in its extreme form can be a profoundly shattering experience.

People in preindustrial cultures typically die in the context of an extended family, clan, or tribe. They thus can receive meaningful emotional support from their close relatives and friends. It is also important to mention psychospiritual help provided by powerful rituals conducted at the time of death. These procedures are designed to assist individuals facing the ultimate transition or even offer specific guidance on the post mortem journey, such as the approach described in the *Bardo Thödol*.

An extremely important factor influencing the attitude toward death and the experience of dying in preindustrial cultures has been the existence of various forms of experiential training for dying involving holotropic states of consciousness. These include:

Shamanic methods
Rites of passage
Mysteries of death and rebirth
Various spiritual practices
Books of the dead

In our earlier discussions of shamanism, we have seen that novice shamans are introduced to the experiential territories of the beyond in their initiatory crises. These occur spontaneously or are induced by various methods during their apprenticeship with older shamans. After they complete the initiation and successfully integrate the psychospiritual transformation involved, they are able to enter holotropic states of their own volition and to guide other members of their tribes on their visionary journeys.

There is general agreement in shamanic literature that the experiential domain one visits in these inner journeys is identical with the territory one traverses during the posthumous journey of the soul. The experiences of shamans and their clients can thus be considered experiential training for dying. As I will show later, we have been able to collect supportive evidence for this thesis in a large project of psychedelic therapy with terminal cancer patients.

Anthropologists conducting field work in native cultures have described in detail many *rites of passage,* powerful ceremonies that these cultures enact repeatedly at the time of important transitions in life. The Dutch anthropologist Arnold van Gennep, who coined the term rites of passage, showed that they are practically ubiquitous among preindustrial peoples (van Gennep 1960). The external symbolism of rites of passage typically revolves around the triad birth-sex-death. The inner experiences of the initiates represent different combinations of perinatal and transpersonal elements and their common denominator is a profound confrontation with death and subsequent transcendence. People living in cultures that conduct rites of passage have thus during their lifetime numerous experiences of psychospiritual death and rebirth before they face their biological demise.

Experiences of psychospiritual death and rebirth, similar to those of shamans and participants in rites of passage, played also the key role in the *ancient mysteries of death and rebirth.* As we have seen earlier, they existed in many parts of the world and were based on mythological stories of deities that symbolize death and rebirth, such as Inanna and Tammuz, Isis and Osiris, Pluto and Persephone, Dionysus, Attis and Adonis, or the Aztec Quetzalcoatl and the Mayan Hero Twins. These mystery religions were widespread and played an important role in the ancient world.

The popularity of the mystery religions is evident from the fact that the number of initiates participating every five years in the mysteries in Eleusis has been estimated to exceed three thousand. This is how the mysteries were praised in an epic poem known as the *Homeric Hymn to Demeter* written around the seventh century B.C. by an unknown author: "Whoever among men who walk the Earth has seen these Mysteries is blessed, but whoever is uninitiated and has not received his share of the rite, he will not have the same lot as the others, once he is dead and dwells in the mould where the sun goes down."

The Greek poet Pindaros wrote about the initiation in Eleusis: "Blessed is he who, having seen these rites, undertakes the way beneath the Earth. He knows the end of life, as well as its divinely granted beginning." Similarly, the testimony of the great Greek tragic poet and playwright Sophocles confirms the deep impact that the awe-inspiring experience of the Eleusinian mysteries had on the initiates: "Thrice happy are those of mortals, who having seen those rites depart for Hades; for them alone is granted to have a true life there. For the rest, all there is evil" (Wasson, Hofmann, and Ruck 1978).

While the Homeric myth and the statements by Pindaros and Sophocles mention the importance of the mysteries for the encounter with death, the famous Roman philosopher, statesman, and lawyer Marcus Tullius Cicero emphasized in *De Legibus* also the impact the experience had on his life and the life of many others: "Nothing is higher than these mysteries. They have sweetened our character and softened our customs; they have made us pass from the condition of savages to true humanity. They have not only shown us the way to live joyfully, but they have taught us to die with hope" (Cicero 1977).

Another important mystery religion of antiquity was the Mithraic cult, the sister religion of Christianity and its very serious competitor for a world religion. At the cult's height, in the third century A.D., its influence reached from the Mediterranean area to the Baltic Sea. Over two thousand *mithraea,* underground sanctuaries in which the Mithraic rituals took place, have been discovered and studied by archeologists. These mithraea could be found from the shores of the Black Sea to the mountains of Scotland and to the border of the Sahara Desert (Ulansey 1989).

Of particular interest for transpersonally oriented researchers are practices of *various mystical traditions* and of the *great spiritual philosophies of the East*—various forms of yoga, Buddhism, Taoism, Sufism, Christian mysticism, Cabala, and many others. These systems developed effective forms of meditation, movement meditations, prayers, breathing exercises, and other effective techniques for inducing holotropic states of consciousness with profoundly spiritual components. Like the experiences of the shamans, initiates in the rites of passage, and neophytes in ancient mysteries, these procedures offered the possibility of confronting one's impermanence and mortality, transcending the fear of death, and radically transforming one's being in the world.

The description of the resources available to dying people in preindustrial cultures would not be complete without mentioning the *books of the dead,* such as the Tibetan *Bardo Thödol,* the Egyptian *Pert em hru,* the Aztec *Codex Borgia,* or the European *Ars moriendi.* When the ancient books of the dead first came to the attention of Western scholars, they were considered to be fictitious descriptions of the posthumous journey of the soul, and as such wishful fabrications of people who were unable to accept the grim reality of death. They were put in the same category as fairy tales, imaginary creations of human fantasy that had definite artistic beauty, but no basis in everyday reality and no practical relevance.

Deeper study of these texts revealed that they had been used as guides in the context of sacred mysteries and of spiritual practice and very likely described the experiences of the initiates and practitioners. From this new perspective, presenting the books of the dead as manuals for the dying appeared to be simply a clever disguise invented by the priests to obscure their real function and protect their deeper esoteric meaning and message from the uninitiated. The remaining problem seemed to be to discover the exact nature of the procedures used by the ancient spiritual systems to induce these states.

Modern research focusing on holotropic states brought unexpected new insights into this problem area. Systematic study of the experiences in psychedelic sessions, powerful nondrug forms of psychotherapy, and spontaneously occurring psychospiritual crises showed that in all these situations, people can encounter an entire spectrum of unusual experiences, including sequences of agony and dying, passing through hell, facing divine judgment, being reborn, reaching the celestial realms, and confronting memories from previous incarnations. These states were strikingly similar to those described in the eschatological texts of ancient and preindustrial cultures.

Timothy Leary, Richard Alpert, and Ralph Metzner were so impressed by the parallels between LSD experiences and the states described in the *Bardo Thödol* that they named their first book on the subject *The Psychedelic Experience: A Manual Based on the Tibetan Book of the Dead* and actually used passages from this book in guiding their LSD subjects (Leary, Alpert, and Metzner 1964). Another missing piece of the puzzle was provided by thanatology, the young scientific discipline specifically studying death and dying. Thanatological studies of near-death states showed that the experiences associated with life-threatening situations bear a deep resemblance to the descriptions from the ancient books of the dead, as well as those reported by subjects in psychedelic sessions and modern experiential psychotherapy. The most remarkable of these findings were repeated observations of the capacity of disembodied consciousness to observe immediate and remote environment.

These observations confirmed a claim of the Tibetan Bardo Thödol that previously seemed fantastic and absurd. According to this text, when we die, we leave the confines of the physical body and inhabit a *bardo body*. In this new form, we can travel unimpeded to any location on earth and, at the same time, maintains its capacity to perceive the environment. Modern consciousness research has thus shown that the ancient eschatological texts are actually maps of the inner territories of the psyche encountered in profound holotropic states, including those associated with biological dying.

It is possible to spend one's entire lifetime without ever experiencing these realms or even being aware of their existence, until one is catapulted into them at the time of biological death. However, some people are able to explore this experiential territory while they are still alive. Among the tools that make this possible are psychedelic substances, powerful forms of experiential psychotherapy, serious spiritual practice, and participation in shamanic rituals. For many people, similar experiences occur spontaneously, without any known triggers, during psychospiritual crises (spiritual emergencies).

All these situations offer the possibility of deep experiential exploration of the inner territories of the psyche at a time when we are healthy and strong, so that the encounter with death does not come as a complete surprise at the time of biological demise. The seventeenth-century German Augustinian monk, Abraham a Sancta Clara, expressed in a succinct way the importance of the experiential practice of dying: "The man who dies before he dies does not die when he dies."

This "dying before dying" has two important consequences: It liberates us from the fear of death and changes our attitude toward it. This eases considerably our experience of actually leaving the body at the time of our biological demise. At the same time, the elimination of the fear of death also transforms our way of being in the world. There is thus no fundamental difference between the preparation for death and the practice of dying, on the one hand, and spiritual practice leading to enlightenment, on the other. For this reason, the ancient books of the dead could be used in both situations.

All factors taken into consideration, many aspects of life in preindustrial cultures made the psychological situation of dying people significantly easier in comparison with the Western technological civilization. Naturally, the question that immediately arises is whether this advantage was due to lack of reliable information about the nature of reality and to wishful self-deception. If that were the case, a significant part of our difficulties in facing death would simply be the toll we have to pay for our deeper knowledge of the universal scheme of things. We might then prefer to bear the uncomfortable consequences of knowing the truth. However, closer examination of the existing evidence shows that this is not the case.

As I have shown in the preceding chapter, the single most important factor responsible for the striking differences between the worldview of Western industrial cultures and all other human groups throughout history is not the superiority of materialistic science over primitive superstition, but our profound ignorance in regard to holotropic states. The only way the monistic materialistic worldview of Western science can be maintained is by systematic suppression or misinterpretation of all the evidence generated by consciousness studies, whether its source is history, anthropology, comparative religion, or various areas of modern research, such as parapsychology, thanatology, psychedelic therapy, biofeedback, sensory deprivation, experiential psychotherapies, or the work with individuals in psychospiritual crises.

Systematic use of various forms of holotropic states that characterizes the ritual and spiritual life of ancient and aboriginal cultures opens experiential access to a rich spectrum of transpersonal experiences. This then inevitably leads to an understanding of the nature of reality and of the relationship between consciousness and matter that is fundamentally different from the belief system of industrial societies. The difference of opinion in regard to the possibility of consciousness after death thus exactly reflects the differences in the attitude toward holotropic states and in the degree of personal experience with them.

Let us now briefly review the observations from various fields of research which challenge the materialistic assumption that biological death represents the final end of existence and of conscious activity of any kind. In any exploration of this kind, it is important to keep an open mind and focus as much as possible on the available facts of observation. An unshakeable a priori commitment to the existing paradigm that characterizes the approach of mainstream scientists to this area is an attitude that is well known from fundamentalist religions.

Unlike scientism of this kind, science in the true sense of the word is open to unbiased investigation of any existing phenomena and of any domain of reality that lends itself to such an enterprise. With this in mind, we can divide the existing evidence into two categories: experiences and observations that challenge the traditional understanding of the nature of consciousness and its relationship to matter and experiences and observations specifically related to survival of consciousness after death.

Experiences and Observations that Challenge the Traditional Understanding of the Nature of Consciousness and Its Relationship to Matter

The work with holotropic states of consciousness has amassed a vast body of evidence that represents a serious challenge for the monistic materialistic worldview created by Western science, particularly its belief in primacy of matter over consciousness. Most of the challenging data have emerged from the study of transpersonal experiences and of the observations associated with them. This material suggests an urgent need for a radical revision of our current concepts of the nature of consciousness and its relationship to matter and to the brain. Since the materialistic paradigm of Western science has been the major obstacle for any objective evaluation of the data associated with dying and death, the study of transpersonal experiences has an indirect relevance for thanatology.

As we have seen, in transpersonal experiences it is possible to transcend the usual limitations of the body-ego, three-dimensional space, and linear time. The disappearance of spatial boundaries can lead to authentic and convincing identifications with other people, animals of different species, plant life, and even inorganic materials and processes. One can also transcend the temporal boundaries and experience episodes from the lives of one's human and animal ancestors, as well as collective, racial, and karmic memories. In addition, transpersonal experiences can take us into the archetypal domains of the collective unconscious and mediate encounters with blissful and wrathful deities of various cultures and visits to mythological realms.

In all these types of experiences, it is possible to access entirely new information about the phenomena involved that by far surpasses anything that we have obtained during this lifetime through the conventional channels. The study of consciousness that can extend beyond the body, maintains its capacity to perceive the environment, and collect experiences—William Roll's "theta consciousness" or the "long body" of the Iroquois Indians—is extremely important for the issue of survival, since it is this part of human personality that would be most likely to survive death.

According to materialistic science, any memory requires a material substrate, such as the neurons in the brain or the DNA molecules of the genes. However, it is impossible to imagine any material medium for the information conveyed by various forms of transpersonal experiences described above. This information clearly has not been acquired during our lifetime through the conventional means; that is, through the mediation of the sensory organs, analysis, and synthesis. It seems to exist independently of matter, possibly in the field of consciousness itself, or in some other type of field that at present cannot be detected by our scientific instruments.

The observations from the study of transpersonal experiences are supported by evidence that comes from other avenues of research. Challenging the basic metaphysical assumptions of Newtonian-Cartesian thinking, some scientists seriously explore such possibilities as "memory without a material substrate" (von Foerster 1965), "morphogenetic fields" that cannot be detected by any of the measuring devices available to modern science (Sheldrake 1981), and the subquantum "psi-field" that contains a complete holographic record of all the events constituting the history of the universe (Laszlo 1993). Of special interest in this regard is Sheldrake's paper "Can Our Memories Survive the Death of Our Brains?" that quite specifically addresses the lack of conclusive evidence that memories are located in the brain (Sheldrake 1990)

Traditional academic science describes human beings as highly developed animals and biological thinking machines. If we take into consideration only experiences and observations from the hylotropic state of consciousness that dominates our everyday life, we appear to be Newtonian objects made of atoms, molecules, cells, tissues, and organs. However, transpersonal experiences in holotropic states of consciousness clearly indicate that each of us can also manifest the properties of a field of consciousness that transcends space, time, and linear causality.

The complete new formula, remotely reminiscent of the wave-particle paradox in modern physics, thus describes humans as paradoxical beings who have two complementary aspects. Depending on circumstances, they can show either the properties of Newtonian objects (the "hylotropic aspect"), or those of infinite fields of consciousness (the "holotropic aspect"). The appropriateness of each of these descriptions depends on the state of consciousness in which these observations are made. Physical death then seems to terminate the hylotropic functioning, while the holotropic potential comes into full expression.

Experiences and Observations Specifically Related to Survival of Consciousness after Death

Phenomena on the Threshold of Death

Researchers have reported a variety of interesting phenomena occurring at the time of death. Here belong, for example, numerous reports of people who, shortly after death, appeared to their relatives, friends, and acquaintances. These apparitions show a statistically significant accumulation within a period of twelve hours around the deaths of the envisioned persons (Sidgwick 1894). There also exist many reports of unexplained physical events occurring in the deceased person's home—watches stopping and starting, bells ringing, or paintings and photographs falling from the wall—that seem to announce his or her death (Bozzano 1948).

Individuals approaching death often experience encounters with their dead relatives, who seem to welcome them to the next world. These deathbed visions are very authentic and convincing. They are often followed by a state of euphoria and seem to ease the transition for the dying. The usual objection is that visions of this kind are reconstructions of the images of relatives and friends from memories and products of imagination. For this reason, researchers have paid much attention to visions in which part of the "welcoming committee" was a person about whose death the dying individual was not aware. In parapsychological literature, these observations have been referred to as "peak in Darien" cases (Cobbe 1877).

Of particular interest are near-death experiences (NDEs) that occur in about one-third of the people who encounter various forms of sudden life-threatening situations, such as car accidents, near drowning, heart attacks, or cardiac arrests during operations. Raymond Moody, Kenneth Ring, Michael Sabom, Bruce Greyson, and others have done extensive research of this phenomenon and have described a characteristic experiential pattern.

It typically begins with an out-of-body experience, various forms of personal life review, and a passage through a dark tunnel. Its transpersonal culmination involves an encounter with a radiant divine being, a sense of judgment with ethical evaluation of one's life, and visits to various transcendental realms. In individual cases some components of this general pattern might be missing. Less frequent are painful, anxiety-provoking, and infernal types of NDEs (Grey 1985; Bache 1999). Christopher Bache suggested that negative NDEs represent a truncated and incomplete variety, in which the regressive life review does not proceed beyond the level of negative perinatal matrices.

In our program of psychedelic therapy with terminal cancer patients, conducted at the Maryland Psychiatric Research Center in Baltimore, we were able to obtain some interesting evidence about the similarity of NDEs with experiences induced by psychedelic substances. We observed several patients who had first psychedelic experiences and later actual NDEs when their disease progressed (e.g., cardiac arrest during an operation aimed at removing a metastatic tumor compressing the ureter). They reported that these two situations were very similar and described the psychedelic sessions as invaluable experiential training for dying (Grof and Halifax 1977).

The most extraordinary and fascinating aspect of NDEs is the occurrence of "veridical" out-of-body experiences (OOBEs). This term is being used for experiences of disembodied consciousness with accurate extrasensory perception of the environment. Thanatological studies have repeatedly confirmed that people who are unconscious or even clinically dead can have OOBEs during which they observe their bodies and the rescue procedures from above or even perceive events in other parts of the same building and in remote locations.

Recently, the research conducted by Ken Ring has added an interesting dimension to these observations. It has shown that congenitally blind people can, during near-death experiences, have visions, including those the veracity of which can be confirmed by consensual validation (Ring and Valarino 1998, Ring and Cooper 1999). Modern thanatological research has thus confirmed classical descriptions of OOBEs that can be found in spiritual literature and philosophical texts of all ages.

The occurrence of veridical OOBEs is not limited to near-death situations, vital emergencies, and episodes of clinical death. They can emerge in sessions of powerful experiential psychotherapy (such as primal therapy, rebirthing, or holotropic breathwork), in the context of experiences induced by psychedelics (particularly the dissociative anesthetic ketamine), and also spontaneously. Such events can represent isolated episodes in the life of the individual, or occur repeatedly as part of a crisis of psychic opening or some other type of spiritual emergency.

The best known researcher of OOBEs was Robert Monroe, who after many years of spontaneous experiences of out-of-body travel developed electronic laboratory techniques for inducing them and founded a special institute in Faber, Virginia, where they could be systematically studied. He described his experiences with these phenomena in a series of books (Monroe 1971, 1985, 1994). The authenticity of OOBEs has been demonstrated in controlled clinical studies, such as the experiments of the well-known psychologist and parapsychologist Charles Tart with Ms. Z. at the University of California in Davis (Tart 1968) and perceptual tests conducted by Karlis Osis and D. McCormick with Alex Tanous (Osis and McCormick 1980).

OOBEs with confirmed extrasensory perception of the environment are of special importance for the problem of consciousness after death, since they demonstrate that consciousness can operate independently of the body. According to the Western materialistic worldview, consciousness is a product of the neurophysiological processes in the brain and it is absurd to consider that it could detach itself from the body, become autonomous, and be capable of extrasensory perception. Yet, this is precisely what occurs in many well-documented cases of OOBEs. Naturally, people who have had OOBE might have come close to death, but did not really die. However, it seems reasonable to infer that if consciousness can function independently of the body during one's lifetime, it could be able to do the same after death.

Past-Life Experiences

A category of transpersonal experiences that has very direct relevance for the problem of survival of consciousness after death involves vivid reliving of episodes from earlier historical periods and from different parts of the world associated with a sense of personal remembering. These experiences have important implications for the understanding of the nature of consciousness and for the theory and practice of psychiatry, psychology, and psychotherapy. There is no doubt that experiential sequences of this kind constitute the empirical basis for the widespread belief in reincarnation. The historical and geographical universality of this belief shows that it is a very important cultural phenomenon.

The concept of karma and reincarnation represents a cornerstone of Hinduism, Buddhism, Jainism, Sikhism, Zoroastrianism, the Tibetan Vajrayana Buddhism, and Taoism. Similar ideas can be found in such geographically, historically, and culturally diverse groups as various African tribes, native Americans, pre-Columbian cultures, the Hawaiian kahunas, practitioners of the Brazilian umbanda, the Gauls, and the Druids. In ancient Greece, several important schools of thought subscribed to it. Among them were the Pythagoreans, the Orphics, and the Platonists. This doctrine was also adopted by the Essenes, the Pharisees, the Karaites, and other Jewish and semi-Jewish groups, and it formed an important part of the cabalistic theology of medieval Jewry. It was also held by the Neoplatonists and Gnostics.

For the Hindus and the Buddhists, as well as open-minded and knowledgeable modern consciousness researchers, reincarnation is not a matter of belief, but an empirical issue, based on very specific experiences and observations. This material has been the subject of numerous articles and books. According to Christopher Bache, the evidence in this area is so rich and extraordinary that scientists who do not think the problem of reincarnation deserves serious study are "either uninformed or bone-headed" (Bache 1988). In view of the theoretical importance of this problem area and its highly controversial nature, it is absolutely imperative to examine carefully and critically the existing evidence before making any conclusions and judgments concerning karma and reincarnation.

Spontaneous past-life memories in children. Important supportive evidence for the concept of reincarnation comes from the study of numerous cases of small children who seem to remember and describe their previous life in another body, another place, and with other people. These memories emerge usually spontaneously shortly after these children begin to talk. This often causes serious problems in the life of these children, and can be associated with "carry-over pathologies," such as phobias and specific psychosomatic symptoms. In many instances, the past-life stories told by these children seem to explain otherwise unexplainable attractions and predilections, strange reactions to certain people and situations, or various idiosyncrasies in these children's present life. Cases of this kind have been studied and described by child psychiatrists. Access to these memories usually disappears between the ages of five and eight.

Ian Stevenson, professor of psychology at the University of Virginia in Charlottesville, Virginia, has conducted meticulous studies of over three thousand such cases and reported them in *Twenty Cases Suggestive of Reincarnation, Unlearned Languages,* and *Children Who Remember Previous Lives* (Stevenson 1966, 1984, and 1987). From this rich material, he selected only several hundred cases, because many others have not met the highest standards he had set for himself in his research. Some of the cases were eliminated, because the family benefited financially, in terms of social prestige, or public attention, others because Stevenson found a connecting person who could have been the psychic link. Additional reasons were inconsistent testimony, false memories (*cryptomnesia*), witnesses of questionable character, or indication of fraud. Only the strongest cases were included in his final reports.

The findings of Stevenson's research were quite remarkable. He was able to confirm by independent investigation, often with incredible details, the stories the children were telling about their previous lifetimes, although he had eliminated in all the reported cases the possibility that they could have obtained the information through the conventional channels. In some cases, he actually took the children into the village or town that they remembered from their previous life. Although they had never been there in their current lifetime, they were familiar with the topography of the place, were able to find the home they had allegedly lived in, recognized the members of their "family" and the villagers, and knew their names.

According to Stevenson, the reason why children remember their previous life might be dramatic circumstances surrounding death, particularly those involving shock that "can possibly break through the amnesia." The fact that the most vivid memories usually involve the events immediately leading up to death seems to support this explanation. Christopher Bache offered a detailed analysis of Stevenson's material in his last book, *Dark Night, Early Dawn: Steps to a Deep Ecology of Mind.* He suggested that the process of dying might have several stages and that in Stevenson's cases this process remained truncated and incomplete. The individuals involved did not succeed in severing fully their ties with the earthly plane and moving on to other dimensions of reality. In all of them, new incarnation happened within a relatively short period of time and in close proximity of the place they had lived before (Bache 1999).

Typically, these children do not know anything about events that occurred in the former personality's life after his or her death. This is an important point in deciding whether they are unconsciously reconstructing the details of this life by telepathically reading the minds of those who knew the deceased or possess these details as genuine memories. Possibly the strongest evidence in support of the reincarnation hypothesis is in Stevenson's last work. It focuses on frequent incidence of striking birthmarks in these children that reflect injuries and other events from the remembered life (Stevenson 1997).

In evaluating this evidence, it is important to emphasize that Stevenson's cases were not only from "primitive" and "exotic" cultures with a priori belief in reincarnation, but also from Western countries, including Great Britain and the United States. His research meets high standards and has received considerable esteem. In the year 1977, the *Journal of Nervous and Mental Diseases* devoted almost an entire issue to this subject and the work was reviewed in *the Journal of the American Medical Association* (*JAMA*).

Spontaneous past-life memories in adults. Spontaneous vivid reliving of past-life memories occurs most frequently during episodes of transpersonal crises (spiritual emergencies). However, various degrees of remembering can also happen in more or less ordinary states of consciousness under the circumstances of everyday life. They range from a sudden feeling of familiarity with a location one has not previously visited in the present lifetime to emergence of complex memories from previously unknown times and places. Academic psychiatry and current theories of personality are based on the "one-timer view." Traditional professionals are aware of the existence of past life experiences, but see and treat them as hallucinations and delusions and thus as indications of serious psychopathology.

Evoked past-life memories in adults. Past-life experiences can be elicited by a wide variety of techniques that mediate access to deep levels of the psyche. Among them are meditation, hypnosis, psychedelic substances, sensory isolation, bodywork, and various powerful experiential psychotherapies, such as primal therapy, rebirthing, or holotropic breathwork. Experiences of this kind often appear unsolicited in sessions with therapists who neither work with past-life memories nor necessarily even believe in them. They can thus come as a shocking surprise, catching these therapists completely off guard. The emergence of past-life memories is also completely independent of the subject's previous philosophical and religious belief system. In addition, these phenomena occur on the same continuum with accurate memories from adolescence, childhood, infancy, birth, and prenatal times, the content of which can often be reliably verified. On occasion, past-life memories coexist or alternate with perinatal phenomena (Grof 1988, 1992).

There are important reasons to assume that past-life experiences are authentic phenomena *sui generis*, which have important implications for psychology and psychotherapy because of their heuristic and therapeutic potential. They can feel extremely real and authentic and often mediate access to accurate information about various periods of history, cultures, and even specific historical events. The nature and quality of this information often transcends the education of the individuals involved and includes details which make it clear that it has not been acquired through the ordinary channels. In some instances, the accuracy of these memories can be objectively verified with astonishing detail.

Karmic material is also often involved in the pathogenesis of various emotional, psychosomatic, and interpersonal problems, as we saw earlier in the case history of Norbert (74–75). Conversely, the reliving of past-life experiences has great therapeutic potential. In many instances, it can resolve difficult symptoms that could not be significantly influenced by therapeutic work focusing on their biographical and perinatal roots. One aspect of past-life memories is particularly extraordinary and surprising: they are often associated with meaningful synchronicities that involve various aspects of everyday existence.

The criteria for verification of the content of past-life experiences are the same as for determining what happened last month or ten years ago. We have to retrieve specific memories with as much detail as possible and secure independent evidence for at least some of them. Naturally, past-life memories are more difficult to verify than memories of events from the present lifetime. They do not always contain specific information that would lend itself to a verification procedure. The evidence is also harder to find, since the events we are trying to verify are much older and involve other countries and cultures. It is important to consider that even the memories from our current lifetime cannot always be corroborated, only some of them. In addition, most evoked past-life memories do not permit the same degree of verification as Stevenson's spontaneous memories, which are typically more recent and rich in detail.

In rare cases, the circumstances allow verification of induced past-life memories in remarkable detail. I have observed and published two cases where the most unusual aspects of these experiences could be verified by historical research. The first one involved Renata, a neurotic patient, who in four consecutive LSD sessions experienced episodes from the life of a Czech aristocrat from the beginning of the seventeenth century. Together with twenty-six other noblemen, this man was publicly executed in the Old Town Square in Prague after the Hapsburgs had defeated the Czech king in the battle of White Mountain. By genealogical search, carried quite independently and without Renata's knowledge, her father was able to trace the family pedigree to one of these unfortunate noblemen (Grof 1975).

In the second case Karl, a participant in our month-long workshop at the Esalen Institute, relived in several consecutive holotropic breathwork sessions a series of memories from the time of Walter Raleigh, when Great Britain was in war with Spain. In his experiences, he was a priest who, together with about four hundred Spanish soldiers, had been besieged by the British army in the fortress Dunanoir on the West Coast of Ireland. After long negotiations, the British promised them free egress if they surrendered. The Spaniards accepted the offer and opened the gates. The British did not keep their word and brutally slaughtered all of them. Their dead bodies were thrown over the ramparts to the beach below and denied burial (Grof 1988).

Being a good artist, Karl portrayed the most important experiences from his self-exploration in a series of drawings and impulsive finger paintings. Among them was the vision of his own hand with a beautiful seal ring that carried the initials of the priest's name. Through meticulous detective work, Karl was able to identify the place and time of the battle and find detailed descriptions of this episode in historical archives. The actual events matched closely the content of his experiences. One detailed document gave the name of the priest and Karl was astounded to find out that the initials of this man's name were identical with those on the picture he had drawn weeks earlier.

Tibetan practices relevant to the problem of reincarnation. Tibetan spiritual literature contains some interesting stories which suggest that highly developed spiritual masters are able to gain far-reaching knowledge related to the process of reincarnation and develop the ability to exert a certain degree of control over it. This includes the possibility of determining the time of their death, predicting or even choosing the time and place of their next incarnation, and maintaining consciousness through the intermediate states between death and the next incarnation (*bardos*).

Conversely, accomplished Tibetan monks can through various clues received in dreams, meditation, and through other channels locate and identify the child who is the reincarnation of a Dalai Lama or a *tulku*. The child is then exposed to a test, during which he has to identify correctly from several sets of similar objects those that belonged to the deceased. Some aspects of this practice could, at least theoretically, be subjected to a rather rigorous testing following Western standards. Other unusual claims of the Tibetan Vajrayana tradition, such as the existence of exercises that can increase the body temperature by many degrees (*tummo*), have already been confirmed by Western specialists (Benson et al. 1982). This research was done with the consent and support of His Holiness the Dalai Lama.

The extraordinary characteristics of past-life experiences have been repeatedly confirmed by independent observers. However, all these impressive facts do not necessarily constitute a definitive proof that we survive death and reincarnate as the same separate unit of consciousness, or the same individual soul. This conclusion is just one possible interpretation of the existing evidence. This is essentially the same situation that we encounter in science, where we have certain facts of observation and look for a theory that would explain them and put them into a coherent conceptual framework.

One of the basic rules in modern philosophy of science is that a theory should never be confused with the reality that it describes. The history of science clearly shows that there always exists more than one way to interpret the available data. In the study of past-life phenomena, as in any other area of exploration, we have to separate facts of observation from the theories that try to make sense of them. For example, the falling of objects is a fact of observation, whereas the theories trying to explain why it happens have changed several times in the course of history and undoubtedly will change again.

The existence of past-life experiences with all their remarkable characteristics is an unquestionable fact that can be verified by any serious researcher who is sufficiently open-minded and interested to check the evidence. It is also clear that there is no plausible explanation for these phenomena within the conceptual framework of mainstream psychiatry and psychology. On the other hand, the interpretation of the existing data is a much more complex and difficult matter. The popular understanding of reincarnation as a repeated cycle of life, death, and rebirth of the same individual is a reasonable conclusion from the available evidence. It certainly is far superior to the attitude most traditional psychologists and psychiatrists assume vis-à-vis this material. They either do not know or ignore the available data and rigidly adhere to the established ways of thinking.

While the observations suggestive of reincarnation are very impressive, it certainly is not difficult to imagine some alternative interpretations of the same data. Naturally, none of them is congruent with the monistic materialistic paradigm of Western science. At least two such alternative explanations can already be found in the spiritual literature. In the Hindu tradition, the belief in reincarnation of separate individuals is seen as a popular and unsophisticated understanding of reincarnation. In the last analysis, there is only one being that has true existence and that is Brahman, or the creative principle itself.

All separate individuals in all the dimensions of existence are just products of infinite metamorphoses of this one immense entity. Since all the divisions and boundaries in the universe are illusory and arbitrary, only Brahman really incarnates. All the protagonists in the divine play of existence are different aspects of this One. When we attain this ultimate knowledge, we are able to see that our past incarnation experiences represent just another level of illusion or *maya*. To see these lives as "our lives" requires perception of the karmic players as separate individuals and reflects ignorance concerning the fundamental unity of everything.

Shri Ramana Maharshi expressed the paradoxical relationship between the creative principle and the elements of the material world in a very succinct way:

> The world is illusory
> Brahman alone is real;
> Brahman is the world

In *Lifecycles: Reincarnation and the Web of Life,* Christopher Bache (1988) discusses another interesting concept of reincarnation found in the books by Jane Roberts (1973) and in the works of other authors. Here the emphasis is neither on the individual separate unit of consciousness nor on God, but on the Oversoul, an entity that lies in between the two. If the term *soul* refers to the consciousness that collects and integrates the experiences of an individual incarnation, the Oversoul or Soul is the name given to the larger consciousness that collects and integrates the experiences of many incarnations. According to this view, it is the Oversoul that incarnates, not the individual unit of consciousness.

Bache points out that if we are extensions of our former lives, we clearly are not the summation of all the experiences that they have contained. The purpose that the Oversoul has for incarnating is to collect specific experiences. A full involvement in a particular life requires severing the connection with the Oversoul and assuming discrete personal identity. At the time of death, the separate individual dissolves in the Oversoul, leaving only a mosaic of unassimilated difficult experiences. These then become assigned to the life of other incarnated beings in a process that can be compared to dealing a handful of cards in a card game.

In this model, there is no true continuity between the lives of the individuals who incarnate at different times. By experiencing undigested parts of other lives, we are not dealing with our personal karma, but actually clearing the field of the Oversoul. The image that Bache uses to illustrate the relationship between the individual soul and the Oversoul is that of a nautilus shell. Here each chamber represents a separate unit and reflects a certain period in the life of the mollusk, but it is also integrated into a larger whole.

We have so far discussed three different ways of interpreting the observations related to past-life phenomena. The incarnating units were described as, respectively, the individual unit of consciousness, the Oversoul, and Absolute Consciousness. However, we have not exhausted all the possibilities of alternative explanations that could account for the observed facts. Because of the arbitrary nature of all boundaries in the universe, we could just as easily define as the incarnating principle a unit larger than the Oversoul, for example, the field of consciousness of the entire human species or that of all life forms.

We could also take our analysis a step further and explore the factors that determine the specific choice of the karmic experiences that are assigned to the incarnating unit of consciousness. For example, some people with whom I have worked had convincing insights that an important factor in the selection process might be the relationship between karmic patterns and the time and place of a particular incarnation with its specific astrological correlates. This notion is in general agreement with the observations from psychedelic sessions, holotropic breathwork, and spontaneous episodes of psychospiritual crises. They show that in all these situations the content and timing of holotropic states are closely correlated with planetary transits An extensive treatment of this subject can be found in Richard Tarnas's meticulously documented study (Tarnas, in press).

Apparitions of the Dead and Communication with Them

We have discussed earlier the experiences of encounter and communication with deceased persons occurring in two situations in which they are particularly frequent. The first of these was the time within several hours of these persons' death, when it is very common for friends and relatives to see apparitions of the deceased. The second one involved the time when the percipients themselves were dying or having a near-death experience and had visions of the "welcoming committee." But the apparitions of deceased persons are not limited to these two situations. They can occur at any time, either spontaneously or in psychedelic sessions, in the course of experiential psychotherapies, or during meditation. Naturally, the data from this area have to be evaluated particularly carefully and critically.

The simple fact of a private experience of this kind does not really amount to very much and can easily be dismissed as a wishful fantasy or hallucination. Some significant additional factors would have to be present should such experiences be considered valid research material. Fortunately, some of the apparitions have certain characteristics that make them very interesting or even challenging for researchers. For example, many cases reported in the literature involve apparitions of persons unknown to the percipient, who were later reliably identified through photographs and verbal descriptions. It also is not uncommon for apparitions to be witnessed collectively by an entire group of people or successively by many different individuals over long periods of time, such as it is the case in "haunted" houses and castles.

In some instances, the apparitions can have distinguishing bodily marks accrued around the time of death unbeknownst to the percipient. Of particular interest are those cases where the apparitions of the deceased convey some specific and accurate new information that can be verified or is linked with an extraordinary synchronicity. I have myself observed in LSD therapy and in holotropic breathwork several remarkable instances of this kind. Here are three examples to illustrate the nature of such observations.

The first of these examples is an event that occurred during LSD therapy of a young, severely depressed patient who had made repeated suicidal attempts.

> In one of his LSD sessions, Richard had a very unusual experience involving a strange and uncanny astral realm. This domain had an eerie luminescence and was filled with discarnate beings who were trying to communicate

with him in a very urgent and demanding manner. He could not see or hear them; however, he sensed their almost tangible presence and was receiving telepathic messages from them. I wrote down one of these messages that was very specific and could be subjected to subsequent verification.

It was a request for Richard to connect with a couple in the Moravian city of Kroměříž and let them know that their son Ladislav was doing all right and was well taken care of. The message included the couple's name and telephone number; all of these data were unknown to me and the patient. This experience was extremely puzzling; it seemed to be an alien enclave in Richard's experience, totally unrelated to his problems and the rest of his treatment.

After the session, I decided to do what certainly would have made me the target of my colleagues' jokes, had they found out. I went to the telephone, dialed the number in Kroměříž, and asked if I could speak with Ladislav. To my astonishment, the woman on the other side of the line started to cry. When she calmed down, she told me with a broken voice: "Our son is not with us anymore; he passed away; we lost him three weeks ago."

The second illustrative example involves a close friend and former colleague, Walter N. Pahnke, who was a member of our psychedelic research team at the Maryland Psychiatric Research Center in Baltimore. He had deep interest in parapsychology, particularly in the problem of consciousness after death, and worked with many famous mediums and psychics, including our joint friend Eileen Garrett, president of the American Parapsychological Association. In addition, he was also the initiator of the LSD program for patients dying of cancer at the Maryland Psychiatric Research Center in Catonsville.

In summer 1971, Walter went with his wife Eva and their children for a vacation in a cabin in Maine, situated right on the ocean. One day, he went scuba diving all by himself and did not return. An extensive and well-organized search failed to find his body or any part of his diving gear. Under these circumstances, Eva found it very difficult to accept and integrate his death. Her last memory was of Walter leaving the cabin, full of energy and in perfect health. It was hard for her to believe that he was not part of her life any more and to start a new chapter of her existence without a sense of closure of the preceding one.

Being a psychologist herself, she qualified for an LSD training session for mental health professionals offered through a special program in our institute. She decided to have a psychedelic experience with the hope of getting some more insights and asked me to be her sitter. In the second half of the session, she had a very powerful vision of Walter and carried on a long and meaningful dialogue with him. He gave her specific instructions concerning each of their three children and released her to start a new life of her own, unencumbered and unrestricted by a sense of commitment to his memory. It was a very profound and liberating experience.

Just as Eva was questioning whether the entire episode was just a wishful fabrication of her own mind, Walter appeared once more for a brief period of time and asked Eva to return a book that he had borrowed from a friend of his. He then proceeded to give her the name of the friend, the room where it was, the name of the book, the shelf, and the sequential order of the book on this shelf. Following the instructions, Eva was actually able to find and return the book, about the existence of which she had had no previous knowledge.

Kurt, one of the psychologists participating in our three-year professional training program in transpersonal psychology and holotropic breathwork had witnessed a wide variety of transpersonal experiences of his colleagues and had had a few of them himself. In spite of it, he continued to be very skeptical about the authenticity of these phenomena. Then, in one of his holotropic sessions, he experienced the following unusual synchronicity which convinced him that he had been too conservative in his approach to human consciousness.

Toward the end of the session, Kurt had a vivid experience of encountering his grandmother, who had been dead for many years. He had been very close to her in his childhood and was deeply moved by the possibility that he might be really communicating with her again. In spite of deep emotional involvement in the experience, he continued to maintain an attitude of professional skepticism about this encounter. Naturally, he had had many real interactions with his grandmother while she was still alive and suspected that his mind might have easily created an imaginary encounter from these old memories.

However, this meeting with his dead grandmother was so emotionally profound and convincing that he simply could not dismiss it as a wishful fantasy. He decided to seek proof that the experience was real and not just his imagination. He asked his grandmother for some form of confirmation that this was really happening and received the following message: "Go to Aunt Anna and look for cut roses." Still skeptical, he decided on the following weekend to visit his Aunt Anna's home and see what would happen.

Upon his arrival, Kurt found his aunt in the garden, surrounded by cut roses. He was astonished. The day of his visit just happened to be the one day of the year that his aunt had decided to do some radical pruning of her roses.

Like the two preceding examples, observations of this kind certainly are not a definitive proof of objective existence of astral realms and discarnate beings. However, the astonishing synchronicities that are sometimes associated with them give us some understanding as to how such beliefs might have originated and why they are so strong and convincing for some people. Current dismissal of these phenomena as products of superstition and wishful thinking simply is not adequate and this fascinating area deserves serious attention of consciousness researchers.

Of special interest is the quasi-experimental evidence suggestive of survival of consciousness after death that comes from the highly charged and controversial area of spiritistic seances and mental or trance mediumship. Although some of the professional mediums, including the famous Eusapia Palladino, have occasionally been caught cheating, others, such as Mrs. Piper, Mrs. Leonard, and Mrs. Verall, withstood all the tests and gained a high esteem of careful and reputable researchers (Grosso 1994). The best media have been able to accurately reproduce in their performances the deceased's voice, speech patterns, gestures, mannerisms, and other characteristic features, even if they did not have any previous knowledge of these persons.

On occasion, the received information was unknown to any of the present persons or even to any living person whatsoever. There also have been instances of sudden intrusion of uninvited "drop-in" entities whose identities were later independently confirmed. In other instances, relevant messages were received in "proxy sittings," in which a distant and uninformed party sought information in lieu of a close relative or friend of the deceased. In the cases of "cross correspondence," bits and pieces of a comprehensive message have been conveyed through several mediums.

An interesting innovation in this area is the procedure described in Raymond Moody's *Reunions: Visionary Encounters with Departed Loved Ones*. Inspired by a Greek underground complex known for offering the opportunity to see dead relatives and friends in a large copper kettle full of water, Moody conducted a systematic literary research of crystal-gazing, scrying, and similar phenomena. He then created a special environment and procedure that, according to his experience, greatly facilitate visionary encounters with the deceased loved ones. Moody described instances in which the apparitions actually emerged from the mirror and freely moved around the room as three-dimensional holographic images (Moody 1993).

Some of the spiritistic reports considerably stretch the mind of an average Westerner, let alone a traditionally trained scientist. For example, the extreme form of spiritistic phenomena, the "physical mediumship," includes among others telekinesis and materializations. Here belong, for example, upward levitation of objects and people, projection of objects through the air, manifestation of ectoplasmic formations, and appearance of writings or objects without explanation ("apports").

In the Brazilian spiritist movement, media perform psychic surgeries using their hands or knives allegedly under the guidance of the spirits of deceased people. These surgeries do not require any anesthesia and the wounds close without sutures. Philippino psychic surgeons, who are also members of the spiritist church, have been known to perform similar extraordinary procedures. Events of this kind have been repeatedly studied and filmed by Western researchers of the stature of Walter Pahnke, Stanley Krippner, and Andrija Puharich.

A particularly intriguing development in the efforts to communicate with the spirits of deceased people is an approach called *instrumental transcommunication* (ITC) that uses for this purpose modern electronic technology. This avenue began in 1959, when the Scandinavian filmmaker Friedrich Juergensen picked up on an audiotape human voices of allegedly dead persons while recording in a silent forest the sounds of passerine birds. Inspired by Juergensen's observation, psychologist Konstantin Raudive conducted a systematic study of this phenomenon and recorded over 100.000 multilingual paranormal voices allegedly communicating messages from the beyond (Raudive 1971).

More recently, a worldwide network of researchers, including Ernest Senkowski, George Meek, Mark Macy, Scott Rogo, Raymond Bayless, and others, have been involved in a group effort to establish interdimensional communication with the use of modern technology. They claim to have received many paranormal messages and pictures from various deceased persons through electronic media, including tape recorders, telephones, FAX machines, computers, and TV screens. Among the spirits communicating from the beyond are supposedly some of the former researchers in this field, such as Juergensen and Raudive (Senkowski 1994). A discarnate entity, who calls himself the Technician, allegedly provides specific technical instructions and advice for construction of electronic devices for optimal reception of messages from the beyond.

As fantastic and unbelievable as all the reports about communicating with the world of spirits might seem, it is certainly unlikely that scores of competent and respectable researchers, including some with impeccable scientific credentials and awards, would get attracted to a field that does not provide any genuine phenomena to observe and study. Among the individuals seriously interested and involved in spiritism were Nobel Prize winning scientists. There is certainly no other area in which the positions and opinions of prominent scientists are so easily dismissed and even ridiculed.

Psychedelic Therapy in Patients with Terminal Diseases

During the last three decades, we have seen a rapid increase of knowledge related to death and dying. Thanatologists have conducted systematic studies of near-death experiences and made the information about them available to professional circles and lay audiences. Consciousness researchers and experiential therapists have demonstrated that memories of life-threatening experiences, particularly of the trauma of birth, play a crucial role in the psychogenesis of emotional and psychosomatic disorders. They also realized that psychological confrontation with death in a therapeutic context can be profoundly healing and transformative.

Much has changed also in the care of terminal patients. The pioneering work of Elisabeth Kübler-Ross brought to the attention of the medical profession the emotional needs of terminal patients and the necessity to provide for them adequate support (Kübler-Ross 1969). The growing network of hospices, the result of an effort to humanize terminal care initiated in 1967 by the work of Cicely Saunders at St. Christopher's in London (Saunders 1967), has greatly improved the situation of many severely ill patients. It has helped to create a more relaxed and informal atmosphere with emphasis on human warmth, compassion, and emotional support.

In the late 1960s and early 1970s, I had the privilege to participate for several years in a research program of psychedelic psychotherapy for terminal cancer patients, which was without a doubt the most radical and interesting attempt to alleviate the suffering of patients with incurable diseases and transform their experience of dying. It was one of the most moving experiences of my life to see how the attitude toward death and the experience of dying of many terminal cancer patients was transformed by profound mystical experiences in psychedelic sessions.

Unfortunately, the political and administrative difficulties resulting from unsupervised use of LSD made it impossible to make this extraordinary procedure available on a large scale for the patients in hospitals and hospices. Hopefully, at some point in time, when the current hysteria concerning psychedelic substances subsides and the administrative policies are more enlightened, terminal patients around the world will be able to take advantage of the findings of the Maryland study and face death with less pain and more equanimity and dignity.

The idea that psychedelics could be useful in the therapy of individuals dying of cancer originated independently in the minds of several researchers. The first suggestion that these substances might be useful in this regard came from the Russian-American pediatrician Valentina Pavlovna Wasson. After years of intensive ethnomycological studies, she and her husband, Gordon Wasson, found in the literature reports about the use of psychedelic mushrooms in pre-Columbian cultures and made several trips to Mexico to pursue these clues.

After several trials, they were able to locate a Mazatec *curandera,* Maria Sabina, who knew the secret of the magic mushrooms. In June 1955, the Wassons became the first Westerners to be admitted to a *velada,* a sacred mushroom ritual. In an interview given two years later, Valentina Pavlovna described her powerful experience and suggested that, as the drug would become better known, medical uses would be found for it in the treatment of mental diseases, alcoholism, narcotic addiction, and terminal diseases associated with severe pain (Wasson 1957).

The second person who suggested that psychedelics could be useful for dying individuals was not a physician, but the philosopher and writer Aldous Huxley. He was deeply interested both in mystical experiences induced by psychedelics and in problems related to death and dying. In 1955, when his first wife Maria was dying of cancer, he used a hypnotic technique to bring her in touch with the memories of several spontaneous ecstatic experiences she had had during her life. The explicit purpose of this experiment was to ease her transition by inducing a mystical state of consciousness. This experience inspired Huxley's description of a similar situation in his novel *Island,* where the *moksha* medicine, a preparation made of psychedelic mushrooms, is used to help Lakshmi, one of the central characters, to face death (Huxley 1963).

In a letter to Humphrey Osmond, a psychiatrist and pioneer in psychedelic research, who introduced him to LSD and mescaline, Huxley wrote: "My own experience with Maria convinced me that the living can do a great deal for the dying, to raise the most purely physiological act of human existence to the level of consciousness and perhaps even spirituality." In another letter to Humphrey Osmond, written as early as 1958, Huxley suggested a number of uses he foresaw for LSD, among them "yet another project—the administration of LSD to terminal cancer cases, in the hope that it would make dying a more spiritual, less strictly physiological process."

In 1963, when Huxley was himself dying of cancer, he demonstrated the seriousness of his proposal. Several hours before his death, he asked his second wife Laura to give him 100 micrograms of LSD to facilitate his dying process. This moving experience was later described in Laura Huxley's book *This Timeless Moment* (Huxley 1968). Aldous Huxley's suggestion, although powerfully illustrated by his personal example, had for several years no influence on medical researchers. The next contribution to this area came from an unexpected source and was unrelated to Huxley's thinking and writing.

In the early 1960s, Eric Kast of the Chicago Medical School studied the effects of various drugs on the experience of pain in search of a good and reliable analgesic. In the course of this study, he became interested in LSD as a possible candidate. In a paper published in 1963, Kast and Collins described the results of a research project, in which the effects of LSD were compared with two established potent narcotic drugs, the opiates Dilaudid and Demerol. Statistical analysis of the results showed that the analgesic effect of LSD was superior to both opiates (Kast 1963, Kast and Collins 1964).

In addition to pain relief, Kast and Collins noticed that some of the patients showed after the LSD experience a striking disregard for the gravity of their situation. They frequently talked about their impending death with an emotional attitude that would be considered atypical in our culture; yet it was obvious that this new perspective was beneficial in view of the situation they were facing. In a later study, the same authors confirmed their initial findings concerning the analgesic effects of LSD. The relief of pain lasted on average twelve hours, but in some patients extended over a period of several weeks. Many of the patients also showed a change in philosophical and spiritual attitudes toward dying, "happy oceanic feelings," and enhanced morale (Kast and Collins 1966).

In the above studies, the patients were given LSD without any previous information about its effects and did not receive any psychological support during the sessions. Kast interpreted the changes in the attitude toward death in psychoanalytical terms, as "regression to the stage of infantile omnipotence" and "psychological denial of the seriousness of the situation," rather than a genuine change of philosophical and spiritual views. In spite of what to an LSD therapist might appear as shortcomings in Kast's studies and his interpretations, the historical value of his pioneering effort is unquestionable. He not only discovered the analgesic value of LSD, but also brought forth the first experimental evidence for Valentina Pavlovna's and Aldous Huxley's ideas.

The encouraging results of Kast and Collins's studies inspired Sidney Cohen, a prominent Los Angeles psychiatrist, friend of Aldous Huxley and one of the pioneers of psychedelic research, to start a program of psychedelic therapy for terminal cancer patients. Cohen confirmed Kast's findings concerning the effect of LSD on severe pain and stressed the importance of developing techniques that would alter the experience of dying (Cohen 1965). His co-worker, Gary Fisher, who continued these studies, emphasized the important role that transcendental experiences play in the treatment of the dying, whether these are spontaneous, resulting from various spiritual practices, or induced by psychedelic substances (Fisher 1970).

Another series of observations that was later integrated into the theory and practice of psychedelic therapy for the dying originated in the Psychiatric Research Institute in Prague, Czechoslovakia, where I headed in the 1960s a research project exploring the therapeutic and heuristic potential of LSD and other psychedelics. In the course of this research, I observed repeatedly that the clinical condition of the patients improved considerably after they had powerful experiences of psychospiritual death and rebirth.

In addition to describing improvement of various emotional and psychosomatic symptoms, these patients often reported that these experiences profoundly changed their image of death and attitude toward it. This included two patients who had suffered from thanatophobia, pathological fear of death. Since these were generally young and healthy individuals, I became very curious whether the same changes would occur in patients with terminal diseases, for whom the prospect of death lay in the immediate future. I conducted LSD sessions with several patients in this category and was very impressed by the results. I was about to start a special study exploring this issue further when I received an offer of a one-year fellowship in the United States.

It came as a big surprise for me when the first meeting of the research team at Spring Grove after my arrival in Baltimore concerned LSD therapy with cancer patients. The idea to start a special research project of this kind was inspired by a misfortune of a staff member. Gloria, a middle-aged woman who was very popular among her colleagues, had been diagnosed with breast cancer. The cancer had metastasized and the prognosis was rather poor. She became very depressed and experienced a strong fear of death.

The Spring Grove team had been conducting a large study with chronic alcoholics that involved therapeutic LSD sessions. The symptoms of these patients that most readily responded to psychedelic therapy, as measured by the Minnesota Multiphasic Personality Inventory (MMPI), were depression and anxiety. Sidney Wolf, one of the LSD therapists, suggested to the staff that it might be worth experimenting to determine whether their colleague's depression and anxiety would respond to LSD therapy even though it was clearly reactive, reflecting a desperate life situation. The result of Sidney Wolf's experiment was so encouraging that the research team now seriously considered to start a special study with a group of selected cancer patients.

The next important step in this endeavor was made in late 1967, when Walter Pahnke joined the Spring Grove team. Walter was instrumental in changing the initial interest of the staff into a pilot study and eventually into a large research project. He was an M.D., graduate of Harvard Medical School, with an additional doctorate in comparative religion and a degree in divinity. It would be difficult to imagine a more ideal background for conducting psychedelic therapy with cancer patients than this combination of medicine, psychology, and religion.

With unusual energy, enthusiasm, and devotion, Walter assumed the role of Principal Investigator in the project, exploring LSD therapy with cancer patients. He was able to obtain funds from the Mary Reynold Babcock Foundation (Winston/Salem cigarettes). Later, he initiated a similar project, in which a short-acting psychedelic dipropyltryptamine (DPT) was used in lieu of LSD. Unfortunately, before the project was completed, Walter disappeared while scuba diving in the Atlantic Ocean near his Maine summer cabin. As I described earlier in this chapter, his body or pieces of diving equipment have never been found and his death has remained a mystery.

After Walter's death, I assumed the leadership of the Spring Grove psychedelic research, with the cancer study my primary research responsibility. The project was extended to include another psychedelic substance, methylene-dioxy-amphetamine (MDA). We were able to complete the studies and I presented the results at the meeting of the Foundation of Thanatology in New York City and later in a book written jointly with Joan Halifax, entitled *The Human Encounter with Death* (Grof and Halifax 1977).

The Spring Grove study of psychedelic therapy with cancer patients was a cooperative effort involving the Maryland Psychiatric Research

Center and the oncological unit of Sinai Hospital in Baltimore. Walter Pahnke and I spent one day a week at Sinai, attending staff conferences and participating in the grand rounds. On these occasions, the Sinai oncologists recommended for our program those patients for whom there was no help along medical lines and who suffered from severe pain, depression, and fear of death. Walter and I then sat down with these patients and explained the program to them. If they were interested, we received from them informed consent and accepted them into the program.

The course of psychedelic therapy consisted of three phases. The first of these was the *preparatory period* that lasted approximately twelve hours. In these initial sessions, we explored the patients' past history and present situation and established good working contact with them and their family. We wanted to know what they had been told about their disease, what was their reaction to the situation, and what impact the disease had on their lives. An important task during the preparation was assessment of the interpersonal situation in the patient's family and of the nature and amount of "unfinished business." The last two hours of the preparatory period were dedicated to a discussion focusing on the psychedelic session—the effects of the drug, the experiences that can emerge, the bodywork that might be necessary, and the ways of communicating about the experience.

The second phase of treatment was the *psychedelic session* itself. Typical dosage for LSD ranged between 300 and 500 micrograms, for dipropyltryptamine (DPT), a shorter-acting LSD-like substance, between 90 and 150 milligrams, and for methylene-dioxy amphetamine (MDA) between 100 and 150 milligrams. LSD sessions typically lasted the entire day, DPT and MDA sessions more than half a day. During this time, the client was attended by a therapist and a co-therapist, always a male-female dyad. The reclining position, the use of eyeshades and headphones, and hi-fi music played throughout most of the session helped the internalization of the process. According to our experience, internalization of the session maximizes the benefit and minimizes the risks of the use of psychedelics.

As the pharmacological effect of the psychedelic substance was wearing off, the patient was encouraged to open the eyes, sit up, and briefly share his or her experience. This was also the time when we conducted bodywork to resolve residual problems, if this was indicated. When the intense inner experiences subsided, we invited into the session relatives or friends of the client's choice. This "family reunion," which lasted for the rest of the session, was a very important part of the procedure. The fact that the patients were at this time still in a holotropic state of consciousness facilitated a more open and honest communication. This made it possible to break through the confusion and distortions that often existed in interpersonal interactions between the dying patient, the family, and the medical staff.

The reunion offered an opportunity to discuss, in many cases for the first time, the feelings the patients and their families had about the disease, about the imminence of death, and about each other. This was followed by a dinner ordered from a nearby Chinese restaurant featuring meals with interesting tastes, colors, and textures. This, together with the warm human environment and music, helped the patients to connect the positive new feelings to various aspects of everyday life. After the dinner, the patients spent the rest of the evening and the night with relatives or friends of their choice. Our treatment suites were self-contained units, equipped with bathrooms and kitchenettes, providing everything that the guests needed.

On the following day and during the next week, we scheduled *post-session interviews* to help the patients integrate the experiences of the session and bring the new insights into their everyday lives. The protocol of our research project allowed us to repeat the session if it seemed necessary or appropriate. Because of the nature of the physical disease, the duration of the study was self-limiting and, unlike in our other projects, no external restrictions as to the number of sessions were imposed on us by the research protocol.

The results were evaluated with the use of psychological tests and a special instrument developed for this purpose by Walter Pahnke and Bill Richards, called the Emotional Condition Rating Scale (ECRS). This scale made it possible to obtain values from minus 6 to plus 6 reflecting the degree of the patients' depression, psychological isolation, anxiety, difficulty in management, fear of death, and preoccupation with death and physical suffering. Ratings were conducted one day before and three days after the psychedelic session by attending physicians, nurses, family members, and LSD therapists.

In the LSD study, about 30 percent of the patients showed dramatic improvement, 40 percent moderate improvement, and the remaining 30 percent were essentially unchanged. In the few cases where the post-session rated lower, the difference was minimal and statistically not significant (Kurland et al. 1968, Richards et al. 1972). In the DPT study, significant results and important trends were found in regard to certain individual scales but, in general, this study did not bring evidence that DPT could successfully replace LSD in psychedelic therapy of cancer patients (Richards 1975). This agreed with the clinical impressions and feelings of the therapists, who almost unanimously preferred to work with LSD.

Important therapeutic changes were observed in several different areas. Least surprising were the positive effects of psychedelic therapy on emotional symptoms such as depression, suicidal tendencies, tension, anxiety, insomnia, and psychological withdrawal, since these were well known from other clinical studies. The Spring Grove study also confirmed earlier reports by Kast and Collins concerning the potential of LSD to alleviate physical pain, even in many cases in which narcotics had been ineffective. The analgesic effect was often dramatic and lasted for several weeks or even months. However, it was not dose related and was not sufficiently predictable to be simple pharmacological analgesia.

This is a very puzzling observation that clearly involves a complicated mechanism and cannot be explained solely by the pharmacological effect of the drug. We tried to account for it by referring to Ronald Melzack's "gate-control theory of pain" (Melzack 1950; Melzack and Wall 1965). According to this theory, pain is a complex phenomenon that includes, besides the sensory message about the tissue damage and the motor reaction to it, also one's history of past pain, emotional evaluation of the sensations, meaning of the suffering involved, and cultural programming.

These factors are naturally significantly different, depending on circumstances—whether pain is experienced in the context of a progressive disease, difficult childbirth, torture in a concentration camp, or the Lakota Sioux sun dance. When LSD is administered, the resulting effect on pain reflects the interaction between its complex effect on the neurophysiological and psychospiritual processes and the equally complex mechanisms of pain. The final result involves many levels and many dimensions and is, therefore, not easily predictable.

The most important and striking effect of LSD in terminal cancer patients was a profound change in the concept of death and significant attenuation of the fear of death. Deep experiences of psychospiritual death and rebirth, cosmic unity, past-life memories, and other transpersonal forms of consciousness seem to render physical death much less frightening. The fact that these experiences can have such a convincing effect on individuals who have only months, weeks, or days to live, deserves serious attention. These experiences occur in a complex psychospiritual, mythological, and philosophical context and cannot be dismissed as momentary delusional self-deceptions resulting from impaired brain functioning.

Psychedelic experiences that reach the perinatal and transpersonal level also typically have profound effect on the patients' hierarchy of values and life strategy. Psychological acceptance of impermanence and death results in realization of the futility and absurdity of grandiose ambitions and attachment to money, status, fame, and power, as well as pursuit of other temporary values. This makes it easier to face the termination of one's secular goals and the impending loss of all worldly possessions. Another important shift occurs in time orientation; the past and future become much less important than the present moment and "living one day at a time."

This is associated with increased zest, as well as a tendency to appreciate and enjoy every moment of life, and to derive pleasure from simple things like nature, food, sex, music, and human company. There is also typically a major increase in spirituality of a mystical, universal, and ecumenical nature, which is not related to any specific church affiliation. We have also seen instances where a dying individual's traditional religious beliefs were illuminated by new dimensions of meaning.

The positive effects of psychedelic therapy extend beyond the dying individual to his or her immediate family and friends. The nature of the grieving and bereavement process is deeply affected by the nature and degree of conflicts in the survivors' relationships with the dying person. Adjustment to the death of a family member can be much more difficult if relatives have negative or mixed feelings about the appropriateness of their behavior toward the dying person and about the way the entire situation was managed.

The absence of the opportunity to express one's love and compassion for the dying, to show one's gratitude for the past, and to find a way to say goodbye leaves survivors with feelings of incompleteness, dissatisfaction, and guilt. If the therapist can enter the system as a catalyzing agent and help to open channels of effective emotional exchange and communication, dying and death can become an event of profound psychospiritual meaning for everybody involved.

I will illustrate the potential of psychedelic therapy for cancer patients by a case history of Joan, a housewife, mother of four children and a former dancer, who at the time of her treatment was forty years old. Two of her children, a seventeen-year-old daughter and an eight-year-old son, were from her first marriage. Joan was also taking care of an adopted boy of nine and a nine-year-old boy from her husband's first marriage. Her cancer, an infiltrating, highly malignant carcinoma, was diagnosed in August 1971, after a long period of vague transitional gastrointestinal disturbances.

Joan decided that she did not want to spend the rest of her life awaiting death. She wanted to get actively involved in the therapeutic process, no matter how little hope there might be in this endeavor. After the physicians had made it clear to her that nothing more could be done for her along medical lines, Joan spent some time looking for faith healers and other unorthodox help. During this time, she heard about the Spring Grove program for persons suffering from cancer and made an appointment with us to see the place, meet the people involved in the project, and get more specific information about the treatment program.

Joan came for the first interview accompanied by her husband Dick. He was an educator, very strongly influenced by all the negative publicity about LSD, and was concerned about the possible adverse effects of LSD. We had to spend some time explaining that in the judicious use of LSD the ratio between benefits and risks is drastically different from that in unsupervised self-experimentation. After this issue had been clarified, both Joan and Dick enthusiastically participated in the LSD program.

The preparation for Joan's first LSD session consisted of several drug-free interviews with her alone and one meeting with her and Dick. Joan was deeply depressed and very anxious. She felt a drastic decrease of zest, as well as a lack of interest in subjects and activities that prior to her disease used to bring her much joy. In the course of her illness, she had become very tense and irritable. During our preliminary discussions, her physical suffering was still tolerable. She felt undifferentiated gastrointestinal discomfort, but her pain had not reached the intensity that, in and of itself, would make her life unbearable.

Joan felt that, by and large, her problem at that time was anxious preoccupation with what the future would bring rather than suffering in the present. She was fully aware of the situation she was facing, as far as diagnosis and prognosis was concerned, and was able to discuss her disease quite openly. Her major concern was to reach a decent and honest closure in her relationship with Dick and all the children. Joan wanted to leave them resolved and with good feelings, without guilt, anger, bitterness, or pathological grief, in a situation where they could continue to live their own lives without having to carry the psychological burden of her death.

First LSD Session

I began the session with considerable apprehension and found it very comforting to hold onto Stan and Jewell's hands. About twenty minutes after the administration of 300 micrograms of LSD, I started having floating and vibrating sensations. As I was listening to Brahms's second piano concerto, I experienced myself standing in a gigantic hall of a futuristic, supersonic airport, waiting for my flight. The hall was crowded with passengers dressed in extremely modern fashion; a strange feeling of excitement and expectation seemed to permeate this unusual crowd.

Suddenly I heard a loud voice through the system of airport speakers: "The event that you are going to experience is Yourself. With some of you, as you may notice, it is already happening." As I looked around at my fellow travelers, I saw strange changes in their faces; their bodies were twitching and assuming unusual postures, as they began their journeys into the inner worlds. At that point, I noticed an intense humming sound of a comforting and soothing quality, like a radio signal, guiding me through the experience and reassuring me. It seemed as if my brain was being burned very slowly, revealing its content in one picture after another.

My father's image appeared with great clarity, and the nature of our relationship was analyzed and explored with the precision of a surgical operation. I perceived my father's need for me to be something or someone that I could not be. I realized that I had to be myself even if it disappoints him. I became aware of a whole network of other people's needs—my husband's, my children's, my friends'. I realized that the needs of other people made it more difficult for me to accept the reality of my impending death and to surrender to the process.

Then the inward journey deepened and I was encountering various terrifying monsters that resembled images from Asian art—vicious demons and lean, hungry, surrealistic creatures, all in strange dayglow green color. It was as if a whole panoply of demons from the *Tibetan Book of the Dead* had been evoked and performed a wild dance in my head. Whenever I moved toward them and into them, the fear would disappear and the picture would change into something else, usually quite pleasant. At one point, when I was looking at some slimy, evil creatures, I realized that they were products of my own mind and extensions of myself. I mumbled: "Uh hum, that's me too all right."

The encounter with demons was accompanied by an intense struggle for breath and feelings of anxiety, but it was of relatively brief duration. When it ended, I felt fantastic amounts of energy streaming through my body. I felt it was so much energy that no single individual could contain it and handle it effectively. It became clear to me that I contained so much energy that in everyday life I had to deny it, misuse it, and project it on other people. I had a flash of myself in various stages of my life, trying on different roles—daughter, lover, young wife, mother, artist—and realized that they could not work since they were inadequate containers for my energy.

The most important aspect of these experiences was their relevance for the understanding of death. I saw the magnificent unfolding of the cosmic design in all its infinite nuances and ramifications. Each individual represented a thread in the beautiful warp of life and was playing a specific role. All these roles were equally necessary for the central energy core of the universe; none of them was more important than others. I saw that after death the life energy underwent a transformation and the roles were recast. I saw my role in this life to be a cancer patient and was able and willing to accept it.

I envisioned and intuitively understood the dynamics of reincarnation. It was represented symbolically as a view of the earth with many paths leading in all directions; they looked like tunnels in a giant ant hill. It became clear to me that there have been many lives before this one and many others will follow. The purpose and task is to experience and explore whatever is assigned to us in the cosmic screenplay. Death is just one episode, one transitional experience within this magnificent perennial drama.

Throughout my session, I had visions of pictures, sculptures, handicraft, and architecture of a number of different countries and cultures—ancient Egypt, Greece, Rome, Persia, as well as pre-Columbian North, South, and Central America. This was accompanied by many insights into the nature of human existence. Through the richness of my experience, I discovered that the dimensions of my being were much greater than I had ever imagined.

Whatever I perceived the world doing—inventing hostile countries, internecine wars, racial hatred and riots, corrupted political schemes, or polluting technology—I saw myself participating in it and projecting on other people the things I denied in myself. I got in touch with what I felt was "pure being" and realized that it could not be comprehended and did not need any justification. With this came the awareness that my only task was to keep the energy flowing and not to "sit on it," as I used to do. The flow of life was symbolized by many beautiful images of moving water, fish and aquatic plants, and delightful dancing scenes, some majestic and ethereal, others down to earth.

As a result of all these experiences and insights, I developed an affirmative attitude toward the totality of existence and the ability to accept whatever happens in life as being ultimately all right. I made many enthusiastic comments about the incredible cosmic wit and humor built into the fabric of existence. As I allowed the energy of life to flow through me and opened up to it, my entire body was vibrating with excitement and delight. After having enjoyed this new way of being for some time, I curled into a comfortable fetal position.

About five hours into the session I decided to take off my eyeshades, sit up, and connect with the environment. I sat on the couch in deep peace and relaxation, listening to Zen meditation music and watching a single rosebud in a crystal vase on a nearby table. Occasionally I closed my eyes and returned to my inner world. As I saw later on the video taken during the session, my face was radiant and had the expression of quiet bliss found in Buddhist sculptures. For a long period of time, I experienced nothing but a beautiful warm, nourishing golden glow, like a transcendental rain of liquid gold. At one point, I noticed a bowl of grapes in the room and decided to taste a few of them. They tasted like ambrosia and the grape stems looked so beautiful that I decided to take some of them home as a souvenir.

Later in the afternoon, Dick joined us in the session room. Immediately after his arrival he and I fell into each other's arms and stayed in a close embrace for a very long time. Dick commented that he sensed an enormous amount of energy radiating from me. He was aware of an almost tangible energy field surrounding my body. We were then given about two hours of absolute privacy, which we enjoyed tremendously. This made it possible for me to share my experiences with Dick. One of my best memories from the session was the shower we took together. I felt unusually tuned into Dick's body, as well as my own, and experienced a sense of exquisite sensuality unlike anything I had known before.

Later we all shared a Chinese dinner. Although the food was brought from a nearby suburban Chinese restaurant and was probably of average quality, I considered it the best meal I had ever tasted. I could not recall ever enjoying food, or myself, more. The only factor that somewhat inhibited my culinary pleasure was my rational awareness that I should be somewhat conservative with the food because of my subtotal gastrectomy.

For the rest of the evening, Dick and I shared quiet time together, lying on the couch and listening to stereophonic music. Dick was very impressed by my openness and all my insights. He was convinced that I was tapping some sources of genuine cosmic wisdom that were closed to him. He admired the depth in my reporting and the spontaneous confidence and authority with which I spoke about my experience.

I was elated, in radiant mood, and felt absolute freedom from anxiety. My ability to enjoy music, tastes, colors, and the shower was greatly enhanced. Dick's conclusion was that I was just pure pleasure to be with. This was such a contagious experience that Dick himself felt and expressed his desire to have a psychedelic session. He decided to explore the possibility of participating in the LSD training program for professionals that was also available at the Maryland Psychiatric Research Center.

I stayed up for a long time talking to Dick and awoke several times during the night. I had one dream about working in a library and hearing others say: "This Zen stuff does not make any sense." I smiled to myself, knowing it was too simple to make sense to them.

> The next morning after the session, I felt refreshed, relaxed, and very much in tune with the world. Dick put Bach's Brandenburger Concerto on the record player and it seemed absolutely perfect. The outside world appeared clear, serene, and beautiful. I saw things I have never seen on the road going home. The trees, grass, colors, sky—all were a real delight to behold.

For about two months after her first LSD session, Joan felt relaxed, elated, and optimistic. The psychedelic experience also seemed to have opened new realms of mystical and cosmic feelings within her. The religious elements that she had experienced in her session transcended the narrow boundaries of the traditional Catholic religion she had been brought up with. She was now precipitating toward the more universal approaches found within Hinduism and Buddhism.

During the weeks following the session, Joan felt so much overflowing energy that it baffled her attending physicians. They found her energetic resources quite incongruent with her serious clinical condition and explicitly expressed their surprise that she was still able to move around on her own and to drive a car. They also voiced their doubt that she would be able to spend the forthcoming summer vacation in California, as the family was planning to do. Joan herself felt very confident and believed that this would be possible. The later course of events justified her feelings when the vacation in California proved to be a very meaningful and rewarding time for the whole family.

This positive development was drastically interrupted in mid-January, when Joan saw her physician because of continued belching and retching. He discovered a new mass in the area of the spleen, which he identified as metastatic growth. Joan was very disappointed when, in spite of this finding, no concrete medical procedure was suggested. She realized that the doctors had given up on her. At this point, both Joan and Dick felt very strongly that Joan should have another psychedelic session and our staff agreed. Joan felt very optimistic about the possibility of the session influencing her emotional condition and deepening her philosophical and spiritual insights. She was also toying with the idea that it might be able to influence the psychosomatic component that she suspected in the etiology of her cancer.

The second LSD session took place in February 1972. Since the dosage of 300 micrograms had had a powerful effect the first time, we decided to use the same quantity in this session. The following is Joan's account of her experience, which summarizes the most important events of the session:

Second LSD Session

This session was a grim one for me. It contrasted with my first in almost every way: black and white rather than color; personal rather than cosmic; sad, not joyous. There was a short time at the beginning when I felt myself in a universal place or space where I knew again that the whole universe was in each of us and that there was a meaning to our lives and deaths. After that the experience narrowed and became much more personal. Death was the main subject of my session.

I experienced several funeral scenes in ornate or traditional church surroundings, sometimes at the cemetery, sometimes inside a church with a choir of many people. I cried often in the course of the several hours. I also asked many questions and answered them; they would lead to ultimate unanswerable problems and then it would seem funny. Early on, I remember thinking: *All that ugliness is really beauty.* In the course of the day, other polarities came to my mind—good and evil, victory and defeat, wisdom and ignorance, life and death.

I experienced my childhood, but not any specific scenes, just a feeling tone, a very sad one. Much of it had to do with very early feelings of frustration and deprivation, hunger, and starvation. It flashed through my mind whether there might have been a connection between these experiences and my peptic ulcer that turned into cancer. I remember once just the feeling of being out in the rain for what seemed like a long time. I recall being with my brothers and being turned away from a show or circus by the man in charge, and feeling very sad as we walked away, not too sure where we were going. The hidden allusion to my present situation is obvious—being denied further participation in the show of life and facing the uncertainty of death.

For what seemed like a fairly long time, I experienced my present family in terms of preparing them for my death. There was a scene in which, after preparing myself for some time, I finally told them. In a sequence of scenes, I was able to say good-bye to my children, my husband, my father, and other relatives, as well as friends and acquaintances. I did it in a very individualized way, with regard to the personality and special sensitivity of each of them.

Tears followed, but after a time, there was warmth and cheer. At the end, they all gathered around me to take care of me. I recall their fixing warm and sweet things to eat. After this, I spent some good bit of time saying goodbye to them and to my husband and realizing that there were caring people who were going to look after them. I said goodbye to them, too, and felt that something of me would live on in them.

There was a happy, warm scene toward the end of my session, which I felt I was observing, not part of, but really enjoyed. It was a scene with adults and children playing outside in the snow. I felt it was in some very northern place. All were bundled up and staying warm in spite of the cold and the snow. The children were being enjoyed and cared for by the grown-ups, and there was laughter and play and general good cheer. Then I remember seeing a whole row of boots, knowing that children's feet were in them and were warm.

In the evening after the session I felt good in some ways—quite responsive and pleased to see Dick, but I found myself crying off and on for the rest of the evening. I felt that I saw myself and my situation realistically, that I could handle it better now, but still felt very sad. I wished that the experience could have gone on for a few more hours and that I might have gone on from the grimness to joy.

The second session proved to be very beneficial for Joan. She became reconciled to her situation and decided to spend her remaining days focusing on her spiritual quest. After a vacation with the family on the West Coast, she decided to say goodbye to her husband and her children. She thought that it would save them from the painful process of watching her progressive deterioration and make it possible for them to remember her full of life and energy. In California, Joan remained in close contact with her father, who was interested in the spiritual path and introduced her to a Vedanta group.

In late summer, Joan became interested in having another LSD experience. She wrote us a letter inquiring about the possibility of arranging the third session in California. We recommended that she approach Sidney Cohen, a Los Angeles psychiatrist who had extensive experience with psychedelic therapy of cancer patients and a license to use LSD. The following is Joan's account of her third LSD session, which she had under Sidney Cohen's auspices. This time, the dosage was increased to 400 micrograms.

Third LSD Session

My first response after the drug took effect was to get cold, colder, and colder. It seemed that no amount of covers could alleviate the bone-penetrating, angular, and greenish freezing cold. It was hard to believe later that so many warm blankets had been put on top of me, for nothing—at the time—seemed to alleviate the cold. I called for hot tea, which I sipped through a glass straw. While holding the hot cup of tea, I went into a very intense experience.

The cup became the universe and all was vividly clear and real. The greenish, brownish color of the tea melted into a swirling vortex. No more questions; life, death, meaning—all were there. I had always been there—

we all were. All was one. Fear did not exist; death, life—all the same thing. The swirling circularity of it all. The intense desire for everyone to realize the universe is in everything. The tear coming down my cheek, the cup, the tea—everything! What harmony, I felt, is there behind the seeming chaos!

Wanting not to lose sight of this, wanting all to share in this experience; then there could be no discord. I was feeling that Dr. Cohen knew with me. Then my father came in and I tried to share with him what I could of the intense earlier experience, trying to express the inexpressible: that there is no fear, no question of fear. We have always been where we are going. Just being is sufficient. No need to worry, ask, question, reason. Just be. I told him the importance of us all in keeping things moving in the everyday world.

I consumed my hot broth and tea, craving for nourishment and warmth. After a break, I got back into myself. This time I experienced bleak and sad scenes of my very early life that I was familiar with from my previous sessions. The pictures took the form of small skeletal creatures floating about in emptiness, looking for, but not finding, nourishment. Emptiness, no fulfillment. Scrawny birds looking for food in an empty nest. Some feeling of me and my brothers alone, looking, nowhere to go.

At some point, I got into my sadness. Sadness as an overriding theme running from early childhood throughout my life. I became aware of the progressive effort to disguise it—to satisfy what others seemed to want instead: "Smile . . . look alive . . . stop daydreaming!" Later in the session, I had the feeling that some are chosen to feel the sadness inherent in the universe. If I am one, fine. I thought of all the children looking for mothers who are not there. Thought of the Stations of the Cross and felt the suffering of Christ or the sadness he had to feel. I realized that others' karma is to feel the gladness, or the strength, or the beauty, whatever. Why not gladly accept the sadness?

At another time, I was on many cushions with many comforters on top of me, warm, secure. Wanting not to be reborn as a person, but perhaps as a rainbow—orangey, reddish, yellowish, soft, beautiful. At some point in the afternoon, I became aware of the centrality of my stomach. So many pictures of people being comforted with food, my earlier craving for the hot tea, broth, always something coming into my stomach. I realized that I am aware of that in my day-to-day life now, always wanting the tit and substituting spoon, straw, cigarette. Never enough!

I became aware of being a child again, dependent, but now having a mother to take care of me, who wants to and likes taking care of me. I found comfort and pleasure in getting what I never had as a child. There were moments to enjoy the smell and feel of the fruit—a beautiful mango, pear, peach, grapes. While looking at them I saw the cellular movement. Much later, I enjoyed the rosebud, velvety, fragrant, and lovely.

> Toward the end of the day, I became suddenly aware that I had found a way to legitimize my lifelong sadness: to become terminally ill. The irony of this situation was that I then found happiness and felt relief in this discovery. I wanted to get into the sources of my sadness. I saw that from very early my mother had not much to give me, that, in fact, she looked to me to give her. I did indeed have more to give her than she me. I experienced this as a heavy burden.
>
> I had much discussion with my father about sadness, what is wrong with it and why it is so discouraged by others. I described to him how much energy I expended pretending to be glad or happy or to smile. I talked about the beauty in sadness—sad sweetness, sweet sadness. Allowing yourself and others to be sad when they feel it. Sadness perhaps is not in vogue, as is joy, spontaneity, or fun. These I expended great energy in acting out. Now I am just being; not being this or that, just being.
>
> Sometimes it is sad, often peaceful, sometimes angry or irritable, sometimes very warm and happy. I am not sad any longer that I am to die. I have many more loving feelings than ever before. All the pressures to be something "other" have been taken off me. I feel relieved from sham and pretense. Much spiritual feeling permeates my everyday life.

A member of our team who visited Joan in California a short time before her death gave us a moving description of her everyday life during her remaining days. She maintained her interest in the spiritual quest and spent several hours a day in meditation. In spite of her rapidly deteriorating physical condition, she appeared to be emotionally balanced and in good spirits. Quite remarkable was her determination not to lose any opportunity to experience the world fully as long as she could.

She insisted that she be served all the meals that others were eating, although the passage through her stomach was now totally obstructed and she could not swallow anything. She chewed the food slowly, savored its taste, and then spat it out into a bucket. The last evening of her life, she was totally absorbed in watching the setting sun. "What a magnificent sunset," were her last words before she retired into her bedroom. That night she died quietly in her sleep.

After Joan's death her relatives and friends on the East Coast received the invitation for a memorial get-together that she had written personally when she was still alive. After they all assembled at the appointed time, they were surprised to be addressed by Joan's voice from a cassette tape. It was much more than an unusual and moving farewell. According to the participants, the content and tone of her speech had a powerful comforting effect on those who had come to this meeting with a sense of tragedy and deep grief. Joan succeeded in imparting to them some of the sense of inner peace and reconciliation that she herself had reached in her sessions.

As we have seen, psychedelic therapy has an extraordinary potential to alleviate, in the dying individuals as well as the survivors, the emotional and physical agony of the potentially most painful crisis in human life. The current political and administrative hindrances that prevent hundreds of thousands of terminal patients from benefitting from this remarkable procedure are unnecessary and not defendable. All the objections that could be raised against the use of psychedelics in other populations, such as patients with emotional and psychosomatic disorders, mental health professionals, artists, and clergy are absurd in a situation that is time limited and in which the problems involved are so serious that even the taboo against the use of narcotics does not apply.

Individual and Social Implications of the Research on Death and Dying

The research of psychological, philosophical, and spiritual aspects of death and dying discussed in this chapter has considerable theoretical and practical implications. The experiences and observations I have explored certainly are not an unequivocal "proof" of survival of consciousness after death, of the existence of astral realms inhabited by discarnate beings, or of reincarnation of the individual unit of consciousness and continuation of its physical existence in another lifetime. It is possible to imagine other types of interpretation of the same data, such as extraordinary paranormal capacities of human consciousness referred to as *superpsi* or the Hindu concept of the universe as *lila,* the divine play of consciousness of the cosmic creative principle.

However, one thing seems to be clear: none of the interpretations based on careful analysis of these data are compatible with the monistic materialistic worldview of Western science. Systematic examination and unbiased evaluation of this material would necessarily result in an entirely new understanding of the nature of consciousness, its role in the universal scheme of things, and its relationship to matter and the brain. Besides their theoretical relevance, the issues discussed in this chapter have also great practical significance.

I have explored earlier the importance of death within the framework of psychiatry, psychology, and psychotherapy. As we saw, our past encounters with death in the form of vital threats during our postnatal history, the trauma of birth, and embryonal existence are deeply imprinted in our unconscious. In addition, the motif of death also plays an important role in the transpersonal domain of the human psyche in connection with powerful archetypal and karmic material. In all these varieties, the theme of death and dying contributes significantly to the development of emotional and psychosomatic disorders.

And, conversely, confronting this material and coming to terms with the fear of death is conducive to healing, positive personality transformation, and consciousness evolution. As we discussed in connection with the ancient mysteries of death and rebirth, this "dying before dying" influences deeply the quality of life and the basic strategy of existence. It reduces irrational drives and increases the ability to live in the present and to enjoy simple life activities.

Another important consequence of freeing oneself from the fear of death is a radical opening to spirituality of a universal and nondenominational type. This tends to occur whether the encounter with death happens during a real brush with death in a near-death experience, or in a purely psychological way, such as in meditation, experiential therapy, or a spontaneous psychospiritual crisis (spiritual emergency).

In conclusion, I would like to mention briefly some of the broadest possible implications of this material. Whether or not we believe in survival of consciousness after death, in reincarnation, and karma will have a profound impact on our behavior. The idea that belief in immortality has profound moral implications can be found already in Plato, who in *Laws* has Socrates say that disconcern for the post mortem consequences of one's deeds would be "a boon to the wicked." Modern authors, such as Alan Harrington (Harrington 1969) and Ernest Becker (Becker 1973) have emphasized that massive denial of death leads to social pathologies that have dangerous consequences for humanity. Modern consciousness research certainly supports this point of view (Grof 1985).

At a time when a combination of unbridled greed, malignant aggression, and existence of weapons of mass destruction threatens the survival of humanity and possibly life on this planet, we should seriously consider any avenue that offers some hope. While this is not a sufficient reason for embracing uncritically the material suggesting survival of consciousness after death, it should be an additional incentive for reviewing the existing data with an open mind and in the spirit of true science.

The same applies to the powerful experiential technologies available these days that make it possible to confront the fear of death and can facilitate deep positive personality changes and spiritual opening. A radical inner transformation and rise to a new level of consciousness might be the only real hope we have in the current global crisis. We will return to this important problem in a later chapter.

CHAPTER EIGHT

The Cosmic Game: Exploration of the Farthest Reaches of Human Consciousness

The preceding chapters of this book focused primarily on the implications of the research of holotropic states of consciousness for psychiatry, psychology, and psychotherapy. However, this work also generates many interesting philosophical, metaphysical, and spiritual insights. Irrespective of the initial motivation of the person involved and his or her background, systematic disciplined self-exploration using holotropic states in a good set and setting sooner or later tends to take the form of a deep philosophical and spiritual quest. I have seen on numerous occasions that people whose primary interest in psychedelic sessions or in the holotropic breathwork was therapeutic, professional, or artistic, suddenly started asking the most fundamental questions about existence when their inner process reached the transpersonal level.

How did our universe come into being? Is the world in which we live merely a product of mechanical processes involving inanimate, inert, and reactive matter? Can material reality be explained solely in terms of its fundamental building blocks and the objective laws that govern their interaction? What is the source of order, form, and meaning in the universe? Is it possible that the creation of a universe like ours and its evolution could have occurred without participation of superior cosmic intelligence? If there is a supreme creative principle, what is our relationship to it?

How can we come to terms with such dilemmas as finiteness of time and space versus eternity and infinity? What is the relationship between life and matter and between consciousness and the brain? How can we explain the existence of evil and its overwhelming presence in the universal scheme of things? Is our existence limited to just one lifetime, spanning the period from conception to death, or does our consciousness survive the biological demise and experience a long series of consecutive incarnations? And what are the practical implications of the answers to the above questions for our everyday life?

In the late 1960s, I decided to analyze the records from my psychedelic research with specific focus on the metaphysical experiences and insights of my clients. I summarized my findings in a paper entitled "LSD and the Cosmic Game: Outline of Psychedelic Ontology and Cosmology" (Grof 1972). To my surprise I found far-reaching agreement among my clients concerning their insights about basic metaphysical issues. The vision of reality that has emerged from the study of holotropic states portrays the universe not as a mechanical Newtonian supermachine, but as an infinitely complex virtual reality created and permeated by superior cosmic intelligence, Absolute Consciousness or the Universal Mind.

The metaphysical insights from psychedelic research and the answers to the basic ontological and cosmological questions that they provided were obviously in sharp conflict with the worldview and philosophy of materialistic science. However, they showed far-reaching parallels with the great mystical traditions of the world, for which Aldous Huxley used the term *perennial philosophy.* They were also surprisingly compatible with the revolutionary advances of modern science that are usually referred to as the *new* or *emerging paradigm.*

In the following years, as I gained extensive experience with holotropic breathwork and with spontaneously occurring episodes of holotropic states (spiritual emergencies), I realized that the metaphysical insights described in my paper were not limited to psychedelic states, but were characteristic for holotropic states in general. In this chapter, I will briefly sketch the basic ideas of the intriguing vision of reality that spontaneously emerges in people who have done systematic work with holotropic states of consciousness. A more comprehensive treatment of this subject can be found in my book *The Cosmic Game: Explorations of the Frontiers of Human Consciousness* (Grof 1998).

The Ensouled Nature and the Archetypal Domain

As we saw earlier, in holotropic states we can have authentic and convincing experiences of conscious identification with animals, plants, and even inorganic materials. Following such experiences, our worldview typically expands and we begin to understand the beliefs of animistic cultures that see the entire universe as being ensouled. From their perspective, not only all the animals, but also the trees, the rivers, the mountains, the sun, the moon, and the stars appear to be conscious beings. Naturally, we would not regress to the world view of any of these cultures in all its aspects and completely forget and ignore all the findings of materialistic science. However, we have to add to our worldview an important empirical fact: everything that we experience in the hylotropic state as an object has in the holotropic state a subjective experiential counterpart.

Holotropic states of consciousness can also provide deep insights into the worldview of the cultures who believe that the cosmos is populated by mythological beings and that it is governed by various blissful and wrathful deities. In these states, we can gain direct experiential access to the archetypal world of gods, demons, legendary heroes, suprahuman entities, and spirit guides. We can visit the domain of mythological realities, fantastic landscapes, and abodes of the beyond. The imagery of such experiences can be drawn from the collective unconscious and can feature mythological figures and themes from any culture in the entire history of humanity.

If we feel embarrassed by our discovery, we might prefer to use modern terminology such as *numinous* instead of *sacred* and *archetypal figures* instead of *deities and demons*. But we can no longer dismiss these experiences as mere hallucinations or fantasies. Deep personal experiences of this realm help us realize that the images of the cosmos found in preindustrial societies are not based on superstition, primitive "magical thinking," or psychotic visions, but on authentic experiences of alternate realities. The research of holotropic states has brought ample evidence that there are transphenomenal dimensions of existence that are ontologically real and that they often can withstand the test of consensual validation. To distinguish these phenomena from hallucinatory or imaginary experiences, which do not have any objective basis, some Jungian psychologists refer to these transphenomenal realities as "imaginal."

In holotropic states we discover that our psyche has access to entire pantheons of mythological figures, as well as domains that they inhabit. A particularly convincing proof of the authenticity of these experiences is the fact that, like other transpersonal phenomena, they can bring us new and accurate information about the figures and realms involved. The nature, scope, and quality of this information often far surpasses our previous intellectual knowledge concerning the respective mythologies. Observations of this kind led C. G. Jung to the assumption that, besides the individual unconscious as described by Sigmund Freud, we also have a collective unconscious that connects us with the entire cultural heritage of all humanity. According to Jung, these are manifestations of primordial universal patterns that represent intrinsic constituents of the collective unconscious (Jung 1959).

The archetypal figures fall into two distinct categories. The first one includes entities embodying various specific universal roles and functions. The most famous of them are the Great Mother Goddess, the Terrible Mother Goddess, the Heavenly Father, the Wise Old Man, the Eternal Youth (Puer Eternus and Puella Eterna), the Lovers, the Grim Reaper, and the Trickster. Jung also discovered that men harbor in their unconscious a generalized representation of the feminine principle that he called Anima. Her counterpart, the generalized representation of the masculine principle in the unconscious of women, is the Animus. The unconscious representation of the dark, destructive aspect of human personality is in Jungian psychology called the Shadow.

The archetypal figures of the second category represent various deities and demons related to specific cultures, geographical areas, and historical periods. For example, instead of a generalized universal image of the Great Mother Goddess, we can experience one of her concrete culture-bound forms, such as Virgin Mary, the Hindu goddesses Lakshmi and Parvati, the Egyptian Isis, the Greek Hera, and many others. Similarly, specific examples of the Terrible Mother Goddess would be the Indian Kali, the pre-Columbian serpent-headed Coatlicue, or the Egyptian lion-headed Sekhmet. It is important to emphasize that these images do not have to be limited to our own racial and cultural heritage. They can be drawn from the mythology of any human group, even those we have never heard about.

The encounters with these archetypal figures are very impressive and often bring new and detailed information that is independent of the subjects' racial, cultural, and educational background and previous intellectual knowledge of the respective mythologies. Depending on the nature of the deities involved, these experiences are accompanied by extremely intense emotions ranging from ecstatic rapture to paralyzing metaphysical terror. People who experience these encounters usually view these archetypal figures with great awe and respect, as beings that belong to a superior order, are endowed with extraordinary energies and power, and have the capacity to shape events in our material world. These subjects thus share the attitude of many preindustrial cultures that believed in the existence of deities and demons.

However, people who have such experiences usually do not confuse the archetypal figures with the supreme principle in the universe, nor do they claim that they have gained ultimate understanding of existence. They typically experience these deities as creations of a superior power that transcends them. This insight echoes Joseph Campbell's idea that the deities should be "transparent to the transcendent." They should function as a bridge to the divine source, but not be confused with it. When we are involved in systematic self-exploration or spiritual practice, it is important to avoid the pitfall of making a particular deity opaque and seeing it as the ultimate cosmic force rather than a window into the Absolute.

Mistaking a specific archetypal image for the ultimate source of creation or for its only true representation leads to idolatry, a divisive and dangerous mistake widespread in the histories of religions and cultures. It might unite the people who share the same belief, but sets this group against another one that has chosen a different representation of the divine. They might then try to convert others or conquer and eliminate them. By contrast, genuine religion is universal, all-inclusive, and all-encompassing. It has to transcend specific culture-bound archetypal images and focus on the ultimate source of all forms. The most important question in the world of religion is thus the nature of the supreme principle in the universe.

Experience of the Supreme Cosmic Principle

Individuals involved in systematic self-exploration with the use of holotropic states repeatedly describe this process as a philosophical and spiritual quest. This inspired me to search the records from psychedelic and holotropic sessions, as well as reports from people who were undergoing spiritual emergency, for experiences that would convey the sense that this quest reached its goal, its final destination. I found out that people who have the experience of the Absolute that fully satisfies their spiritual longing typically do not see any specific figurative images. When they feel that they have attained the goal of their mystical and philosophical quest, their descriptions of the supreme principle are highly abstract and strikingly similar.

Those who report such an ultimate revelation show quite remarkable agreement in describing the experiential characteristics of this state. They report that the experience of the Supreme involved transcendence of all the limitations of the analytical mind, all rational categories, and all the constraints of ordinary logic. This experience was not bound by the usual limitations of three-dimensional space and linear time, as we know them from everyday life. It also contained all conceivable polarities in an inseparable amalgam and thus transcended dualities of any kind.

Time after time, people compared the Absolute to a radiant source of light of unimaginable intensity, though they emphasized that it also differed in some significant aspects from any form of light that we know in the material world. To describe the Absolute as light, as much as it seems appropriate in a certain sense, entirely misses some of its essential characteristics, particularly the fact that it also is an immense and unfathomable field of consciousness endowed with infinite intelligence and creative power. Another attribute that is regularly mentioned is an exquisite sense of humor ("cosmic humor").

The supreme cosmic principle can be experienced in two different ways. Sometimes, all personal boundaries dissolve or are drastically obliterated and we completely merge with the divine source, becoming one with it and indistinguishable from it. Other times, we maintain the sense of separate identity, assuming the role of an astonished observer who is witnessing, as if from outside, the *mysterium tremendum* of existence. Or, like some mystics, we might feel the ecstasy of an enraptured lover experiencing the encounter with the Beloved. Spiritual literature of all ages abounds in descriptions of both types of experiences of the divine.

The encounter with Absolute Consciousness or identification with it is not the only way to experience the supreme principle in the cosmos or the ultimate reality. The second type of experience that seems to satisfy those who search for ultimate answers is particularly surprising, since it has no specific content. It is the identification with Cosmic Emptiness and Nothingness described in the mystical literature as the Void. It is important to emphasize that not every experience of emptiness that we can encounter in holotropic states qualifies as the Void. People very often use this term to describe an unpleasant sense of lack of feeling, initiative, or meaning. To deserve the name Void, this state has to meet very specific criteria.

When we encounter the Void, we feel that it is primordial emptiness of cosmic proportions and relevance. We become pure consciousness aware of this absolute nothingness; however, at the same time, we have a strange paradoxical sense of its essential fullness. This cosmic vacuum is also a plenum, since nothing seems to be missing in it. While it does not feature anything in a concrete manifest form, it seems to contain all of existence in a potential form. The Void transcends the usual categories of time and space. It is unchangeable, and lies beyond all dichotomies and polarities, such as light and darkness, good and evil, stability and motion, microcosm and macrocosm, agony and ecstasy, singularity and plurality, form and emptiness, and even existence and nonexistence.

Some people call it the Supracosmic and Metacosmic Void, indicating that this primordial emptiness and nothingness appears to be the principle that underlies the phenomenal world as we know it and, at the same time, is supraordinated to it. This metaphysical vacuum, pregnant with potential for everything there is, appears to be the cradle of all being, the ultimate source of existence. The creation of all phenomenal worlds is then the realization and concretization of its preexisting inherent potentialities. It is impossible to convey in words how experientially convincing and logical are these paradoxical answers to the most basic and profound questions about existence. Full understanding of these extraordinary states requires direct personal experience

The Beyond Within

In systematic spiritual practice involving holotropic states of consciousness, we can repeatedly transcend the ordinary boundaries of the body-ego. In this process, we discover that any boundaries in the material universe and in other realities are ultimately arbitrary and negotiable. By shedding the limitations of the rational mind and the straitjacket of common sense and everyday logic, we can break through many separating barriers, expand our consciousness to unimaginable proportions, and eventually experience union and identity with the transcendental source of all being, known from the spiritual literature by many different names.

When we reach experiential identification with the Absolute, we realize that our own being is ultimately commensurate with the entire cosmic network, with all of existence. The recognition of our own divine nature, our identity with the cosmic source, is the most important discovery we can make during the process of deep self-exploration. This is the essence of the famous statement found in the ancient Indian scriptures, the Upanishads: *Tat tvam asi.* The literal translation of this sentence is "Thou art That" meaning "you are of divine nature," or "you are Godhead." It reveals that our everyday identification with the "skin-encapsulated ego," embodied individual consciousness, or "name and form" (*namarupa*) is an illusion and that our true nature is that of cosmic creative energy (Atman-Brahman).

This revelation concerning the identity of the individual with the divine is the ultimate secret that lies at the core of all great spiritual traditions, although it might be expressed in somewhat different ways. I have already mentioned that in Hinduism Atman, the individual consciousness, and Brahman, the universal consciousness, are one. The followers of Siddha Yoga hear in many variations the basic tenet of their school: "God dwells within you as you." In Buddhist scriptures, we can read: "Look within, you are the Buddha." In the Confucian tradition, we are told that "heaven, earth, and human are one body."

The same message can be found in the words of Jesus Christ: "Father, you, and I are one." And St. Gregory Palamas, one of the greatest theologians of the Christian Orthodox Church, declared: "For the kingdom of heaven, nay rather, the King of Heaven, is within us." Similarly, the great Jewish sage, cabalist Avraham ben Shemu'el Abulafia, taught that "He and we are one." According to Mohammed, "whoso knoweth himself knoweth his Lord." Mansur al-Hallaj, the Sufi ecstatic and poet known as "the martyr of mystical love," described it in this way: "I saw my Lord with the Eye of the Heart. I said: 'Who art thou?' He answered: 'Thou.'" Al-Hallaj was imprisoned and sentenced to death for his statement: "Ana'l Haqq—I am God, the Absolute Truth, the True Reality."

Words for the Ineffable

The supreme principle can be directly experienced in holotropic states of consciousness, but it eludes any attempts at adequate description or explanation. The language that we use to communicate about matters of daily life simply is not adequate for this task. Individuals who have had this experience seem to agree that it is ineffable. Words and the structure of our language are painfully inappropriate tools to describe its nature and dimensions, particularly to those who have not had it.

Any attempts at description of transcendental experiences have to rely on words of everyday language that has been developed to denote objects and activities in the material world as it is experienced in the ordinary state of consciousness in our daily life. For this reason, language proves to be inappropriate and inadequate when we want to communicate about the experiences and insights encountered in various holotropic states of consciousness. This is particularly true when our experiences focus on the ultimate problems of existence, such as the Void, Absolute Consciousness, and creation.

Those who are familiar with the Eastern spiritual philosophies often resort to words from various Asian languages when describing their spiritual experiences and insights. They use Sanskrit, Tibetan, Chinese, or Japanese terms. These languages were developed in cultures with high sophistication in regard to holotropic states and spiritual realities. Unlike the Western languages, they contain many technical terms specifically describing nuances of the mystical experiences and related issues. Ultimately even these words can be fully understood only by those who have had the corresponding experiences.

Poetry, although still a highly imperfect tool, seems to be a more adequate and appropriate means for conveying the essence of spiritual experiences and for communicating about transcendental realities. For this reason, many of the great visionaries and religious teachers resorted to poetry while sharing their metaphysical insights. Many people who have experienced transcendental states recall and quote corresponding passages from various visionary poems.

The Process of Creation

People who in their holotropic states of consciousness experience the cosmic creative principle often try to understand the impulse that leads to the creation of experiential worlds. Their insights into the "motivation" of the Divine to generate phenomenal realities contain some interesting contradictions. One important category of these insights emphasizes the fantastic inner richness and inconceivable creative potential of Absolute Consciousness. The cosmic source is so overabundent and overflowing with possibilities that it simply has to give expression to it in the creative act.

Another group of revelations suggests that, in the process of creation, Absolute Consciousness also seeks something that it lacks and misses in its original pristine state. From an ordinary perspective, these two categories of insights might seem to contradict each other. In holotropic states, this conflict disappears and the two seeming opposites can easily coexist and actually complement each other.

The impulse to create is often described as an elemental force that reflects the unimaginable inner richness and abundance of the Divine. The creative cosmic source is so immense and bursting with limitless possibilities that it cannot contain itself and has to express its full hidden potential. Other descriptions stress the immense desire of the Universal Mind to get to know itself and to explore and experience its full potential. This can only be done by exteriorization and manifestation of all its latent possibilities in the form of a concrete creative act. It requires polarization into subject and object, the experiencer and the experienced, the observer and the observed. Similar ideas can be found in medieval cabalistic scriptures, according to which the motive for creation is that "God wants to see God."

Additional important dimensions of the creative process that are often emphasized are the playfulness, self-delectation, and cosmic humor of the Creator. These are elements that have best been described in ancient Hindu texts which talk about the universe and existence as *lila,* or Divine Play. According to this view, creation is an intricate, infinitely complex cosmic game that the godhead, Brahman, creates from himself and within himself.

Creation can also be viewed as a colossal experiment that expresses the immense curiosity of Absolute Consciousness, a passion that is analogous to the infatuation of a scientist who dedicates his or her life to exploration and research. Some people who have experienced insights into the "motives" for creation also emphasize its esthetic side. From this perspective, the universe we live in and all the experiential realities in other dimensions also appear to be ultimate works of art and the impulse to create them can be likened to the inspiration and creative passion of the supreme artist.

As I said earlier, sometimes the insights concerning the forces underlying creation do not reflect overflowing abundance, richness, ultimate self-sufficiency, and mastery of the cosmic creative principle, but rather a certain sense of deficiency, need, or want. For example, it is possible to discover that, in spite of the immensity and perfection of its state of being, Absolute Consciousness realizes that it is alone. This Loneliness finds its expression in an abysmal yearning for partnership, communication, and sharing, a kind of Divine Longing. The most powerful force behind creation is then described as the need of the creative principle to give and receive Love.

Another critical dimension of the creative process that has occasionally been reported in this category seems to be the primordial craving of the divine source for the experiences that characterize the material world. According to these insights, Spirit has a profound desire to experience what is opposite and contrary to its own nature. It wants to explore all the qualities that in its pristine nature it does not have and to become everything that it is not.

Being eternal, infinite, unlimited, and ethereal, it longs for the ephemeral, impermanent, limited by time and space, solid, tangible, and corporeal. Another important "motive" for creation that is occasionally mentioned is the element of Monotony. However immense and glorious the experience of the divine might appear from the human perspective, for the divine it is always the same and, in that sense, monotonous. Creation can then be seen as a titanic effort expressing a transcendental longing for change, action, movement, drama, and surprise.

All those who have been fortunate to experience such profound insights into the cosmic laboratory of creation seem to agree that anything that can be said about this level of reality cannot possibly do justice to what they have witnessed. The monumental impulse of unimaginable proportions that is responsible for creating the worlds of phenomena seems to contain all the above elements, however contradictory and paradoxical they might appear to our everyday sensibility and common sense, and many more. It is clear that, in spite of all our efforts to comprehend and describe creation, the nature of the creative principle and of the process of creation remains shrouded in unfathomable mystery.

Besides the revelations concerning the motives or reasons for creation (the "why" of creation), the experiences in holotropic states often bring illuminating insights into the specific dynamics and mechanisms of the creative process (the "how" of creation). These are related to the "technology of consciousness" that generates experiences with different sensory characteristics and by orchestrating them in a systematic and coherent way creates virtual realities. Although the descriptions of these insights vary in terms of details, language, and metaphors used to illustrate them, they typically distinguish two interrelated and mutually complementary processes that are involved in creating the worlds of phenomena.

The first of these is the activity that splits the original undifferentiated unity of Absolute Consciousness into infinite numbers of derived units of consciousness. The Universal Mind engages in a creative play that involves complicated sequences of divisions, fragmentations, and differentiations. This finally results in experiential worlds that contain countless separate entities endowed with specific forms of consciousness and possess selective self-awareness. There seems to be general agreement that these come into being by multiple divisions and subdivisions of the originally undivided field of cosmic consciousness. The divine thus does not create something outside of itself, but by transformations within the field of its own being.

The second important element in the process of creation is a unique form of partitioning, dissociation, or forgetting through which the filial conscious entities progressively and increasingly lose contact with their original source and the awareness of their pristine nature. They also develop a sense of individual identity and absolute separateness from each other. In the final stages of this process, intangible but relatively impermeable screens exist between these split-off units and also between each of them and the original undifferentiated pool of Absolute Consciousness.

The relationship between Absolute Consciousness and its parts is unique and complex and cannot be understood in terms of conventional thinking and ordinary logic. Our common sense is telling us that a part cannot simultaneously be the whole and that the whole, being an assembly of its parts, has to be larger than any of its components. In the universal fabric, separate units of consciousness, in spite of their individuality and specific differences, remain on another level essentially identical with their source and with each other. They have a paradoxical nature, being wholes and parts at the same time. The invention of optical holography has provided a useful model for a scientific approach to these otherwise incomprehensible aspects of creation.

The insights from the research of holotropic states of consciousness portray existence as an astonishing play of the cosmic creative principle that transcends time, space, linear causality, and polarities of any kind. From this perspective, the worlds of phenomena, including the material world, appear to be "virtual realities" generated by technology of consciousness—by an infinitely complex orchestration of experiences. They exist on many different levels of reality, ranging from the undifferentiated Absolute Consciousness through rich pantheons of archetypal beings to countless individual units constituting the world of matter, all seemingly taking place within undifferentiated Consciousness itself.

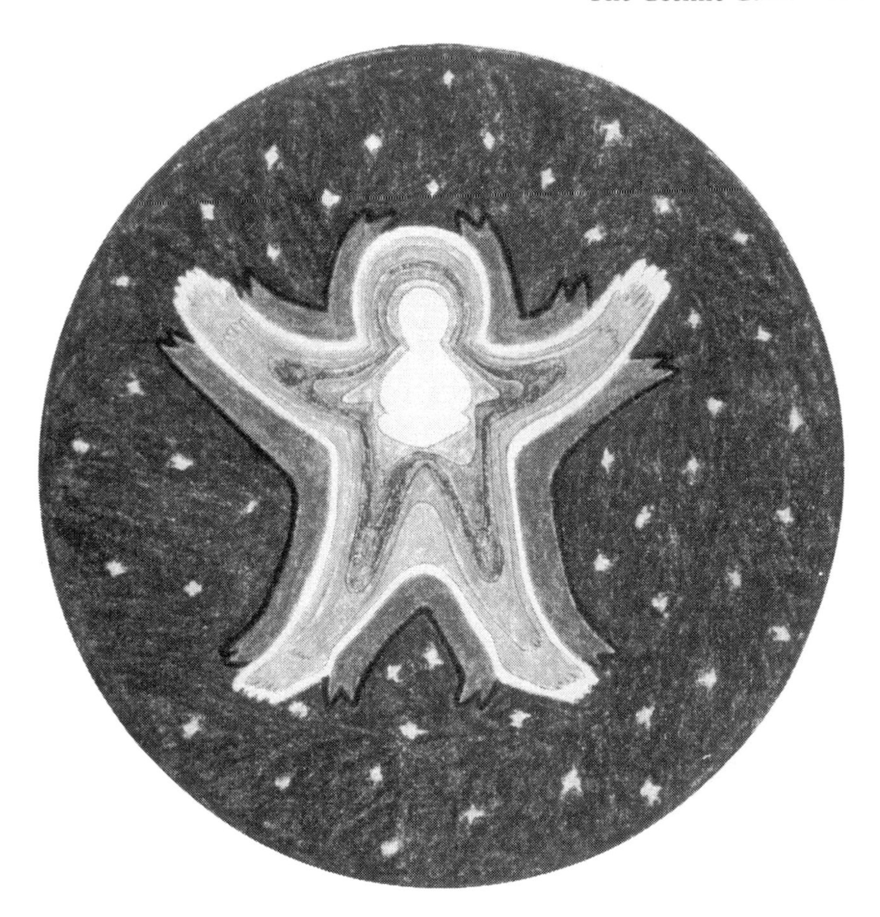

Painting reflecting an experience from a holotropic breathwork session, which involved breaking out of the state of encapsulation and isolation, transcending the veils that separate us from our divine nature, and connecting with the cosmos.

The Ways to Reunion

The process of successive divisions combined with increasing separation and alienation represents only one half of the cosmic cycle. The insights from holotropic states repeatedly reveal another part of this process consisting of events in consciousness that reflect a movement in the opposite direction, from the worlds of plurality and separation toward increasing dissolution of boundaries and merging into ever larger wholes.

These insights parallel the descriptions and discussions of these two cosmic movements described in various spiritual and philosophical systems. For example Plotinus, the founder of Neoplatonism, talked about them as *efflux* and *reflux* (Plotinus 1991). In the East, similar concepts found their most articulate expression in the writings of the Indian mystic and philosopher Shri Aurobindo under the names of *involution* and *evolution* of consciousness (Aurobindo 1965). Modern discussion of the dynamics of *descent* and *ascent* in the cosmic process can be found in the writings of Ken Wilber (Wilber 1980, 1995).

According to the insights from holotropic states, the universal process offers not only an infinite number of possibilities for becoming a separate individual, but also an equally rich and ingenious range of opportunities for dissolution of boundaries and fusion that mediate experiential return to the source. The unitive experiences make it possible for the individual monads of consciousness to overcome their alienation and free themselves from the delusion of their separateness. This transcendence of what earlier appeared to be absolute boundaries and the resulting progressive merging creates larger and larger experiential units. In its farthest reaches, this process dissolves all the boundaries and brings about a reunion with Absolute Consciousness. The sequences of fusions occurring in many forms and on many different levels complete the overall cyclical pattern of the cosmic dance.

The most frequent trigger of spontaneous unitive experiences is exposure to wonders of nature, such as the Grand Canyon, tropical islands, or sunsets over the Pacific Ocean. Exquisite artistic creations of extraordinary beauty can have a similar effect, whether they are musical masterpieces, great paintings and sculptures, or monumental architecture. Additional frequent sources of unitive experiences are athletic activity, sexual union, and in women delivery and nursing. Their occurrence can be facilitated by a variety of ancient, aboriginal, and modern "technologies of the sacred" that were discussed in the introductory chapter of this book.

While unitive experiences happen most likely in emotionally positively charged situations, they can also occur under circumstances which are highly unfavorable, threatening, and critical for the individual. In this case, the ego consciousness is shattered and overwhelmed rather than dissolved and transcended. This happens during severe acute or chronic stress, at the time of intense emotional and physical suffering, or when the integrity or survival of the body are seriously threatened.

Many people discover the mystical realms during near-death experiences at the time of accidents, injuries, dangerous diseases, and operations.

Traditional psychiatrists, who do not distinguish between mysticism and psychosis, consider unitive experiences to be manifestations of mental illness. The credit for demonstrating that this is a serious error belongs to Abraham Maslow, the founder of humanistic and transpersonal psychology. He has shown in a study of many hundreds of individuals that these "peak experiences" are supernormal rather than abnormal phenomena. Under favorable circumstances, they can result in superior emotional and physical health and be conducive to what Maslow called "self-realization" or "self-actualization" (Maslow 1964).

The Taboo Against Knowing Who You Are

If it is true that our deepest nature is divine and that we are identical with the creative principle of the universe, how do we account for the intensity of our conviction that we are physical bodies existing in a material world? What is the nature of this fundamental ignorance concerning our true identity, this mysterious veil of forgetting that Alan Watts called "the taboo against knowing who you are"? How is it possible that an infinite and timeless spiritual entity creates from itself and within itself a virtual facsimile of a tangible reality populated by sentient beings who experience themselves as separate from their source and from each other? How can the actors in the world drama be deluded into believing in the objective existence of their illusory reality?

The best explanation I have heard from the people with whom I have worked is that the cosmic creative principle traps itself by its own perfection. The creative intention behind the divine play is to call into being experiential realities that would offer the best opportunities for adventures in consciousness, including the illusion of the material world. To meet this requirement, these realities have to be convincing and believable in all details. We can use here as an example works of art such as theater plays or movies. These can occasionally be enacted and performed with such perfection that they make us forget that the events we are witnessing are illusory and react to them as if they were real. Also a good actor and actress can sometimes lose their true identity and temporarily merge with the characters they are portraying.

The world in which we live has many characteristics that the supreme principle in its pure form is missing, such as plurality, polarity, density and physicality, change, and impermanence. The project of creating a facsimile of a material reality endowed with these properties is executed with such artistic and scientific perfection that the split-off units of the Universal Mind find it entirely convincing and mistake it for reality. In the extreme expression of its artistry, represented by the atheist, the divine actually succeeds in bringing forth arguments not only against its involvement in creation, but against its very existence.

One of the important ploys that help to create the illusion of an ordinary material reality is the existence of the trivial and ugly. If we all were radiant ethereal beings, drawing our life energy directly from the sun and living in a world where all the landscapes would look like the Himalayas, the Grand Canyon, and unspoiled Pacific islands, it would be too obvious to us that we are part of a divine reality. Similarly, if all the buildings in our world looked like Alhambra, the Taj Mahal, Xanadu, or the Cathedral in Chartres, and we were surrounded by Michelangelo's sculptures, listening to Beethoven's or Bach's music, the divine nature of our world would be easily discernible.

The fact that we have physical bodies with all their secretions, excretions, odors, imperfections, and pathologies, as well as a gastrointestinal system with its repulsive contents, certainly effectively obscures and confuses the issue of our divinity. Various physiological functions like vomiting, burping, passing gas, defecating, and urinating, together with the final decomposition of the human body further complicate the picture. Similarly, the existence of unattractive natural sceneries, junkyards, polluted industrial areas, foul-smelling toilets with obscene graffiti, urban ghettoes, and millions of funky houses make it very difficult to realize that our life is a divine play. The existence of evil and the fact that the very nature of life is predatory makes this task almost impossible for an average person. For educated Westerners, the worldview created by materialistic science is an additional serious hurdle.

There exists another important reason why it is so difficult to free ourselves from the illusion that we are separate individuals living in a material world. The ways to reunion with the divine source are fraught with many hardships, risks, and challenges. The divine play is not a completely closed system. It offers the protagonists the possibility to discover the true nature of creation, including their own cosmic status. However, the ways leading out of self-deception to enlightenment and to reunion with the source present serious problems and most of the potential loopholes in creation are carefully covered. This is absolutely necessary for the maintenance of stability and balance in the cosmic scheme. These vicissitudes and pitfalls of the spiritual path represent an important part of the "taboo against knowing who we are."

All the situations that provide opportunities for spiritual opening are typically associated with a variety of strong opposing forces. Some of the obstacles that make the way to liberation and enlightenment extremely difficult and dangerous are intrapsychic in nature. Here belong terrifying experiences that can deter less courageous and determined seekers, such as encounters with dark archetypal forces, fear of death, and the specter of insanity. Even more problematic are various interferences and interventions that come from the external world. In the Middle Ages, many people who had spontaneous mystical experiences were risking torture, trial, and execution by the Holy Inquisition. In our time, stigmatizing psychiatric labels and drastic therapeutic measures replaced accusations of witchcraft, tortures, and *autos-da-fe*. Materialistic scientism of the twentieth century has ridiculed and pathologized any spiritual effort, no matter how well founded and sophisticated.

The authority that materialistic science enjoys in modern society makes it difficult to take mysticism seriously and pursue the path of spiritual discovery. In addition, the dogmas and activities of mainstream religions tend to obscure the fact that the only place where true spirituality can be found is inside the psyche of each of us. At its worst, organized religion can actually function as a grave impediment for any serious spiritual search, rather than an institution that can help us connect with the divine. By denigrating its members, it makes it difficult to believe that the divine is within them. It might also cultivate in the followers the false belief that regular attendance of formal divine service, prayer, and financial contributions to the church are adequate and sufficient spiritual activities.

The technologies of the sacred developed by various aboriginal cultures have in the West been dismissed as products of magical thinking and primitive superstitions of the savages. The spiritual potential of sexuality that finds its expression in Tantra is by far outweighed by the pitfalls of sex as a powerful animal instinct. The advent of psychedelics that have the capacity to open wide the gates to the transcendental dimension was soon followed by irresponsible secular misuse of these compounds and the threats of insanity, chromosomal damage, and legal sanctions.

The Problem of Good and Evil

One of the most challenging tasks of the spiritual journey is to come to terms with the existence of evil. Final understanding and philosophical acceptance of evil always seems to involve the recognition that it has an important or even necessary role in the cosmic process. For example, deep experiential insights into ultimate realities that become available in holotropic states might reveal that cosmic creation has to be symmetrical, since it is *creatio ex nihilo*. Everything that emerges into existence has to be counterbalanced by its opposite. From this perspective, the existence of polarities of all kinds is an absolutely indispensable prerequisite for creation of the phenomenal worlds.

It was also mentioned earlier that one of the 'motives' for creation seems to be the "need" of the creative principle to get to know itself, so that "God can see God" or "Face can behold Face." To the extent to which the divine creates to explore its own inner potential, not expressing the full range of this potential would mean incomplete self-knowledge. And if Absolute Consciousness is also the ultimate Artist, Experimenter, and Explorer, it would compromise the richness of creation to leave out some significant options. Artists do not limit their topics to those that are beautiful, ethical, and uplifting. They portray any aspects of life that can render interesting images or promise intriguing stories.

The existence of the shadow side of creation enhances its light aspects by providing contrast and gives extraordinary richness and depth to the universal drama. The conflict between good and evil in all the domains and on all the levels of existence is an inexhaustible source of inspiration for fascinating stories. A disciple once asked Shri Ramakrishna, the great Indian visionary, saint, and spiritual teacher: "Swamiji, why is evil in the world?" After a short deliberation, Ramakrishna replied succinctly: "To thicken the plot." This answer might appear cynical in view of the nature and scope of suffering in the world, seen in a concrete form of millions of children dying of starvation or various diseases, the insanity of wars throughout history, countless sacrificed and tortured victims, and the desolation of natural disasters.

However, when we conduct a mental experiment in which we eliminate from the universal scheme all that we consider bad or evil, such as diseases and violence, we will start seeing things differently. We quickly realize that such an act of ethical sanitation will also eliminate from the world many aspects of existence that we value and appreciate enormously—the history of medicine, all those who dedicated their lives to alleviate suffering, the heroism of freedom fighters, and the triumphs of victory over evil forces, as well as all the works of art inspired by the conflicts of good and evil. Such radical purging of the universal shadow would strip creation of its immense depth and richness and would result in a very colorless and uninteresting world.

This way of looking at ethical issues can be very disturbing, in spite of the fact that it is based on very convincing personal experiences in holotropic states. The problems become obvious as we start thinking about the practical consequences that such a perspective has for our life and our everyday conduct. At first sight, seeing the material world as "virtual reality" and comparing human existence to a movie seems to trivialize life and make light of the depth of human misery. It might appear that such a perspective denies the seriousness of human suffering and fosters an attitude of cynical indifference, where nothing really matters. Similarly, accepting evil as an integral part of creation and seeing its relativity could easily be seen as a justification for suspending any ethical constraints and for unlimited pursuit of egotistical goals. It might also seem to sabotage any effort to actively combat evil in the world.

Before we can fully appreciate the ethical implications that deep transcendental insights can have for our behavior, we have to take into consideration some additional factors. Experiential exploration that makes such profound insights available typically reveals important biographical, perinatal, and transpersonal sources of violence and greed in our unconscious. Psychological work on this material leads to a significant reduction of aggression and to an increase of tolerance. We also encounter a large spectrum of transpersonal experiences in which we identify with various aspects of creation. This results in deep reverence for life and empathy with all sentient beings. The same process through which we are discovering the emptiness of forms and the relativity of ethical values thus also significantly reduces our proclivity to immoral and antisocial behavior and teaches us love and compassion.

We develop a new system of values that is not based on conventional norms, precepts, commandments, and fear of punishment, but on our knowledge and understanding of the universal order. We realize that we are an integral part of creation and that by hurting others we would be hurting ourselves. In addition, deep self-exploration leads to the experiential discovery of reincarnation and of the law of karma. This brings us awareness of the possibility of serious experiential repercussions of harmful behaviors, including those that escape societal retributions.

Practical experience also shows that the awareness of the emptiness behind all forms is not at all incompatible with genuine appreciation and love for all creation. Transcendental experiences leading to profound metaphysical insights into the nature of reality actually engender reverence toward all sentient beings and responsible engagement in the process of life. Our compassion does not require objects that have material substance. It can just as easily be addressed to sentient beings who are units of consciousness.

Playing the Cosmic Game

For many religions, the recipe for dealing with the hardships of life is to play down the importance of the earthly plane and to focus on the transcendental realms. The religious systems with this orientation portray the material world as an inferior domain that is imperfect, impure, and conducive to suffering and misery. They recommend a shift in attention and emphasis from the material world to other realities. From their point of view, physical reality appears to be a valley of tears and incarnate existence a curse or a quagmire of death and rebirth.

These creeds and their officials offer their dedicated followers the promise of a more desirable domain or a more fulfilling state of consciousness in the Beyond. In more primitive forms of popular beliefs, these are various forms of abodes of the blessed, paradises, or heavens. These become available after death for those who meet the necessary requirements defined by their respective theology. For more sophisticated and refined systems of this kind, heavens and paradises are only stages of the spiritual journey and its final destination is dissolution of personal boundaries and union with the divine, reaching the state of a pristine monad uncontaminated by biology, or extinguishing the fire of life and disappearance into the nothingness.

However, other spiritual orientations embrace nature and the material world as containing or embodying the Divine. Let us take a look at this dilemma using the insights from holotropic states. What can we gain from moving away from life and escaping from the material plane into transcendental realities? And, conversely, what is the value of embracing wholeheartedly the world of everyday reality? Many spiritual systems define the goal of the spiritual journey as dissolution of personal boundaries and reunion with the Divine. However, those people who have actually experienced in their inner explorations identification with Absolute Consciousness, realize that defining the final goal of the spiritual journey as the experience of oneness with the supreme principle of existence involves a serious problem.

They become aware of the fact that the undifferentiated Absolute Consciousness/Void represents not only the end of the spiritual journey, but also the source and the beginning of creation. The Divine is the principle offering reunion for the separated, but also the agent responsible for the division and separation of the original unity. If this principle were complete and self-fulfilling in its pristine form, there would not be any reason for it to create and the other experiential realms would not exist. Since they do, the tendency of Absolute Consciousness to create clearly expresses a fundamental "need." The worlds of plurality thus represent an important complement to the undifferentiated state of the Divine. In the terminology of the Cabala, "people need God and God needs people."

The overall scheme of the cosmic drama involves a dynamic interplay of two fundamental forces, one of which is centrifugal (*hylotropic,* or matter oriented) and the other centripetal (*holotropic,* or aiming for wholeness) in relation to the creative principle. The undifferentiated Cosmic Consciousness shows an elemental tendency to create worlds of plurality that contain countless separate beings. We have discussed earlier some of the possible reasons or motives for this propensity to generate virtual realities. And conversely, the individualized units of consciousness experience their separation and alienation as painful and manifest a strong need to return to the source and reunite with it. Identification with the embodied self is fraught, among others, with the problems of emotional and physical suffering, spatial and temporal limitations, impermanence, and death.

If it is true that our psyche is governed by these two powerful cosmic forces, the hylotropic and the holotropic, and that these two are in fundamental conflict with each other, is there an approach to existence that can adequately cope with this situation? Since neither separate existence nor undifferentiated unity is fully satisfactory in and of itself, what is the alternative? Clearly, the solution is not to reject embodied existence as inferior and worthless and try to escape from it. We have seen that experiential worlds, including the world of matter, represent not only an important and valuable, but absolutely necessary, complement to the undifferentiated state of the creative principle. At the same time, our efforts to reach fulfillment and peace of mind will necessarily fail, and possibly backfire, if they involve only objects and goals in the material realm. Any satisfactory solution will thus have to embrace both the earthly and the transcendental dimensions, both the world of forms and the Formless.

The material universe as we know it offers countless possibilities for extraordinary adventures in consciousness. As embodied selves, we can witness the spectacle of the heavens with its billions of galaxies and the natural wonders on earth. Only in the physical form and on the material plane can we fall in love, enjoy the ecstasy of sex, have children, listen to Beethoven's music, or admire Rembrandt's paintings. The opportunities for the explorations of the microworld and the macroworld are virtually unlimited. In addition to the experiences of the present, there is also the adventure of probing the mysterious past, from the ancient civilizations and the antidiluvian world to the events during the first microseconds of the Big Bang.

To participate in the phenomenal world and to be able to experience this rich spectrum of adventures requires a certain degree of identification with the embodied self and acceptance of the world of matter. However, when our identification with the body-ego is absolute and our belief in the material world as the only reality unshatterable, it is impossible to fully enjoy our participation in creation. The specters of personal insignificance, impermanence, and death can completely overshadow the positive side of life and rob it of its zest. We also have to add to it the frustration associated with repeated futile attempts to realize our full divine potential within the constraints imposed on us by the limitations of our bodies and of the material world.

To find the solution to this dilemma, we have to turn inside, to a systematic inner quest. As we keep discovering and exploring various hidden dimensions of ourselves and of reality, our identification with the body-ego becomes progressively looser and less compelling. We continue to identify with the "skin-encapsulated ego" for pragmatic purposes, but this orientation becomes increasingly more tentative and playful. If we have sufficient experiential knowledge of the transpersonal dimensions of existence, including our own true identity and cosmic status, everyday life becomes much easier and more rewarding.

As our inner search continues, we also sooner or later discover the essential emptiness behind all forms. As the Buddhist teachings suggest, knowledge of the virtual nature of the phenomenal world and its voidness can help us achieve freedom from suffering. This includes the recognition that belief in any separate selves in our life, including our own, is ultimately an illusion. In Buddhist texts, the awareness of the essential emptiness of all forms and the ensuing realization that there are no separate selves is referred to as *anatta* (*anatman*), literally "no-self."

Awareness of our divine nature and of the essential emptiness of all things, which we discover in our transpersonal experiences, form the foundations of a metaframework that can help us considerably to cope with the complexity of everyday existence. We can fully embrace the experience of the material world and enjoy all that it has to offer, the beauty of nature, human relationships, love making, family, works of art, sports, culinary delights, and countless other things. However, no matter what we do, life will bring obstacles, challenges, painful experiences, and losses. When things get too difficult and devastating, we can call on the broader cosmic perspective that we have discovered in our inner quest.

The connection with higher realities and the liberating knowledge of *anatta* and the emptiness behind all forms makes it possible to tolerate what otherwise might be unbearable. With the help of this transcendental awareness we might be able to experience fully the entire spectrum of life, or "the whole catastrophe," as Zorba the Greek called it. The ability to successfully reconcile and integrate the material and spiritual aspects of existence, or the hylotropic and the holotropic dimensions of life, belongs to the loftiest aspirations of the mystical traditions.

A person whose existence is limited to the pedestrian level of everyday consciousness and who has not had experiential access to the transcendental and numinous dimensions of reality will find it very difficult to overcome deep-seated fear of death and find deeper meaning in life. Under these circumstances, much of the daily behavior is motivated by the needs of the false ego and significant aspects of life are reactive and inauthentic. For this reason, it is essential to complement our everyday practical activities with some form of systematic spiritual practice that provides experiential access to transcendental realms. In preindustrial societies, this opportunity existed in the form of shamanic rituals, rites of passage, healing ceremonies, ancient mysteries, mystical schools, and the meditation practices of the great religions of the world.

In recent decades, the Western world has seen a significant revival of the ancient spiritual practices and aboriginal "technologies of the sacred." In addition, modern depth psychology and experiential psychotherapy have developed effective new approaches that can facilitate spiritual opening. These tools are available to all those who are interested in psychospiritual transformation and consciousness evolution. C. G. Jung, the forefather of transpersonal psychology, described in his writings a life strategy that addresses both the secular and cosmic dimensions of ourselves and of existence. He suggested that whatever we do in our everyday life should be complemented by systematic self-exploration, by an inner search reaching into the deepest hidden recesses of our psyche. This makes it possible to connect to a higher aspect of ourselves that Jung called the Self and receive its guidance on the way to "individuation."

If we follow Jung's advice, important decisions in our life will be based on a creative synthesis integrating the pragmatic knowledge of the material world with the wisdom drawn from the collective unconscious. This idea of the great Swiss psychiatrist is in general agreement with the insights and observations from holotropic states that have been reported by people with whom I had the privilege to work in the last four decades.

It is my personal belief that this strategy of existence would not only greatly enhance the quality of our individual lives but, practiced on a sufficiently large scale, could also significantly improve our chances for overcoming the current global crisis that threatens survival of life on this planet. This is an issue of such importance that we will explore it at some length in the closing chapter of this book.

CHAPTER NINE

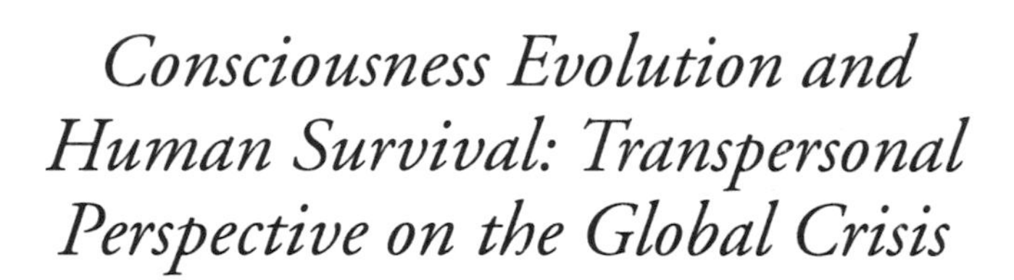

Consciousness Evolution and Human Survival: Transpersonal Perspective on the Global Crisis

The research of holotropic states of consciousness has important implications not only for each of us individually, but also for the future of humanity and survival of life on this planet. In this chapter, I will explore how the experiences and observations from consciousness research can help us understand the nature and roots of the global crisis we are all facing. I will also discuss some new strategies for coping with this critical situation that have emerged from this work. We will pay special attention to the psychospiritual roots of two elemental forces that have driven human history since time immemorial, the proclivity to violence and insatiable greed. We will also take a look at the role that the monistic materialistic worldview of Western science has played in technological progress and in the loss of spiritual values.

Violence and Greed in Human History

The number and degree of atrocities that have been committed throughout the ages in various countries of the world, many of them in the name of God, are truly unimaginable and indescribable. Millions of soldiers and civilians have been killed in wars and revolutions of all times or in other forms of atrocities. In ancient Rome, countless Christians were sacrificed in the arenas to provide a highly sought-after spectacle for the masses. Hundreds of thousands of innocent victims were tortured, killed, or burned alive in the autos-da-fe by the medieval Inquisition.

In Mesoamerica, the soldiers of the tribes defeated by the Aztecs, who had not died in the battle, were slaughtered on sacrificial altars. The Aztec cruelty found its match in the bloody ventures of the Spanish conquistadores. Genghis Khan's Mongolian hordes swept through Asia killing, pillaging, and burning towns and villages. During his unparalleled military campaign, Alexander the Great conquered all the countries between Macedonia and India. Secular and religious ambitions from the expansion of the Roman Empire to the spread of Islam and the Christian Crusades found their expression in the use of sword and fire. The colonialism of Great Britain and other European countries and the Napoleonic wars are additional examples of violence and relentless greed.

This trend has continued in an unmitigated fashion in the twentieth century. The loss of life in World War I was estimated at ten million soldiers and twenty million civilians. Additional millions died from war-spread epidemics and famine. In World War II, approximately twice as many lives were lost. This century saw the expansionism of Nazi Germany and the horrors of the Holocaust, Stalin's reckless domination of Eastern Europe and his Gulag Archipelago, and the civil terror in Communist China. We can add to it the victims of South American dictatorships, the atrocities and genocide committed by the Chinese in Tibet, and the cruelties of the South African Apartheid. The war in Korea and Vietnam, the wars in the Middle East, and the slaughter in Yugoslavia and Rwanda are some more examples of the senseless bloodshed we have witnessed during the last hundred years.

The human greed has also found new, less violent forms of expression in the philosophy and strategy of capitalist economy emphasizing increase of the gross national product, "unlimited growth," reckless plundering of nonrenewable natural resources, conspicuous consumption, and "planned obsolescence." Moreover, much of this wasteful economic policy that has disastrous ecological consequences has been oriented toward production of weapons of increasing destructive power.

Doomsday Scenarios Threatening Life on Our Planet

In the past, violence and greed had tragic consequences for the individuals involved in the internecine encounters and for their immediate families.

However, they did not threaten the evolution of the human species as a whole and certainly did not represent a danger for the eco system and for the biosphere of the planet. Even after the most violent wars, nature was able to recycle all the aftermath and completely recover within a few decades. This situation has changed very radically in the course of the twentieth century. Rapid technological progress, exponential growth of industrial production, massive population explosion, and particularly the discovery of atomic energy have forever changed the equations involved.

In the course of this century, we have witnessed more major scientific and technological breakthroughs within a single decade, or even a single year, than people in earlier historical periods experienced in an entire century. However, these astonishing intellectual successes have brought modern humanity to the brink of a global catastrophe, since they were not matched by a comparable growth of emotional and moral maturity. We have the dubious privilege of being the first species in natural history that has achieved the capacity to eradicate itself and destroy in the process all life on this planet.

The intellectual history of humanity is one of incredible triumphs. We have been able to learn the secrets of nuclear energy, send spaceships to the moon and all the planets of the solar system, transmit sound and color pictures all around the globe and across cosmic space, crack the DNA code, and begin experimenting with cloning and genetic engineering. At the same time, these superior technologies are being used in the service of primitive emotions and instinctual impulses that are not very different from those that drove the behavior of the people in the Stone Age.

Unimaginable sums of money have been wasted in the insanity of the arms race, and the use of even a minuscule fraction of the existing arsenal of atomic weapons would destroy all life on earth. Tens of millions of people have been killed in the two world wars and in countless other violent confrontations occurring for ideological, racial, religious, or economic reasons. Hundreds of thousands have been bestially tortured by the secret police of various totalitarian systems. Insatiable greed is driving people to hectic pursuit of profit and acquisition of personal property beyond any reasonable limits. This strategy has resulted in a situation where, besides the specter of a nuclear war, humanity is threatened by several less spectacular, but insidious and more predictable doomsday scenarios.

Among these are industrial pollution of soil, water, and air; the threat of nuclear waste and accidents; destruction of the ozone layer; the greenhouse effect; possible loss of planetary oxygen through reckless deforestation and poisoning of the ocean plankton; and the dangers of toxic additives in our food and drinks. To this we can add a number of developments that are of less apocalyptic nature, but equally disturbing, such as species extinction proceeding at an astronomical rate, homelessness and starvation of a significant percentage of the world's population, deterioration of family and crisis of parenthood, disappearance of spiritual values, absence of hope and positive perspective, loss of meaningful connection with nature, and general alienation. As a result of all the above factors, humanity now lives in chronic anguish on the verge of a nuclear and ecological catastrophe, while in possession of fabulous technology approaching the world of science fiction.

Modern science has developed effective means that could solve most of the urgent problems in today's world—combat the majority of diseases, eliminate hunger and poverty, reduce the amount of industrial waste, and replace destructive fossil fuels by renewable sources of clean energy. The problems that stand in the way are not of economical or technological nature; their deepest sources lie inside the human personality. Because of them, unimaginable resources have been wasted in the absurdity of the arms race, power struggle, and pursuit of "unlimited growth." They also prevent a more appropriate distribution of wealth among individuals and nations, as well as a reorientation from purely economic and political concerns to ecological priorities that are critical for survival of life on this planet.

Psychospiritual Roots of the Global Crisis

Diplomatic negotiations, administrative and legal measures, economic and social sanctions, military interventions, and other similar efforts have had very little success; as a matter of fact, they have often produced more problems than they solved. It is becoming increasingly clear why they had to fail. The strategies used to alleviate this crisis are rooted in the same ideology that created it in the first place. In the last analysis, the current global crisis is basically a psychospiritual crisis; it reflects the level of consciousness evolution of the human species. It is, therefore, hard to imagine that it could be resolved without a radical inner transformation of humanity on a large scale and its rise to a higher level of emotional maturity and spiritual awareness.

The task of imbuing humanity with an entirely different set of values and goals might appear too unrealistic and utopian to offer any real hope.

Considering the paramount role of violence and greed in human history, the possibility of transforming modern humanity into a species of individuals capable of peaceful coexistence with their fellow men and women regardless of race, color, and religious or political conviction, let alone with other species, certainly does not seem very plausible. We are facing the necessity to instill humanity with profound ethical values, sensitivity to the needs of others, acceptance of voluntary simplicity, and a sharp awareness of ecological imperatives. At first glance, such a task appears too fantastic even for a science-fiction movie.

However, although serious and critical, the situation might not be as hopeless as it appears. After more than forty years of intensive study of holotropic states of consciousness, I have come to the conclusion that the theoretical concepts and practical approaches developed by transpersonal psychology, a discipline that is trying to integrate spirituality with the new paradigm emerging in Western science, could help alleviate the crisis we are all facing. These observations suggest that radical psychospiritual transformation of humanity is not only possible, but is already underway. The question is only whether it can be sufficiently fast and extensive to reverse the current self-destructive trend of modern humanity.

Three Poisons of Tibetan Buddhism

Let us take a look at the theoretical insights from the research of holotropic states and their practical implications for our everyday life. Can the new knowledge be used in a way that would make our life more fulfilling and rewarding? How could systematic self-exploration using holotropic states improve our emotional and physical well-being and bring about positive personality transformation and beneficial changes of the worldview and system of values? And, more specifically, how could this strategy contribute to alleviation of the global crisis and survival of life on this planet?

Spiritual teachers of all ages seem to agree that pursuit of material goals, in and of itself, cannot bring us fulfillment, happiness, and inner peace. The rapidly escalating global crisis, moral deterioration, and growing discontent accompanying the increase of material affluence in the industrial societies bear witness to this ancient truth. There seems to be general agreement in the mystical literature that the remedy for the existential malaise that besets humanity is to turn inside, look for the answers in our own psyche, and undergo a deep psychospiritual transformation.

It is not difficult to understand that an important prerequisite for successful existence is general intelligence—the ability to learn and recall, think and reason, and adequately respond to our material environment. More recent research emphasized the importance of "emotional intelligence," the capacity to adequately respond to our human environment and skillfully handle our interpersonal relationships (Goleman 1996). Observations from the study of holotropic states confirm the basic tenet of perennial philosophy that the quality of our life ultimately depends on what can be called "spiritual intelligence."

Spiritual intelligence is the capacity to conduct our life in such a way that it reflects deep philosophical and metaphysical understanding of reality and of ourselves. This, of course, brings questions about the nature of the psychospiritual transformation that is necessary to achieve this form of intelligence, the direction of the changes that we have to undergo, and the means that can facilitate such development. A very clear and specific answer to these questions can be found in different schools of Mahayana Buddhism.

We can use here as the basis for our discussion a famous Tibetan screen painting (*thangka*) portraying the cycle of life, death, and reincarnation. It depicts the Wheel of Life held in the grip of the horrifying Lord of Death. The wheel is divided into six segments representing the different *lokas,* or realms into which we can be reborn. The celestial domain of gods (*devas*) is shown as being challenged from the adjacent segment by the jealous warrior gods, or *asuras.* The region of hungry ghosts is inhabited by *pretas,* pitiful creatures representing insatiable greed. They have giant bellies, enormous appetites, and mouths the size of a pinhole. The remaining sections of the wheel depict the world of human beings, the realm of the wild beasts, and hell. Inside the wheel are two concentric circles. The outer one shows the ascending and descending paths along which souls travel. The innermost circle contains three animals—a pig, a snake, and a rooster.

The animals in the center of the wheel represent the "three poisons" or forces that, according to the Buddhist teachings, perpetuate the cycles of birth and death and are responsible for all the suffering in our life. The pig symbolizes the *ignorance* concerning the nature of reality and our own nature, the snake stands for *anger and aggression,* and the rooster depicts *desire and lust* leading to attachment. The quality of our life and our ability to cope with the challenges of existence depend critically on the degree to which we are able to eliminate or transform these forces that run the world of sentient beings. Let us now look from this perspective at the process of systematic self—exploration involving holotropic states of consciousness.

Practical Knowledge and Transcendental Wisdom

The most obvious benefit that we can obtain from deep experiential work is access to extraordinary knowledge about ourselves, other people, nature, and the cosmos. In holotropic states, we can reach deep understanding of the unconscious dynamics of our psyche. We can discover how our perception of ourselves and of the world is influenced by forgotten or repressed memories from childhood, infancy, birth, and prenatal existence. In addition, in transpersonal experiences we can identify with other people, various animals, plants, and elements of the inorganic world. Experiences of this kind represent an extremely rich source of unique insights about the world we live in and can radically transform our worldview.

In recent years, many authors have pointed out that a significant factor in the development of the global crisis has been the Newtonian-Cartesian paradigm and monistic materialism that have dominated Western science for the last three hundred years. This way of thinking involves a sharp dichotomy between mind and nature and portrays the universe as a giant, fully deterministic supermachine governed by mechanical laws. The image of the cosmos as a mechanical system has led to the erroneous belief that it can be adequately understood by dissecting it and studying all its parts. This has been a serious obstacle for viewing problems in terms of their complex interactions and from a holistic perspective.

In addition, by elevating matter to the most important principle in the cosmos, Western science reduces life, consciousness, and intelligence to its accidental by-products. In this context, humans appear to be nothing more than highly developed animals. This led to the acceptance of antagonism, competition, and the Darwinian "survival of the fittest" as the leading principles of human society. In addition, the description of nature as unconscious provided the justification for its exploitation by humans, following the program very eloquently formulated by Francis Bacon (Bacon 1870).

Psychoanalysis has painted a pessimistic picture of human beings as creatures whose primary motivating forces are bestial instincts. According to Freud, if we were not afraid of societal repercussions and controlled by the superego (internalized parental prohibitions and injunctions), we would kill and steal indiscriminately, commit incest, and be involved in unbridled promiscuous sex (Freud 1961). This image of human nature relegated such concepts as complementarity, synergy, mutual respect, and peaceful cooperation into the domain of temporary opportunistic strategies or naive utopian fantasies. It is not difficult to see how these concepts and the system of values associated with them have helped to create the crisis we are facing.

Insights from holotropic states have brought convincing support for a radically different understanding of the cosmos, nature, and human beings. They brought experiential confirmation for the concepts formulated by pioneers of information theory and the theory of systems, which have shown that our planet and the entire cosmos represent a unified and interconnected web of which each of us is an integral part (Bateson 1979, Capra 1996). In holotropic states, we can thus gain a considerable amount of knowledge that can be useful in our everyday life. However, the ignorance symbolized in the Tibetan thangkas by the pig is not the absence or lack of knowledge in the ordinary sense. It does not mean simply inadequate information about various aspects of the material world, but ignorance of a much deeper and more fundamental kind.

The form of ignorance that is meant here (*avidya*) is a fundamental misunderstanding and confusion concerning the nature of reality and our own nature. The only remedy for this kind of ignorance is transcendental wisdom (*prajña paramita*). From this point of view, it is essential that the inner work involving holotropic states offers more than just increase, deepening, and correction of our knowledge about the material universe. It is also a unique way of gaining insights about issues of transcendental relevance, as we have seen throughout this book.

In the light of this evidence, consciousness is not a product of the physiological processes in the brain, but a primary attribute of existence. The deepest nature of humanity is not bestial, but divine. The universe is imbued with creative intelligence and consciousness is inextricably woven into its fabric. Our identification with the separate body-ego is an illusion and our true identity is the totality of existence. This understanding provides a natural basis for reverence for life, cooperation and synergy, concerns for humanity and the planet as a whole, and deep ecological awareness.

Anatomy of Human Destructiveness

Let us now look from the same perspective at the second "poison," human propensity to aggression. Modern study of aggressive behavior started with Charles Darwin's epoch-making discoveries in the field of evolution in the middle of the nineteenth century (Darwin 1952). The attempts to explain human aggression from our animal origin generated such theoretical concepts as Desmond Morris's image of the "naked ape" (Morris 1967), Robert Ardrey's idea of the "territorial imperative" (Ardrey 1961), Paul MacLean's "triune brain" (MacLean 1973), and Richard Dawkins's sociobiological explanations interpreting aggression in terms of genetic strategies of the "selfish genes" (Dawkins 1976). More refined models of behavior developed by pioneers in ethology, such as Konrad Lorenz, Nikolaas Tinbergen, and others, complemented mechanical emphasis on instincts by the study of ritualistic and motivational elements (Lorenz 1963, Tinbergen 1965).

Any theories suggesting that the human tendency to violence simply reflects our animal origin are inadequate and unconvincing. With rare exceptions, such as the occasional violent group raids of the chimpanzees (Wrangham and Peterson 1996), animals exhibit aggression when they are hungry, defend their territory, or compete for sex. The nature and scope of human violence—Erich Fromm's "malignant aggression"—has no parallels in the animal kingdom (Fromm 1973). The realization that human aggression can not be adequately explained as a result of phylogenetic evolution led to the formulation of psychodynamic and psychosocial theories that consider a significant part of human aggression to be learned phenomena. This trend began in the late 1930s and was initiated by the work of Dollard and Miller (Dollard et al. 1939).

Biographical Sources of Aggression

Psychodynamic theories attempt to explain the specifically human aggression as a reaction to frustration, abuse, and lack of love in infancy and childhood. However, explanations of this kind fall painfully short of accounting for extreme forms of individual violence, such as serial murders of the Boston Strangler and Jeffrey Dahmer or the indiscriminate multiple killing of the "running amok" type. Current psychodynamic and psychosocial theories are even less convincing when it comes to bestial acts committed by entire groups, like the Sharon Tate murders or atrocities that occur during prison uprisings. They fail completely when it comes to mass societal phenomena such as Nazism, Communism, bloody wars, revolutions, genocide, and concentration camps.

In the last several decades, psychedelic research and deep experiential psychotherapies have been able to throw much light on the problem of human aggression. This work has revealed that the roots of this problematic and dangerous aspect of human nature are much deeper and more formidable than traditional psychology ever imagined. However, this work has also discovered extremely effective approaches that have the potential to neutralize and transform these violent elements in human personality. In addition, these observations indicate that malignant aggression does not reflect true human nature. It is connected with a domain of unconscious dynamics that separates us from our deeper identity. When we reach the transpersonal realms that lie beyond this screen, we realize that our true nature is divine rather than bestial.

Perinatal Roots of Violence

There is no doubt that "malignant aggression" is connected with traumas and frustrations in childhood and infancy. However, modern consciousness research has revealed additional significant roots of violence in deep recesses of the psyche that lie beyond postnatal biography and are related to the trauma of biological birth. The vital emergency, pain, and suffocation experienced for many hours during biological delivery generate enormous amounts of anxiety and murderous aggression that remain stored in the organism. As we saw earlier, the reliving of birth in various forms of experiential psychotherapy involves not only concrete replay of the original emotions and sensations, but is typically associated with a variety of experiences from the collective unconscious portraying scenes of unimaginable violence. Among these are often powerful sequences depicting wars, revolutions, racial riots, concentration camps, totalitarianism, and genocide.

The spontaneous emergence of this imagery during the reliving of birth is often associated with convincing insights concerning perinatal origin of such extreme forms of human violence. Naturally, wars and revolutions are extremely complex phenomena that have historical, economic, political, religious, and other dimensions. The intention here is not to offer a reductionistic explanation replacing all the others, but to add some new insights concerning the psychological and spiritual dimensions of these forms of social psychopathology that have been neglected or received only superficial treatment in earlier theories.

The images of violent sociopolitical events accompanying the reliving of biological birth tend to appear in very specific connection with the consecutive stages of the birth process and the dynamics of the basic perinatal matrices (BPMs). While reliving episodes of undisturbed intrauterine existence (BPM I), we typically experience images from human societies with an ideal social structure, from cultures living in complete harmony with nature, or from future utopian societies where all major conflicts have been resolved. Disturbing intrauterine memories, such as those of a toxic womb, imminent miscarriage, or attempted abortion, are accompanied by images of human groups living in industrial areas where nature is polluted and spoiled, or in societies with insidious social order and all-pervading paranoia.

Regressive experiences related to the first clinical stage of birth (BPM II), during which the uterus periodically contracts but the cervix is not open, present a diametrically different picture. They portray oppressive and abusive totalitarian societies with closed borders, victimizing their populations, and "choking" personal freedom, such as Czarist or Communist Russia, Hitler's Third Reich, South American dictatorships, and the African Apartheid), or bring specific images of the inmates in Nazi concentration camps and Stalin's Gulag Archipelago. While experiencing these scenes of living hell, we identify exclusively with the victims and feel deep sympathy for the down-trodden and the underdog.

The experiences accompanying reliving of the second clinical stage of delivery (BPM III), when the cervix is dilated and continued contractions propel the fetus through the narrow passage of the birth canal, feature a rich panoply of violent scenes—bloody wars and revolutions, human or animal slaughter, mutilation, sexual abuse, and murder. These scenes often contain demonic elements and repulsive scatological motifs. Additional frequent concomitants of BPM III are visions of burning cities, launching of rockets, and explosions of nuclear bombs. Here we are not limited to the role of victims, but can participate in three roles—that of the victim, of the aggressor, and of an emotionally involved observer.

The events characterizing the third clinical stage of delivery (BPM IV), the actual moment of birth and the separation from the mother, are typically associated with images of victory in wars and revolutions, liberation of prisoners, and success of collective efforts, such as patriotic or nationalistic movements. At this point, we can also experience visions of triumphant celebrations and parades or of exciting postwar reconstruction.

In 1975, I described these observations, linking sociopolitical upheavals to stages of biological birth, in *Realms of the Human Unconscious* (Grof 1975). Shortly after its publication, I received a letter from Lloyd de Mause, a New York psychoanalyst and journalist. De Mause is one of the founders of psychohistory, a discipline that applies the findings of depth psychology to history and political science. Psychohistorians study such issues as the relationship between the childhood history of political leaders and their system of values and process of decision making, or the influence of child-rearing practices on the nature of revolutions of that particular historical period. Lloyd de Mause was very interested in my findings concerning the trauma of birth and its possible sociopolitical implications, because they provided independent support for his own research.

For some time, de Mause had been studying the psychological aspects of the periods preceding wars and revolutions. It interested him how military leaders succeed in mobilizing masses of peaceful civilians and transforming them practically overnight into killing machines. His approach to this problem was very original and creative. In addition to analysis of traditional historical sources, he drew data of great psychological importance from caricatures, jokes, dreams, personal imagery, slips of the tongue, side comments of speakers, and even doodles and scribbles on the edge of the rough drafts of political documents. By the time he contacted me, he had analyzed in this way seventeen situations preceding the outbreak of wars and revolutionary upheavals, spanning many centuries since antiquity to most recent times (de Mause 1975).

He was struck by the extraordinary abundance of figures of speech, metaphors, and images related to biological birth that he found in this material. Military leaders and politicians of all ages describing a critical situation or declaring war typically used terms that equally applied to perinatal distress. They accused the enemy of choking and strangling their people, squeezing the last breath out of their lungs, or constricting them and not giving them enough space to live (Hitler's "Lebensraum").

Equally frequent were allusions to dark caves, tunnels, and confusing labyrinths, dangerous abysses into which one might be pushed, and the threat of engulfment by treacherous quicksand or a terrifying whirlpool. Similarly, the offer of the resolution of the crisis comes in the form of perinatal images. The leader promises to rescue his nation from an ominous labyrinth, to lead it to the light on the other side of the tunnel, and to create a situation where the dangerous aggressor and oppressor will be overcome and everybody will again breathe freely.

Lloyd de Mause's historical examples at the time included such famous personages as Alexander the Great, Napoleon, Samuel Adams, Kaiser Wilhelm II, Hitler, Khrushchev, and Kennedy. Samuel Adams talking about the American Revolution referred to "the child of Independence now struggling for birth." In 1914, Kaiser Wilhelm stated that "the Monarchy has been seized by the throat and forced to choose between letting itself be strangled and making a last ditch effort to defend itself against attack."

During the Cuban missile crisis Krushchev wrote to Kennedy, pleading that the two nations not "come to a clash, like blind moles battling to death in a tunnel." Even more explicit was the coded message used by Japanese ambassador Kurusu when he phoned Tokyo to signal that negotiations with Roosevelt had broken down and that it was all right to go ahead with the bombing of Pearl Harbor. He announced that the "birth of the child was imminent" and asked how things were in Japan: "Does it seem as if the child might be born?" The reply was: "Yes, the birth of the child seems imminent." Interestingly, the American intelligence listening in recognized the meaning of the "war-as-birth" code.

Particularly chilling was the use of perinatal language in connection with the explosion of the atomic bomb in Hiroshima. The airplane was given the name of the pilot's mother, Enola Gay, the atomic bomb itself carried a painted nickname "The Little Boy," and the agreed-upon message sent to Washington as a signal of successful detonation was "The baby was born." It would not be too far-fetched to see the image of a newborn also behind the nickname of the Nagasaki bomb, Fat Man. Since the time of our correspondence, Lloyd de Mause collected many additional historical examples and refined his thesis that the memory of the birth trauma plays an important role as a source of motivation for violent social activity.

The issues related to nuclear warfare are of such relevance that I would like to elaborate on them using the material from a fascinating paper by Carol Cohn entitled "Sex and Death in the Rational World of the Defense Intellectuals" (Cohn 1987). The defense intellectuals (DIs) are civilians who move in and out of government, working sometimes as administrative officials or consultants, sometimes at universities and think tanks. They create the theory that informs and legitimates U.S. nuclear strategic practice—how to manage the arms race, how to deter the use of nuclear weapons, how to fight a nuclear war if the deterrence fails, and how to explain why it is not safe to live without nuclear weapons.

Carol Cohn had attended a two-week summer seminar on nuclear weapons, nuclear strategic doctrine, and arms control. She was so fascinated by what had transpired there that she spent the following year immersed in the almost entirely male world of defense intellectuals (except for secretaries). She collected some extremely interesting facts confirming the perinatal dimension in nuclear warfare. In her own terminology, this material confirms the importance of the motif of "male birth" and "male creation" as important psychological forces underlying the psychology of nuclear warfare. She uses the following historical examples to illustrate her point of view:

In 1942, Ernest Lawrence sent a telegram to a Chicago group of physicists developing the nuclear bomb that read: "Congratulations to the new parents. Can hardly wait to see the new arrival." At Los Alamos, the atom bomb was referred to as "Oppenheimer's baby." Richard Feynman wrote in his article "Los Alamos from Below" that when he was temporarily on leave after his wife's death, he received a telegram that read: "The baby is expected on such and such a day."

At Lawrence Livermore laboratories, the hydrogen bomb was referred to as "Teller's baby," although those who wanted to disparage Edward Teller's contribution claimed he was not the bomb's father, but its mother. They claimed that Stanislaw Ulam was the real father, who had all the important ideas and "conceived it"; Teller only "carried it" after that. Terms related to motherhood were also used to the provision of "nurturance"—the maintenance of the missiles.

General Grove sent a triumphant coded cable to Secretary of War Henry Stimson at the Potsdam conference reporting the success of the first atomic test: "Doctor has just returned most enthusiastic and confident that the little boy is as husky as his big brother. The light in his eyes discernible from here to Highhold and I could have heard his screams from here to my farm." Stimson, in turn, informed Churchill by writing him a note that read: "Babies satisfactorily born."

William L. Laurence witnessed the test of the first atomic bomb and wrote: "The big boom came about a hundred seconds after the great flash—the first cry of a new-born world." Edward Teller's exultant telegram to Los Alamos, announcing the successful test of the hydrogen bomb "Mike" at the Eniwetok atoll in Marshall Islands read "It's a boy." The Enola Gay, "Little Boy," and "The baby was born" symbolism of the Hiroshima bomb, and the "Fat Man" symbolism of the Nagasaki bomb were already mentioned earlier. According to Carol Cohn, "male scientists gave birth to a progeny with the ultimate power of domination over female Nature."

Carol Cohn also mentions in her paper abundance of overtly sexual symbolism in the language of defense intellectuals. The nature of this material, linking sex to aggression, domination, and scatology shows a deep similarity to the imagery occurring in the context of birth experiences (BPM III). Cohn used the following examples: American dependence on nuclear weapons was explained as irresistible, because "you get more bang for the buck." A professor's explanation, why the MX missiles should be placed in the silos of the newest Minutemean missiles, instead of replacing the older, less accurate ones: "You are not going to take the nicest missile you have and put it into a crummy hole." At one point, there was a serious concern that "we have to harden our missiles, because the Russians are a little harder than we are." One military adviser to the National Security Council referred to "releasing 70 to 80 percent of our megatonnage in one orgasmic whump."

Lectures were filled with terms like vertical erector launchers, thrust-to-weight ratios, soft lay-downs, deep penetration, and the comparative advantages of protracted versus spasm attacks. Another example was the popular and widespread custom of patting the missiles practiced by the visitors to nuclear submarines, which Carol Cohn saw as an expression of phallic supremacy and also homoerotic tendencies. In view of this material, it clearly is quite appropriate for feminist critics of nuclear policies to refer to "missile envy" and "phallic worship."

Further support for the pivotal role of the perinatal domain of the unconscious in war psychology can be found in Sam Keen's excellent book *The Faces of the Enemy* (Keen 1988). Keen brought together an outstanding collection of distorted and biased war posters, propaganda cartoons, and caricatures from many historical periods and countries. He demonstrated that the way the enemy is described and portrayed during a war or revolution is a stereotype that shows only minimal variations and has very little to do with the actual characteristics of the country and culture involved.

He was able to divide these images into several archetypal categories according to the prevailing characteristics (e.g., Stranger, Aggressor, Worthy Opponent, Faceless, Enemy of God, Barbarian, Greedy, Criminal, Torturer, Rapist, Death). According to Keen, the alleged images of the enemy are essentially projections of the repressed and unacknowledged shadow aspects of our own unconscious. Although we would certainly find in human history instances of just wars, those who initiate war activities are typically substituting external targets for elements in their own psyches that should be properly faced in personal self-exploration.

Sam Keen's theoretical framework does not specifically include the perinatal domain of the unconscious. However, the analysis of his picture material reveals preponderance of symbolic images that are characteristic of BPM II and BPM III. The enemy is typically depicted as a dangerous octopus, a vicious dragon, a multiheaded hydra, a giant venomous tarantula, or an engulfing Leviathan. Other frequently used symbols include vicious predatory felines or birds, monstrous sharks, and ominous snakes, particularly vipers and boa constrictors. Scenes depicting strangulation or crushing, ominous whirlpools, and treacherous quicksands also abound in pictures from the time of wars, revolutions, and political crises. Juxtaposition of pictures from holotropic states of consciousness that depict perinatal experiences with the historical pictorial documentation collected by Lloyd de Mause and Sam Keen represents strong evidence for the perinatal roots of human violence.

According to the new insights, provided jointly by observations from consciousness research and the findings of psychohistory, we all carry in our deep unconscious powerful energies and emotions associated with the trauma of birth that we have not adequately mastered and assimilated. For some of us, this aspect of our psyche can be completely unconscious, until and unless we embark on some in-depth self-exploration with the use of psychedelics or some powerful experiential techniques of psychotherapy, such as the holotropic breathwork or rebirthing. Others can have varying degrees of awareness of the emotions and physical sensations stored on the perinatal level of the unconscious.

As we have seen in an earlier chapter, activation of this material can lead to serious individual psychopathology, including unmotivated violence. It seems that, for unknown reasons, the awareness of the perinatal elements can increase simultaneously in a large number of people. This creates an atmosphere of general tension, anxiety, and anticipation. The leader is an individual who is under a stronger influence of the perinatal energies than the average person. He also has the ability to disown his unacceptable feelings (the Shadow in Jung's terminology) and to project them on an external situation. The collective discomfort is blamed on the enemy and a military intervention is offered as a solution.

The war provides an opportunity to overcome the psychological defenses that ordinarily keep the dangerous perinatal tendencies in check. Freud's superego, a psychological force which demands restraint and civilized behavior, is replaced by the "war superego." We receive praise and medals for murder, indiscriminate destruction, and pillaging, the same behaviors that in peacetime are unacceptable and would land us in prison. Similarly, sexual violence has been a common practice during wartime and has been generally tolerated. As a matter of fact, military leaders have often promised their soldiers unlimited access to women in the conquered territory to motivate them for battle.

Once the war erupts, the destructive and self-destructive perinatal impulses are freely acted out. The themes that we normally encounter in a certain stage of the process of inner exploration and transformation (BPM II and III) now become parts of our everyday life, either directly or in the form of TV news. Various no exit situations, sadomasochistic orgies, sexual violence, bestial and demonic behavior, unleashing of enormous explosive energies, and scatology, which belong to standard perinatal imagery, are all enacted in wars and revolutions with extraordinary vividness and power.

Witnessing scenes of destruction and acting out of violent unconscious impulses, whether it occurs on the individual scale or collectively in wars and revolutions, does not result in healing and transformation as would an inner confrontation with these elements in a therapeutic context. The experience is not generated by our own unconscious, lacks the element of deep introspection, and does not lead to insights. The situation is fully externalized and connection with the deep dynamics of the psyche is missing. And, naturally, there is no therapeutic intention and motivation for change and transformation. Thus the goal of the underlying birth fantasy, which represents the deepest driving force of such violent events, is not achieved, even if the war or revolution has been brought to a successful closure. The most triumphant external victory does not deliver what was expected and hoped for—an inner sense of emotional liberation and psychospiritual rebirth.

After the initial intoxicating feelings of triumph comes at first a sober awakening and later bitter disappointment. And it usually does not take a long time and a facsimile of the old oppressive system starts emerging from the ruins of the dead dream, since the same unconscious forces continue to operate in the deep unconscious of everybody involved. This seems to happen again and again in human history, whether the event involved is the French Revolution, the Bolshevik Revolution in Russia, the communist revolution in China, or any of the other violent upheavals associated with great hopes and expectations.

Since I conducted for many years deep experiential work in Prague at the time when Czechoslovakia had a Marxist regime, I was able to collect some fascinating material concerning the psychological dynamics of Communism. The issues related to communist ideology typically emerged in the treatment of my clients at the time when these were struggling with perinatal energies and emotions. It soon became obvious that the passion the revolutionaries feel toward the oppressors and their regimes receives a powerful reinforcement from their revolt against the inner prison of their perinatal memories. And, conversely, the need to coerce and dominate others is an external displacement of the need to overcome the fear of being overwhelmed by one's own unconscious. The murderous entanglement of the oppressor and the revolutionary is thus an externalized replica of the situation experienced in the birth canal.

The communist vision contains an element of psychological truth that has made it appealing to large numbers of people. The basic notion that a violent experience of a revolutionary nature is necessary to terminate suffering and oppression and institute a situation of greater harmony is correct when understood as a process of inner transformation. However, it is dangerously false when it is projected on the external world as a political ideology of violent revolutions. The fallacy lies in the fact that what on a deeper level is essentially an archetypal pattern of spiritual death and rebirth takes the form of an atheistic and antispiritual program.

Communist revolutions have been extremely successful in their destructive phase but, instead of the promised brotherhood and harmony, their victories have bred regimes where oppression, cruelty, and injustice ruled supreme. Today, when the economically ruined and politically corrupt Soviet Union has collapsed and the communist world has fallen apart, it is obvious to all people with sane judgment that this gigantic historical experiment, conducted at the cost of millions of human lives and unimaginable human suffering, has been a colossal failure. If the above observations are correct, no external interventions have a chance to create a better world, unless they are associated with a profound transformation of human consciousness.

The observations from modern consciousness research also throw some important light on the psychology of concentration camps. Over a number of years, professor Bastians in Leyden, Holland, has been conducting LSD therapy for people suffering from the "concentration camp syndrome," a condition that develops in former inmates of these camps many years after the incarceration. Bastians has also worked with former kapos on their issues of profound guilt. An artistic description of this work can be found in the book *Shivitti* written by a former inmate, Ka-Tzetnik 135633, who underwent a series of therapeutic sessions with Bastians (Ka-Tzetnik 135633 1989).

Bastians himself wrote a paper describing his work, entitled "Man in the Concentration Camp and Concentration Camp in Man." There he pointed out, without specifying it, that the concentration camps are a projection of a certain domain which exists in the human unconscious: "Before there was a man in the concentration camp, there was a concentration camp in man" (Bastians 1955). Study of holotropic states of consciousness makes it possible to identify the realm of the psyche Bastians was talking about. Closer examination of the general and specific conditions in the Nazi concentration camps reveals that they are a diabolical and realistic enactment of the nightmarish atmosphere that characterizes the reliving of biological birth.

The barbed-wire barriers, high-voltage fences, watch towers with submachine guns, minefields, and packs of trained dogs certainly created a hellish and almost archetypal image of an utterly hopeless and oppressive no exit situation that is so characteristic of the first clinical stage of birth (BPM II). At the same time, the elements of violence, bestiality, scatology, and sexual abuse of women and men, including rape and sadistic practices, all belong to the phenomenology of the second stage of birth (BPM III), familiar to people who have relived their birth.

In the concentration camps, the sexual abuse existed on a random individual level, as well as in the context of the "houses of dolls," institutions providing "entertainment" for the officers. The only escape out of this hell was death—by a bullet, by hunger, disease, or suffocation in the gas chambers. The books by Ka-Tzetnik 135633, *House of Dolls* and *Sunrise Over Hell* (Ka-Tzetnik 1955 and 1977), offer a shattering description of the life in concentration camps.

The bestiality of the SS seemed to be focused particularly on pregnant women and little children, which brings further support for the perinatal hypothesis. The most powerful passage from Terence Près's book *The Survivor* is, without a doubt, the description of a truck full of babies dumped into fire, followed by a scene, in which pregnant women are beaten with clubs and whips, torn by dogs, dragged around by the hair, kicked in the stomach, and then thrown into the crematorium while still alive (Près 1976).

The perinatal nature of the irrational impulses manifesting in the camps is evident also in the scatological behavior of the *kapos* (guard). Throwing eating bowls into the latrines and asking the inmates for their retrieval and forcing the inmates to urinate into each other's mouth were practices that besides their bestiality brought the danger of epidemics. Had the concentration camps been simply institutions providing isolation of political enemies and cheap slave labor, maintenance of hygienic rules would have been a primary concern of the organizers, as it is the case in any facility accommodating large numbers of people. In Buchenwald alone, as a result of these perverted practices, twenty-seven inmates drowned in feces in the course of a single month.

The intensity, depth, and convincing nature of all the experiences of collective violence associated with the perinatal process suggests that they are not individually fabricated from such sources as adventure books, movies, and TV shows, but originate in the collective unconscious. When our experiential self-exploration reaches the memory of the birth trauma, we connect to an immense pool of painful memories of the human species and gain access to experiences of other people who once were in a similar predicament. It is not hard to imagine that the perinatal level of our unconscious that "knows" so intimately the history of human violence is actually partially responsible for wars, revolutions, and similar atrocities.

The intensity and quantity of the perinatal experiences portraying various brutalities of human history is truly astonishing. Christopher Bache, after having carefully analyzed various aspects of this phenomenon, made an interesting conclusion. He suggested that the memories of the violence perpetrated throughout ages in human history contaminated the collective unconscious in the same way in which the traumas from our infancy and childhood polluted our individual unconscious. According to Bache, it might then be possible that when we start experiencing these collective memories, our inner process transcends the framework of personal therapy and we participate in the healing of the field of species consciousness (Bache 1999).

The role of the birth trauma as a source of violence and self-destructive tendencies has been confirmed by clinical studies. For example, there seems to be an important correlation between difficult birth and criminality. In a similar way, aggression directed inward, particularly suicide, seems to be psychogenetically linked to difficult birth. According to an article published in the British journal *Lancet,* resuscitation at birth is conducive to higher risk of committing suicide after puberty. The Scandinavian researcher Bertil Jacobson found a close correlation between the form of self-destructive behavior and the nature of birth. Suicides involving asphyxiation were associated with suffocation at birth, violent suicides with mechanical birth trauma, and drug addiction leading to suicide with opiate and/or barbiturate administration during labor (Jacobsen et al. 1987).

The circumstances of birth play an important role in creating a disposition to violence and self-destructive tendencies or, conversely, to loving behavior and healthy interpersonal relationships. French obstetrician

Michel Odent has shown how the hormones involved in the birth process and in nursing and maternal behavior participate in this imprinting. The catecholamines (adrenaline and noradrenaline) played an important role in evolution as mediators of the aggressive/protective instinct of the mother at the time when birth was occurring in unprotected natural environments. Oxytocine, prolactine, and endorphins are known to induce maternal behavior in animals and foster dependency and attachment. The busy, noisy, and chaotic milieu of many hospitals induces anxiety, engages unnecessarily the adrenaline system, and imprints the picture of a world that is potentially dangerous and requires aggressive responses. This interferes with the hormones that mediate positive interpersonal imprinting. It is, therefore, essential to provide for birthing a quiet, safe, and private environment (Odent 1995).

Transpersonal Origins of Violence

The above material shows that a conceptual framework limited to postnatal biography and the Freudian unconscious does not adequately explain extreme forms of human aggression on the individual and collective scale. However, it seems that the roots of human violence reach even deeper than to the perinatal level of the psyche. Consciousness research has revealed significant additional sources of aggression in the transpersonal domain, such as archetypal figures of demons and wrathful deities, complex destructive mythological themes, and past-life memories of physical and emotional abuse.

C. G. Jung believed that the archetypes of the collective unconscious have a powerful influence not only on the behavior of individuals but also on the events of human history. From this point of view, entire nations and cultural groups might be enacting in their behavior important mythological themes. In the decade preceding the outbreak of World War II, Jung found in the dreams of his German patients many elements from the Nordic myth of Ragnarok, or the twilight of the gods. On the basis of these observations, he concluded that this archetype was emerging in the collective psyche of the German nation and that it would lead to a major catastrophe, which would ultimately turn out to be self-destructive.

In many instances, leaders of nations specifically use not only perinatal, but also archetypal images and spiritual symbolism to achieve their political goals. The medieval crusaders were asked to sacrifice their lives for

Jesus in a war that would recover the Holy Land from the Mohammedans. Adolf Hitler exploited the mythological motifs of the supremacy of the Nordic race and of the millenial empire, as well as the ancient Vedic symbols of the swastika and the solar eagle. Ayatollah Khomeini and Saddam Hussein ignited the imagination of their Moslem followers by references to *jihad,* the holy war against the infidels.

Carol Cohn discussed in her paper not only the perinatal but also the spiritual symbolism associated with the language of nuclear weaponry and doctrine. The authors of the strategic doctrine refer to members of their community as the "nuclear priesthood." The first atomic test was called Trinity—the unity of Father, Son, and Holy Ghost, the male forces of creation. From her feminist perspective, Cohn saw this as an effort of male scientists to appropriate and claim ultimate creative power (Cohn 1987). The scientists who worked on the atomic bomb and witnessed the test described it in the following way: "It was as though we stood at the first day of creation." And Robert Oppenheimer thought of Krishna's words to Arjuna in the Bhagavad Gita: "I am become Death, the Shatterer of Worlds."

Biographical Determinants of Insatiable Greed

This brings us to the third poison of Tibetan Buddhism, a powerful psychospiritual force that combines the qualities of lust, desire, and insatiable greed. Together with "malignant aggression," these qualities are certainly responsible for some of the darkest chapters in human history. Western psychologists link various aspects of this force to the libidinal drives described by Sigmund Freud. Psychoanalytic interpretation of the insatiable human need to achieve, to possess, and to become more than one is, attributes this psychological force to sublimation of lower instincts.

According to Freud, "What appears as . . . an untiring impulse toward further perfection can easily be understood as a result of the instinctual repression upon which is based all that is most precious in human civilization. The repressed instinct never ceases to strive for complete satisfaction, which would consist in the repetition of a primary experience of satisfaction. No substitutive or reactive formations and no sublimations will suffice to remove the repressed instinct's persisting tension" (Freud 1955).

More specifically, Freud saw greed as a phenomenon related to problems during the nursing period. According to him, frustration or overindulgence during the oral phase of libidinal development can reinforce the primitive infantile need to incorporate objects to such an extent that it is in adulthood transferred in a sublimated form to a variety of other objects and situations. When the acquisitive drive focuses on money, psychoanalysts attribute it to the fixation on the anal stage of libidinal development. Insatiable sexual appetite is then considered to be the result of phallic fixation. Many other unrelenting human pursuits are then interpreted in terms of sublimation of such phallic instinctual urges. Modern consciousness research has found these interpretations to be superficial and inadequate. It discovered significant additional sources of acquisitiveness and greed on the perinatal and transpersonal levels of the unconscious.

Perinatal Sources of Insatiable Greed

In the course of biographically oriented psychotherapy, many people discover that their life has been inauthentic in certain specific sectors of interpersonal relations. For example, problems with parental authority can lead to specific patterns of difficulties with authority figures, repeated dysfunctional patterns in sexual relationships can be traced to parents as models for sexual behavior, sibling issues can color and distort future peer relationships, and so on.

When the process of experiential self-exploration reaches the perinatal level, we typically discover that our life up to that point has been largely inauthentic in its totality, not just in certain partial segments. We find out to our surprise and astonishment that our entire life strategy has been misdirected and therefore incapable of providing genuine satisfaction. The reason for this is the fact that it was primarily motivated by the fear of death and by unconscious forces associated with biological birth, which have not been adequately processed and integrated. In other words, during biological birth, we completed the process anatomically, but not emotionally.

When our field of consciousness is strongly influenced by the underlying memory of the struggle in the birth canal, it leads to a feeling of discomfort and dissatisfaction with the present situation. This discontent can focus on a large spectrum of issues—unsatisfactory physical appearance, inadequate resources and material possessions, low social position and influence, insufficient amount of power and fame, and many others. Like the child stuck in the birth canal, we feel a strong need to get to a better situation that lies somewhere in the future.

Whatever is the reality of the present circumstances, we do not find it satisfactory. Our fantasy keeps creating images of future situations that appear more fulfilling than the present one. It seems that, until we reach it, life will be only preparation for a better future, not yet "the real thing." This results in a life pattern that has been described as a "treadmill" or "rat-race" type of existence. The existentialists talk about "auto-projecting" into the future. This strategy is a basic fallacy of human life. It is essentially a loser strategy, since it does not deliver the satisfaction that is expected from it. From this perspective, it is irrelevant whether or not it brings fruit in the material world.

When the goal is not reached, the continuing dissatisfaction is attributed to the fact that we have failed to reach the corrective measures. When we succeed in reaching the goal of our aspirations, it typically does not have much influence on our basic feelings. The continuing dissatisfaction is then blamed either on the fact that the choice of the goal was not correct or that it was not ambitious enough. The result is either substitution of the old goal with a different one or amplification of the same type of ambitions.

In any case, the failure is not correctly diagnosed as being an inevitable result of a fundamentally wrong strategy, which is in principle incapable of providing satisfaction. This fallacious pattern applied on a large scale is responsible for reckless irrational pursuit of various grandiose goals that results in much suffering and many problems in the world. It can be played out on any level of importance and affluence, since it never brings true satisfaction. The only strategy that can significantly reduce this irrational drive is full conscious reliving and integration of the trauma of birth in systematic inner self-exploration.

Transpersonal Causes of Insatiable Greed

Modern consciousness research and experiential psychotherapy have discovered that the deepest source of our dissatisfaction and striving for perfection lies even beyond the perinatal domain. This insatiable craving that drives human life is ultimately transpersonal in nature. In Dante Alighieri's words, "The desire for perfection is that desire which always makes every pleasure appear incomplete, for there is no joy or pleasure so great in this life that it can quench the thirst in our soul" (Dante 1990).

In the most general sense, the deepest transpersonal roots of insatiable greed can best be understood in terms of Ken Wilber's concept of the

Atman Project (Wilber 1980). Our true nature is divine—God, Cosmic Christ, Allah, Buddha, Brahma, the Tao—and although the process of creation separates and alienates us from our source, the awareness of this fact is never completely lost. The deepest motivating force in the psyche on all the levels of consciousness evolution is to return to the experience of our divinity. However, the constraining conditions of the consecutive stages of development prevent a full experience of liberation in and as God.

Real transcendence requires death of the separate self, dying to the exclusive subject. Because of the fear of annihilation and because of grasping onto the ego, the individual has to settle for Atman substitutes or surrogates, which are specific for each particular stage. For the fetus and the newborn, this means the satisfaction experienced in the good womb or on the good breast. For an infant, this is satisfaction of age-specific physiological needs. For the adult the range of possible Atman projects is large; it includes besides food and sex also money, fame, power, appearance, knowledge, and many others.

Because of our deep sense that our true identity is the totality of cosmic creation and the creative principle itself, substitutes of any degree and scope—the Atman Projects—will always remain unsatisfactory. Only the experience of one's divinity in a holotropic state of consciousness can ever fulfill our deepest needs. Thus the ultimate solution for the insatiable greed is in the inner world, not in secular pursuits of any kind and scope. The Persian mystic and poet Rumi made it very clear:

> All the hopes, desires, loves, and affections that people have for different things—fathers, mothers, friends, heavens, the earth, palaces, sciences, works, food, drink—the saint knows that these are desires for God and all those things are veils. When men leave this world and see the King without these veils, then they will know that all were veils and coverings, that the object of their desire was in reality that One Thing (Hines 1996).

Technologies of the Sacred and Human Survival

The finding that the roots of human violence and insatiable greed reach far deeper than academic psychiatry ever suspected and that their reservoirs in the psyche are truly enormous could in and of itself be very discouraging. However, it is balanced by the exciting discovery of new therapeutic mechanisms and transformative potentials that become available in holotropic states on the perinatal and transpersonal levels of the psyche.

I have seen over the years profound emotional and psychosomatic healing, as well as radical personality transformation, in many people who were involved in serious and systematic inner quest. Some of them were meditators and had regular spiritual practice, others had supervised psychedelic sessions or participated in various forms of experiential psychotherapy and self-exploration. I have also witnessed profound positive changes in many people who received adequate support during spontaneous episodes of psychospiritual crises.

As the content of the perinatal level of the unconscious emerged into consciousness and was integrated, these individuals underwent radical personality changes. The level of aggression typically decreased considerably and they became more peaceful, comfortable with themselves, and tolerant of others. The experience of psychospiritual death and rebirth and conscious connection with positive postnatal or prenatal memories reduced irrational drives and ambitions. It caused a shift of focus from the past and future to the present moment and enhanced the ability to enjoy simple circumstances of life, such as everyday activities, food, love-making, nature, and music. Another important result of this process was emergence of spirituality of a universal and mystical nature that was very authentic and convincing, because it was based on deep personal experience.

The process of spiritual opening and transformation typically deepened further as a result of transpersonal experiences, such as identification with other people, entire human groups, animals, plants, and even inorganic materials and processes in nature. Other experiences provided conscious access to events occurring in other countries, cultures, and historical periods and even to the mythological realms and archetypal beings of the collective unconscious. Experiences of cosmic unity and one's own divinity lead to increasing identification with all of creation and brought the sense of wonder, love, compassion, and inner peace.

What had begun as psychological probing of the unconscious psyche automatically became a philosophical quest for the meaning of life and a journey of spiritual discovery. People who connected to the transpersonal domain of their psyche tended to develop a new appreciation for existence and reverence for all life. One of the most striking consequences of various forms of transpersonal experiences was spontaneous emergence and development of deep humanitarian and ecological concerns and need to get involved in service for some common purpose. This was based on an almost cellular awareness that the boundaries in the universe are arbitrary and that each of us is identical with the entire web of existence.

It was suddenly clear that we cannot do anything to nature without simultaneously doing it to ourselves. Differences among people appeared to be interesting and enriching rather than threatening, whether they were related to sex, race, color, language, political conviction, or religious belief. It is obvious that a transformation of this kind would increase our chances for survival if it could occur on a sufficiently large scale.

Lessons from Holotropic States for the Psychology of Survival

Some of the insights of people experiencing holotropic states of consciousness are directly related to the current global crisis and its relationship with consciousness evolution. They show that we have exteriorized in the modern world many of the essential themes of the perinatal process that a person involved in deep personal transformation has to face and come to terms with internally. The same elements that we would encounter in the process of psychological death and rebirth in our visionary experiences make our evening news today. This is particularly true in regard to the phenomena that characterize BPM III.

We certainly see the enormous unleashing of the aggressive impulse in the many wars and revolutionary upheavals in the world, in the rising criminality, terrorism, and racial riots. Equally dramatic and striking is the lifting of sexual repression and freeing of the sexual impulse in both healthy and problematic ways. Sexual experiences and behaviors are taking unprecedented forms, as manifested in the sexual freedom of youngsters, gay liberation, general promiscuity, open marriages, high divorce rate, overtly sexual books, plays and movies, sadomasochistic experimentation, and many others.

The demonic element is also becoming increasingly manifest in the modern world. Renaissance of satanic cults and witchcraft, popularity of books and horror movies with occult themes, and crimes with satanic motivations attest to that fact. The scatological dimension is evident in the progressive industrial pollution, accumulation of waste products on a global scale, and rapidly deteriorating hygienic conditions in large cities. A more abstract form of the same trend is the escalating corruption and degradation in political and economic circles.

Many of the people with whom we have worked saw humanity at a critical crossroad facing either collective annihilation or an evolutionary jump in consciousness of unprecedented proportions. Terence McKenna put it very succinctly: "The history of the silly monkey is over, one way or another" (McKenna 1992). It seems that we all are collectively involved in a process that parallels the psychological death and rebirth that so many people have experienced individually in holotropic states of consciousness. If we continue to act out the problematic destructive and self-destructive tendencies originating in the depth of the unconscious, we will undoubtedly destroy ourselves and life on this planet. However, if we succeed in internalizing this process on a large enough scale, it might result in an evolutionary progress that can take us as far beyond our present condition as we now are from primates. As utopian as the possibility of such a development might seem, it might be our only real chance.

Let us now look into the future and explore how the concepts that have emerged from consciousness research, from the transpersonal field, and from the new paradigm in science could be put into action in the world. Although the past accomplishments are very impressive, the new ideas still form a disjointed mosaic rather than a complete and comprehensive worldview. Much work has to be done in terms of accumulating more data, formulating new theories, and achieving a creative synthesis. In addition, the existing information has to reach much larger audiences before a significant impact on the world situation can be expected.

But even a radical intellectual shift to a new paradigm on a large scale would not be sufficient to alleviate the global crisis and reverse the destructive course we are on. This would require a deep emotional and spiritual transformation of humanity. Using the existing evidence, it is possible to suggest certain strategies that might facilitate and support such a process. Efforts to change humanity would have to start with psychological prevention at an early age. The data from prenatal and perinatal psychology indicate that much could be achieved by changing the conditions of pregnancy, delivery, and postnatal care. This would include improving the emotional preparation of the mother during pregnancy, practicing natural childbirth, creating a psychospiritually informed birth environment, and cultivating emotionally nourishing contact between the mother and the child in the postpartum period.

Much has been written about the importance of child rearing, as well as disastrous emotional consequences of traumatic conditions in infancy and childhood. Certainly this is an area where continued education and guidance is necessary. However, to be able to apply the theoretically known principles, the parents have to reach sufficient emotional stability and maturity themselves. It is well known that emotional problems are passed like curse from generation to generation. We are facing here a very complex problem of the chicken and the egg.

Humanistic and transpersonal psychologies have developed effective experiential methods of self-exploration, healing, and personality transformation. Some of these come from the therapeutic traditions, others represent modern adaptations of ancient spiritual practices. There exist approaches with a very favorable ratio between professional helpers and clients and others that can be practiced in the context of self-help groups. Systematic work with them can lead to a spiritual opening, a move in a direction that is sorely needed on a collective scale for our species to survive. It is essential to spread the information about these possibilities and get enough people personally interested in pursuing them.

We seem to be involved in a dramatic race for time that has no precedent in the entire history of humanity. What is at stake is nothing less than the future of life on this planet. If we continue the old strategies which in their consequences are clearly extremely self-destructive, it is unlikely that the human species will survive. However, if a sufficient number of people undergo a process of deep inner transformation, we might reach a level of consciousness evolution when we deserve the proud name we have given to our species: *homo sapiens.*

REFERENCES

Abraham, K. 1927. *A Short Study of the Development of the Libido.* Selected Papers London: Institute of Psychoanalysis and Hogarth Press.

Adler, A. 1932. *The Practice and Theory of Individual Psychology.* New York: Harcourt, Brace & Co.

Alexander, F. 1931. "Buddhist Training As Artificial Catatonia." *Psychoanalyt. Rev.* 18:129.

———. 1950. *Psychosomatic Medicine.* New York: W. W.Norton.

Anonymous. 1975. *A Course in Miracles.* New York: Foundation for Inner Peace.

Ardrey, R. 1961. *African Genesis.* New York: Atheneum.

Assagioli, R. 1976. *Psychosynthesis.* New York: Penguin Books.

———. 1977. "Self-Realization and Psychological Disturbances." *Synthesis* 3–4. Also in S. Grof and C. Grof (eds). *Spiritual Emergency: When Personal Transformation Becomes a Crisis.* Los Angeles: J. P. Tarcher.

Aurobindo, Shri. 1977. *The Life Divine.* New York: India Library Society.

Bache, C. M. 1988. *Lifecycles: Reincarnation and the Web of Life.* New York: Paragon House.

Bache, C. 1999. *Dark Night, Early Dawn: Steps to a Deep Ecology of Mind.* Albany: State University of New York Press.

Bacon, F. 1870. De Dignitate and The Great Restauration, vol. 4., *The Collected Works of Francis Bacon* (J. Spedding, L. Ellis, and D. D. S. Heath, eds.). London: Longmans Green.

Bastians, A. 1955. "Man in the Concentration Camp and the Concentration Camp in Man." Unpublished manuscript, Leyden, Holland.

Bateson, G. 1979. *Mind and Nature: A Necessary Unity.* New York: E. P. Dutton.

Becker, E. 1973. *The Denial of Death.* New York: Free Press.

Benson, H. et al. 1982. "Body Temperature Changes during the Practice of g Tummo Yoga." *Nature* 295:232.

Blanck, G., and R. Blanck, 1974. *Ego Psychology I: Theory and Practice.* New York: Columbia University Press.

———. 1979. *Ego Psychology II: Psychoanalytic Developmental Psychology.* New York: Columbia University Press.

Bohm, D. 1980. *Wholeness and the Implicate Order.* London: Routledge and Kegan Paul.

Bolen, J. S. 1984. *Goddesses in Everywoman. A New Psychology of Women.* San Francisco: Harper and Row.

———. 1989. *Gods in Everyman: A New Psychology of Men's Lives and Loves.* San Francisco: Harper and Row.
Bozzano, E. 1948. *Dei Fenomeni di Telekinesia in Rapporto con Eventi di Morti (Phenomena of Telekinesis Related to Events Involving the Dead).* Casa Editrice Europa.
Brun, A. 1953. Ueber Freuds Hypothese vom Todestrieb (Apropos of Freud's Theory of the Death Instinct). *Psyche* 17:81.
Campbell, J. 1968. *The Hero with A Thousand Faces.* Princeton: Princeton University Press.
———. 1972. *Myths to Live By.* New York: Bantam.
———. 1984. *The Way of the Animal Powers.* New York: Harper and Row.
Capra, F. 1996. *The Web of Life: A New Scientific Understanding of Living Systems.* New York: Doubleday.
Cicero, M. T. 1977. *De Legibus.* Libri Tres. New York: Georg Olms.
Cobbe, F. P. 1877. "The Peak in Darien: The Riddle of Death." *Linell's Living Age and New Quarterly Review* 134:374.
Cohen, S. 1965. "LSD and the Anguish of Dying." *Harper's Magazine* 231: 69, 77.
Cohn, C. 1987. "Sex and Death in the Rational World of the Defense Intellectuals." *Journal of Women in Culture and Society* 12:687–718.
Dalman, C. et al. 1999. "Obstetric Complications and the Risk of Schizophrenia: A Longitudinal Study of a National Birth Cohort." *Arch. Gen. Psychiatry* 56: 234–240.
Dante, A. 1990. *Il Convivio.* (R. H. Lansing, transl.). New York: Garland.
Darwin, C. 1952. *The Origin of Species and the Descent of Man.* In Great Books of the Western World. Encyclopaedia Britannica. Chicago. (Original work published 1859.)
Dawkins, R. 1976. *The Selfish Gene.* New York: Oxford University Press.
Delacour, J. B. 1974. *Glimpses of the Beyond.* New York: Delacorte Press.
Dollard, J. et al. 1939. *Frustration and Aggression.* New Haven, Conn. Yale University Press.
Eliade, M. 1964. *Shamanism: The Archaic Techniques of Ecstasy.* New York: Pantheon Books.
Fenichel, O. 1945. *The Psychoanalytic Theory of Neurosis.* New York: W. W. Norton.
Fisher, G. 1970. "Psychotherapy for the Dying: Principles and Illustrative Cases with Special Reference to the Use of LSD." *Omega* 1:3.
Foerster, H. von. 1965. "Memory without a Record." In *The Anatomy of Memory* (D. P. Kimble, ed.). Palo Alto: Science and Behavior Books.
Flynn, C. P. 1986. *After the Beyond: Human Transformation and the Near-Death Experience.* Englewood Cliffs, N.J.: Prentice-Hall.
Freud, S. 1953. *Three Essays on the Theory of Sexuality.* Standard Edition, vol. 7. London: Hogarth Press and Institute of Psychoanalysis.
———. 1955. *Beyond the Pleasure Principle.* The Standard Edition of the Complete Works of Sigmund Freud, vol. 18 (J. Strachey, ed.). London: Hogarth Press and Institute of Psychoanalysis.
———. 1961. *Civilization and Its Discontents.* Standard Edition, vol. 21. London: Hogarth Press and Institute of Psychoanalysis.
———. 1964. *An Outline of Psychoanalysis.* Standard Edition, vol. 23. London: Hogarth Press and Institute of Psychoanalysis.
——— and Breuer, J. 1936. *Studies in Hysteria.* New York: Nervous and Mental Diseases.
Fried, R. 1987. *The Hyperventilation Syndrome: Research and Clinical Treatment.* Baltimore: Johns Hopkins Series in Contemporary Medicine and Mental Health.

Fromm, E. 1973. *Anatomy of Human Destructiveness.* New York: Holt, Rinehart and Winston.

Gennep, A. van. 1960. *The Rites of Passage.* Chicago: University of Chicago Press.

Goleman, D. 1996. *Spiritual Intelligence: Why It Can Matter More Than IQ.* New York: Bantam.

Gormsen, K., and J. Lumbye 1979. "A Comparative Study of Stanislav Grof's and L. Ron Hubbard's Models of Consciousness." Presented at the Fifth International Transpersonal Conference, Boston, November, 1979.

Green, E. E., and A. M. Green. 1978. *Beyond Biofeedback.* New York: Delacorte Press.

Grey, M. 1985. *Return from Death: An Exploration of the Near-Death Experience.* London: Arcana.

Greyson, B., and C. P. Flynn (eds.). 1984. *The Near-Death Experience: Problems, Prospects, Perspectives.* Springfield, Ill.: Charles C. Thomas.

Grof, C. 1993. *The Thirst for Wholeness: Attachment, Addiction, and the Spiritual Path.* San Francisco: Harper.

Grof, C., and S. Grof. 1990. *The Stormy Search for the Self: A Guide to Personal Growth through Transformational Crisis.* Los Angeles: J. P. Tarcher.

Grof, S. 1972. "LSD and the Cosmic Game: Outline of Psychedelic Cosmology and Ontology." *Journal for the Study of Consciousness* 5:165.

———. 1975. *Realms of the Human Unconscious.* New York: Viking Press.

——— and Halifax, J. 1977. *The Human Encounter with Death.* New York: E. P. Dutton.

———. 1980. *LSD Psychotherapy.* Pomona, Calif.: Hunter House.

———. 1985. *Beyond the Brain: Birth, Death, and Transcendence in Psychotherapy.* Albany: State University of New York Press.

———. 1987. "Spirituality, Addiction, and Western Science." *Re-Vision Journal* 10:5–18.

——— 1988. *The Adventure of Self-Discovery.* Albany: State University of New York Press.

———. 1994. *Books of the Dead.* London: Thames and Hudson.

———. 1998. *The Cosmic Game: Explorations of the Frontiers of Human Consciousness.* Albany: State University of New York Press.

Grof, S., and C. Grof (eds.) 1989. *Spiritual Emergency: When Personal Transformation Becomes a Crisis.* Los Angeles: J. P. Tarcher.

Grof, S., and Grof, C. 1982. *Beyond Death.* London: Thames & Hudson.

Grof, S. (with H. Z. Bennett). 1992. *The Holotropic Mind.* San Francisco: Harper.

Grosso, M. . 1994. "The Status of Survival Research: Evidence, Problems, Paradigms." A paper presented at the Institute of Noetic Sciences Symposium "The Survival of Consciousness After Death," Chicago, July 1994.

Group for the Advancement of Psychiatry, Committee on Psychiatry and Religion. 1976. "Mysticism: Spiritual Quest or Psychic Disorder?" Washington, D.C.

Harman, W. 1984. *Higher Creativity: Liberating the Unconscious for Breakthrough Insights.* Los Angeles: Tarcher.

Harner, M. 1980. *The Way of the Shaman: A Guide to Power and Healing.* New York: Harper and Row.

Harrington, A. 1969. *The Immortalist.* Milbrae, Calif.: Celestial Arts.

Hines, B. 1996. *God's Whisper, Creation's Thunder: Echoes of Ultimate Reality in the New Physics.* Brattleboro, Vt.: Threshold.

Hubbard, L. R. 1950. *Dianetics: The Modern Science of Mental Health.* East Grinstead, Sussex, England: Hubbard College of Scientology.

Huxley, A. 1945. *Perennial Philosophy.* New York and London: Harper.
———. 1963. *Island.* New York: Bantam.
Huxley, L. A. 1968. *This Timeless Moment.* New York: Farrar, Straus, and Giroux.
Jacobson, B. et al. 1987. "Perinatal Origin of Adult Self-Destructive Behavior." *Acta psychiat. Scand.* 76:364–71.
James, W. 1961. *The Varieties of Religious Experience.* New York: Collier.
Janus, S., B. Bess, and C. Saltus. 1977. *A Sexual Profile of Men in Power.* Englewood Cliffs, N.J.: Prentice-Hall.
Jilek, W. G. 1974. *Salish Indian Mental Health and Culture Change: Psychohygienic and Therapeutic Aspects of the Guardian Spirit Ceremonial.* Toronto and Montreal: Holt, Rinehart, and Winston of Canada.
Jung, C. G. 1956. *Symbols of Transformation.* Collected Works, vol. 5, Bollingen Series 20. Princeton: Princeton University Press.
———. 1958. "Psychological Commentary on the Tibetan Book of the Great Liberation." *Collected Works,* vol. 11. Bollingen Series 20. Princeton: Princeton University Press.
———. 1959. *The Archetypes and the Collective Unconscious.* Collected Works, vol. 9, 1. Bollingen Series 20. Princeton: Princeton University Press.
———. 1960a. "Synchronicity: An Acausal Connecting Principle." *Collected Works,* vol. 8, Bollingen Series 20. Princeton: Princeton University Press.
——— 1960b. A Review of the Complex Theory. *Collected Works,* vol. 8, Bollingen Series 20. Princeton: Princeton University Press.
———. 1960c. *The Psychogenesis of Mental Disease.* Collected Works, vol. 3. Bollingen Series 20. Princeton: Princeton University Press.
———. 1964. "Flying Saucers: A Modern Myth of Things Seen in the Skies." In *Collected Works,* vol. 10. Bollingen Series 20. Princeton: Princeton University Press.
———. 1996. *The Psychology of Kundalini Yoga: Notes on the Seminars Given in 1932 by C. G. Jung* (Soma Shamdasani, ed.). Bollingen Series 99. Princeton: Princeton University Press.
Kane, J. M. 1999. "Schizophrenia: How Far Have We Come?" *Current Opinion in Psychiatry* 12:17.
Kaplan, H. S., and H. I. Kaplan. 1967. "Current Concepts of Psychosomatic Medicine." In *Comprehensive Textbook of Psychiatry.* Baltimore: Williams and Wilkins.
Kast, E. C. 1963. "The Analgesic Action of Lysergic Acid Compared with Dihydromorphinone and Meperidine." *Bull. Drug Addiction Narcotics, App.* 27:3517.
Kast, E. C., and V. J. Collins. 1964. "A Study of Lysergic Acid Diethylamid as an Analgesic Agent." *Anaesth. Analg. Curr. Res.* 43:285.
———. 1966. "LSD and the Dying Patient." *Chicago Med. Sch. Quart.* 26:80.
Katz, R. 1976. "The Painful Ecstasy of Healing." *Psychology Today,* December.
Ka-Tzetnik 135633. 1955. *The House of Dolls.* New York: Pyramid.
———. 1977. *Sunrise over Hell.* London: W. A. Allen.
———. 1989. *Shivitti: A Vision.* San Francisco: Harper and Row.
Keen, S. 1988. *Faces of the Enemy: Reflections of the Hostile Imagination.* San Francisco: Harper.
Kübler-Ross, E. 1969. *On Death and Dying.* London: Collier-Macmillan Ltd.
Kučera, O. 1959. "On Teething." *Dig. Neurol. Psychiat.* 27:296.
Kurland, A. A., W. N. Pahnke, S. Unger, C. Savage, and L. E. Goodman. 1968. "Psychedelic Psychotherapy (LSD) in the Treatment of the Patient with A Malignancy." Excerpta

Medica International Congress Series No. 180. *The Present Status of Psychotropic Drugs 180.* Proceedings of the Sixth International Congress of the CINP in Tarragona, Spain (April).

LaBerge, S. 1985. *Lucid Dreaming: Power of Being Awake and Aware in Your Dreams.* New York: Ballantine.

Laszlo, E. 1993. *The Creative Cosmos.* Edinburgh: Floris Books.

Lavin, T. 1987. "Jungian Perspectives on Alcoholism and Addiction." Paper presented at the month-long seminar "The Mystical Quest, Attachment, and Addiction" at the Esalen Institute, Big Sur, Calif.

Lawson, A. 1984. "Perinatal Imagery In UFO Abduction Reports." *Journal of Psychohistory* 12:211.

Leary, T., R. Alpert, and R. Metzner. 1964. *Psychedelic Experience: Manual Based on the Tibetan Book of the Dead.* New Hyde Park, N.Y.: University Books.

Lee, R. B. and I. DeVore (eds). 1976. *Kalahari Hunter-Gatherers: Studies of !Kung San and Their Neighbors.* Cambridge: Harvard University Press.

Leuner, H. 1962. *Experimentelle Psychose.* Berlin: Springer Series 95.

Lilly, J. C. 1977. *Deep Self: Profound Relaxation and the Tank Isolation Technique.* New York: Simon and Schuster.

Lorenz, K. 1963. *On Aggression.* New York: Harcourt, Brace and World.

Mack, J. 1994. *Abductions: Human Encounters with Aliens.* New York: Charles Scribner Sons.

———. 1999. *Passport to the Cosmos: Human Transformation and Alien Encounters.* New York: Crown Publishers.

MacLean, P. 1973. "A Triune Concept of the Brain and Behavior. Lecture I. Man's Reptilian and Limbic Inheritance"; Lecture II. "Man's Limbic System and the Psychoses"; Lecture III. "New Trends in Man's Evolution." In *The Hincks Memorial Lectures* (T. Boag and D. Campbell, eds.). Toronto: University of Toronto Press.

Mahler, M. 1961. "On Sadness and Grief in Infancy and Childhood: Loss and Restoration of the Symbiotic Love Object." *The Psychoanalytic Study of the Child.* 16:332–351.

Maslow, A. 1962. *Toward a Psychology of Being.* Princeton: Van Nostrand.

———. 1964. *Religions, Values, and Peak Experiences.* Cleveland: Ohio State University.

———. 1969. "A Theory of Metamotivation: The Biological Rooting of the Value of Life." In *Readings in Humanistic Psychology* (A .J. Sutich and M .A. Vich, eds.). New York: Free Press.

Mause, L. de. 1975. "The Independence of Psychohistory." In *The New Psychohistory.* New York: Psychohistory Press.

McGee, D. et al. 1984. "Unexperienced Experience: A Critical Reappraisal of the Theory of Repression and Traumatic Neurosis." *Irish Journal of Psychotherapy* 3:7.

Mc Kenna, T. 1992. *Food of the Gods: The Search for the Original Tree of Knowledge.* New York: Bantam Books.

Melzack, R. 1950. *The Puzzle of Pain.* New York: Basic Books.

Melzack, R. and P. D. Wall. 1965. "Pain Mechanisms: A New Theory." *Science* 150:971.

Monroe, R. A. 1971. *Journeys Out of the Body.* New York: Doubleday.

———. 1985. *Far Journeys.* New York: Doubleday.

———. 1994. *Ultimate Journey.* New York: Doubleday.

Moody, R. A. 1975. *Life after Life.* New York: Bantam.

———. *Reunions: Visionary Encounters with Departed Loved Ones.* New York: Villard Books.

Mookerjee, A., and M. Khanna. 1977. *The Tantric Way.* London: Thames and Hudson.
Morris, D. 1967. *The Naked Ape.* New York: McGraw-Hill.
Neher, A. 1961. "Auditory Driving Observed with Scalp Electrodes in Normal Subjects." *Electroencephalography and Clinical Neurophysiology* 13:449.
———. 1962. "A Physiological Explanation of Unusual Behavior Involving Drums." *Human Biology* 34:151.
Odent, M. 1995. "Prevention of Violence or Genesis of Love? Which Perspective?" Presentation at the Fourteenth International Transpersonal Conference in Santa Clara, California, June.
Origenes Adamantius (Father Origen) 1973. *De Principiis (On First Principles).* G.T. Butterworth (trans.), Gloucester, Mass.: Peter Smith.
Osis, K. et al. 1961. *Deathbed Observations of Physicians and Nurses.* New York: Parapsychology Foundation.
Osis, K. and D. McCormick. 1980. "Kinetic Effects at the Ostensible Location of an Out-of-Body Projection during Perceptual Testing." *Journal of the American Society for Psychical Research.* 74:319–24.
Pahnke, W. N., and W. E. Richards. 1966. "Implications of LSD and Experimental Mysticism." *Journal of Religion and Health.* 5:175.
Pahnke, W. N., A. A. Kurland, S. Unger, C. Savage, and S. Grof. 1970. "The Experimental Use of Psychedelic (LSD) Psychotherapy." *J. Amer. Med. Assoc.* 212:1856.
Perls, F. 1976. *Gestalt Therapy Verbatim.* New York: Bantam Books.
Perry, J. W. 1953. *The Self in the Psychotic Process.* Dallas: Spring.
———. 1966. *Lord of the Four Quarters.* New York: Braziller.
———. 1974. *The Far Side of Madness.* Englewood Cliffs, N.J.: Prentice Hall.
———. 1976. *Roots of Renewal in Myth and Madness.* San Francisco: Jossey-Bass.
Plotinus. 1991. *The Enneads.* London: Penguin Books.
Près, T. des. 1976. *The Survivor: An Anatomy of Life in the Death Camp.* Oxford: Oxford University Press.
Pribram, K. 1981. "Non-Locality and Localization: A Review of the Place of the Holographic Hypothesis of Brain Function in Perception and Memory." Preprint for the Tenth ICUS, November.
Rank, O. 1929. *The Trauma of Birth.* New York: Harcourt Brace.
Rappaport, M. et al. 1978. "Are There Schizophrenics for Whom Drugs Might Be Unnecessary or Contraindicated?" *International Pharmacopsychiatry* 13:100.
Raudive, K. 1971. *Breakthrough.* New York: Lancer.
Reich, W. 1949. *Character Analysis.* New York: Noonday Press.
———. 1961. *The Function of the Orgasm: Sex-Economic Problems of Biological Energy.* New York: Farrar, Strauss and Giroux.
———. 1970. *The Mass Psychology of Fascism.* New York: Simon & Schuster.
Richards, W. A. 1975. "Counseling, Peak Experiences, and the Human Encounter with Death: An Empirical Study of the Efficacy of DPT-Assisted Counseling in Enhancing the Quality of Life of Persons with Terminal Cancer and Their Closest Family Members." Ph.D. Dissertation, School of Education, Catholic University of America, Washington, D.C.
Richards, W. A., S. Grof, L. E. Goodman, and A. A. Kurland. 1972. "LSD-Assisted Psychotherapy and the Human Encounter with Death." *J. Transpersonal Psychol.* 4:121.
Riedlinger, T. 1982. "Sartre's Rite of Passage." *Journal of Transpersonal Psychol.* 14: 105.

Ring, K. 1982. *Life at Death: A Scientific Investigation of the Near-Death Experience.* New York: Quill.

———. 1985. *Heading toward Omega: In Search of the Meaning of the Near-Death Experience.* New York: Quill.

Ring, K., and E. E. Valarino. 1998. *Lessons from the Light: What We Can Learn from the Near-Death Experience.* New York: Plenum Press.

Ring, K. and Cooper, S. 1999. *Mindsight: Near-Death and Out-of-Body Experiences in the Blind.* Palo Alto, Calif.: William James Center for Consciousness Studies.

Roberts, J. 1973. *The Education of Oversoul 7.* Englewood Cliffs, N.J.: Prentice-Hall.

Ross, C. A. 1989. *Multiple Personality Disorder: Diagnosis, Clinical Features, and Treatment.* New York: John Wiley.

Sabom, Michael. 1982. *Recollections of Death: A Medical Investigation.* New York: Harper and Row.

Sannella, L. 1987. *The Kundalini Experience: Psychosis or Transcendence?* Lower Lake, Calif.: Integral.

Saunders, C. M. 1967. *The Management of Terminal Illness.* London: Hospital Medicine Publications.

Savage, C., and O. L. McCabe. 1971. "Psychedelic (LSD) Therapy of Drug Addiction." In *The Drug Abuse Controversy* (C. C. Brown and C. Savage, eds.) Baltimore: Friends of Medical Science Research Center.

Schultes, R. E., and A. Hofmann. 1979. *Plants of the Gods: Origin of Hallucinogenic Use.* New York: McGraw Hill.

Senkowski, E. 1994. "Instrumental Transcommunication (ITC)." An Institute for Noetic Sciences lecture at the Corte Madera Inn, Corte Madera, Calif., July.

Sheldrake, R. 1981. *A New Science of Life.* Los Angeles: Tarcher.

———. 1990. "Can Our Memories Survive the Death of Our Brains?" In *What Survives? Contemporary Explorations of Life After Death.* (G. Doore, ed.). Los Angeles: Tarcher.

Sidgwick, H. et al. 1894. *Report on the Census of Hallucinations.* Proc. S.P.R., vol. 10, 245–51.

Silverman, J. 1967. "Shamans and Acute Schizophrenia." *American Anthropologist* 69: 21.

Sparks, T. 1993. *The Wide Open Door: The Twelve Steps, Spiritual Tradition, and the New Psychology.* Center City, Minn.: Hazelden Educational Materials.

Stevenson, I. 1966. *Twenty Cases Suggestive of Reincarnation.* Charlottesville: University of Virginia Press.

———. 1984. *Unlearned Languages.* Charlottesville: University of Virginia Press.

———. 1987. *Children Who Remember Previous Lives.* Charlottesville: University of Virginia Press.

———. 1997. *Reincarnation and Biology: A Contribution to the Etiology of Birthmarks and Birth Defects.* Westport, Conn.: Praeger.

Tafoya, T. 1994. "Completing the Circle: One Heart, Two Spirits, and Beyond." Lecture at the Annual Conference of the Association for Transpersonal Psychology, August, Asilomar, California.

Tarnas, R. 1991. *The Passion of the Western Mind.* New York: Harmony Books.

———. 1995. *Prometheus the Awakener: An Essay on the Archetypal Meaning of the Planet Uranus.* Woodstock, Conn.: Spring.

———. in press. *Psyche and Cosmos: Intimations of a New World View.* New York: Random House.

Tart, C. 1968. "A Psychophysiological Study of Out-of-Body Phenomena." *Journal of the Society for Psychical Research* 62:3–27.
Tausk, V. 1933. "On the Origin of the Influencing Machine in Schizophrenia." *Psychoanalyt. Quart.* 11.
Tinbergen, N. 1965. *Animal Behavior.* New York: Time-Life.
Tomatis, A. A. 1991. *The Conscious Ear.* Barrytown, N.Y.: Station Hill Press.
Ulansey, D. 1989. *Origins of the Mithraic Mysteries: Cosmology and Salvation in the Ancient World.* Oxford: Oxford University Press.
Vaughan, F. 1979. "Transpersonal Psychotherapy: Context, Content, and Process." *Journal of Transpersonal Psychology* 11:101–110.
Verdoux, H., and R. M. Murray. 1998. "What Is the Role of Obstetric Complications in Schizophrenia?" *Harv. Ment. Health Lett.*
Verny, T., and J. Kelly. 1981. *The Secret Life of the Unborn Child.* Toronto: Collins.
Vithoulkas, G. 1980. *The Science of Homeopathy.* New York: Grove Press.
Warner, R. 1999. "New Directions for Environmental Intervention in Schizophrenia: I. The Individual and the Domestic Level." *Mental Health Services* 83:61–70.
Wasson, R. G., A. Hofmann, and C. A. P. Ruck. 1978. *The Road to Eleusis: Unveiling the Secret of the Mysteries.* New York: Harcourt, Brace Jovanovich.
Wasson, V. P. 1957. An interview in *This Week,* Baltimore, May 19.
Watts, A. 1966. *The Book about the Taboo against Knowing Who You Are.* New York: Vintage Books.
Weil, A. 1972. *The Natural Mind.* Boston: Houghton Mifflin.
Weisse, J. E. 1972. *The Vestibule.* Port Washington, N.Y.: Ashley Books.
Whitwell, G. E. 1999. *Life Before Birth: Prenatal Sound and Music.* Internet column reviewing the literature on prenatal effects of sound, http://www.birthpsychology.com.
Wilber, K. 1977. *The Spectrum of Consciousness.* Wheaton, Ill.: Theosophical Publishing House.
———. 1980. *The Atman Project: A Transpersonal View of Human Development.* Wheaton, Ill.: Theosophical Publishing House.
———. 1995. *Sex, Ecology, and Spirituality: The Spirit of Evolution.* Boston: Shambhala.
Wilson, W., and C. G. Jung. 1963. Letters republished in S. Grof (ed.): "Mystical Quest, Attachment, and Addiction." Special edition of the *Re-Vision Journal* 10 (2):1987.
Wrangham, R., and D. Peterson. 1996. *Demonic Males: Apes and the Origins of Human Violence.* New York: Houghton Mifflin Company.
Wright, P. et al. 1998. Maternal Influenza, Obstetric Complications, and Schizophrenia. *Amer. J. Psychiat.* 154: 292.

ABOUT THE AUTHOR

Stanislav Grof, M.D., is a psychiatrist with over forty years of research experience in nonordinary states of consciousness. He was born in Prague, Czechoslovakia, where he also received his scientific training—an M.D. degree from the Charles University School of Medicine and a Ph.D. (Doctor of Philosophy in Medicine) degree from the Czechoslovakian Academy of Sciences. His early research was in the clinical uses of psychoactive drugs conducted at the Psychiatric Research Institute in Prague. There he was Principal Investigator of a program systematically exploring the heuristic and therapeutic potential of LSD and other psychedelic substances.

In 1967, he was invited to be Clinical and Research Fellow at the Johns Hopkins University in Baltimore. After completion of this two-year fellowship, he remained in the United States and continued his research as Chief of Psychiatric Research at the Maryland Psychiatric Research Center and as Assistant Professor of Psychiatry at the Henry Phipps Clinic of Johns Hopkins University. In 1973, he became Scholar-in-Residence at the Esalen Institute in Big Sur, California, where he lived until 1987. He spent this time writing books and articles, giving seminars and lectures, and developing, with his wife Christina, holotropic breathwork, an innovative form of experiential psychotherapy. He also served on the Board of Trustees of the institute.

Stanislav Grof is one of the founders and chief theoreticians of transpersonal psychology and founding president of the International Transpersonal Association (ITA). In this function, he has organized large international conferences in the United States, India, Australia, Czechoslovakia, and Brazil. At present, he is Professor of Psychology at the California Institute of Integral Studies (CIIS), teaching in the Department of Philosophy, Cosmology, and Consciousness. He lives in Mill Valley, California, writes books, conducts training seminars for professionals in holotropic breathwork and transpersonal psychology (Grof Transpersonal Training), and gives lectures and seminars all over the world.

Among his publications are over 100 articles in professional journals and books.

Books

Realms of the Human Unconscious: Observations from LSD Research. Viking Press, New York, 1975. Paperback: E. P. Dutton, New York, 1976.

The Human Encounter with Death. E. P. Dutton, New York, 1977 (with Joan Halifax).

LSD Psychotherapy. Hunter House, Pomona, California, 1980.

Beyond Death: Gates of Consciousness. Thames and Hudson, London, 1980 (with Christina Grof).

Ancient Wisdom and Modern Science. State University of New York Press, Albany, 1984 (ed.).

Beyond the Brain: Birth, Death, and Transcendence in Psychotherapy. State University of New York Press, Albany, 1985.

The Adventure of Self-Discovery. State University of New York Press, Albany, 1987.

Human Survival and Consciousness Evolution. State University of New York Press, Albany, 1988 (ed.).

Spiritual Emergency: When Personal Transformation Becomes a Crisis. J. P. Tarcher, Los Angeles, 1989 (ed. with Christina Grof).

The Stormy Search for the Self: A Guide to Personal Growth Through Transformational Crises. J. P. Tarcher, Los Angeles, 1991 (with Christina Grof).

The Holotropic Mind: The Three Levels of Consciousness and How They Shape Our Lives. Harper Collins, San Francisco, 1992 (with Hal Zina Bennett).

Books of the Dead: Manuals for Living and Dying. Thames and Hudson, London, 1994.

The Cosmic Game: Explorations of the Frontiers of Human Consciousness. State University of New York Press, Albany, 1998.

The Transpersonal Vision: The Healing Potential of Nonordinary States of Consciousness. Sounds True, Boulder, Colo., 1998.

The Consciousness Revolution: A Transatlantic Dialogue. Element Books, Rockport, Mass., 1999 (with E. Laszlo and P. Russell).

Psychology of the Future: Lessons from Modern Consciousness Research. State University of New York Press, Albany, 2000.

For information on holotropic breathwork workshops and facilitator training, please contact

Grof Transpersonal Training, www.holotropic.com
PMB 516 phone: 415 383-8779
38 Miller Avenue fax: 415 383-0965
Mill Valley, CA 94941 email: gtt@dnai.com

INDEX